Maternal Morbidity and Mortality

Edited by

Allan B MacLean and James Neilson

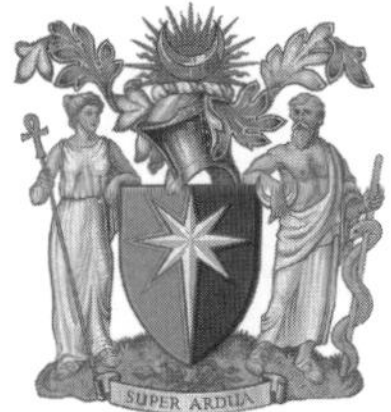

RCOG Press

It was not possible to refer all the material back to the authors or discussants but it is hoped that the proceedings have been reported fairly and accurately.

Allan B MacLean MD FRCOG
Professor of Obstetrics and Gynaecology, Royal Free & University College Medical School, Royal Free Campus, Rowland Hill Street, Hampstead, London NW3 2PF, UK

James Neilson MD FRCOG
Professor of Obstetrics and Gynaecology, University of Liverpool, Liverpool Women's Hospital, Crown Street, Liverpool, L8 7SS, UK

Published by the **RCOG Press** at the
Royal College of Obstetricians and Gynaecologists
27 Sussex Place, Regent's Park
London
NW1 4RG

www.rcog.org.uk

Registered Charity No. 213280

First published 2002

ISBN 1 900364 76 X

DECLARATION OF INTEREST

All contributors to the Study Group were invited to make a specific Declaration of Interest in relation to the subject of the Study Group. This was undertaken and all contributors complied with this request. Professor Wendy Graham is the grant-holder for a number of charity, foundation and Government-funded research projects on maternal morbidity and mortality and Professor Ian Greer is a member of INATE, an international multidisciplinary group of investigators aiming to improve management of venous thrombosis.

RCOG Editor: Sophie Leighton
Typeset and printed by FiSH Books, London

MATERNAL MORBIDITY AND MORTALITY

RCOG Press

Since 1973 the Royal College of Obstetricians and Gynaecologists has regularly convened Study Groups to address important growth areas within obstetrics and gynaecology. An international group of eminent scientists and clinicians from various disciplines is invited to present the results of recent research and to take part in in-depth discussions. The resulting volume, containing the papers presented and also edited transcripts of the discussions, is published within a few months of the meeting and provides a summary of the subject that is both authoritative and up-to-date.

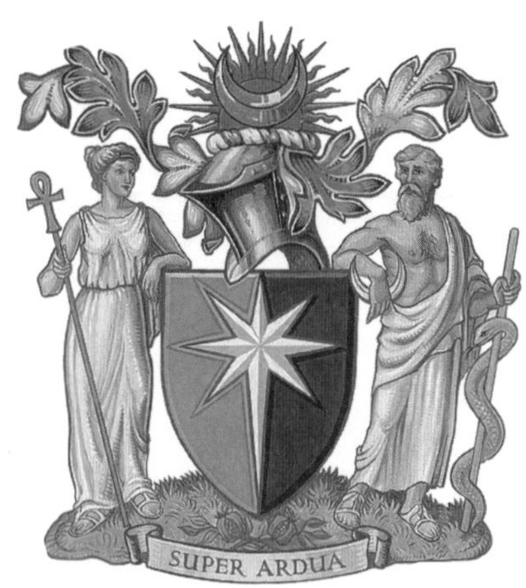

Some previous Study Group publications available

Infertility
Edited by A.A. Templeton and J.O. Drife

Intrapartum Fetal Surveillance
Edited by J.A.D. Spencer and R.H.T. Ward

Early Fetal Growth and Development
Edited by R.H.T. Ward, S.K. Smith and D. Donnai

Ethics in Obstetrics and Gynaecology
Edited by S. Bewley and R.H.T. Ward

The Biology of Gynaecological Cancer
Edited by R. Leake, M. Gore and R.H.T. Ward

Multiple Pregnancy
Edited by R.H.T. Ward and M. Whittle

The Prevention of Pelvic Infection
Edited by A.A. Templeton

Down Syndrome in the First Trimester
Edited by J.G. Grudzinskas and R.H.T. Ward

Problems in Early Pregnancy: Advances in Diagnosis and Management
Edited by J.G. Grudzinskas and P.M.S. O'Brien

Gene Identification, Manipulation and Treatment
Edited by S.K. Smith, E.J. Thomas and P.M.S. O'Brien

Evidence-based Fertility Treatment
Edited by A.A. Templeton, I.D. Cooke and P.M.S. O'Brien

Fetal Programming: Influences on Development and Disease in Later Life
Edited by P.M.S. O'Brien, T. Wheeler and D.J.P. Barker

Hormones and Cancer
Edited by P.M.S. O'Brien and A.B. MacLean

The Placenta: Basic Science and Clinical Practice
Edited by J.C.P. Kingdom, E.R.M. Jauniaux and P.M.S. O'Brien

Disorders of the Menstrual Cycle
Edited by P.M.S. O'Brien, I.T. Cameron and A.B. MacLean

Infection and Pregnancy
Edited by A.B. MacLean, L. Regan and D. Carrington

Pain in Obstetrics and Gynaecology
Edited by A.B. MacLean, R.W. Stones and S. Thornton

Incontinence in Women
Edited by A.B. MacLean and L. Cardozo

Contents

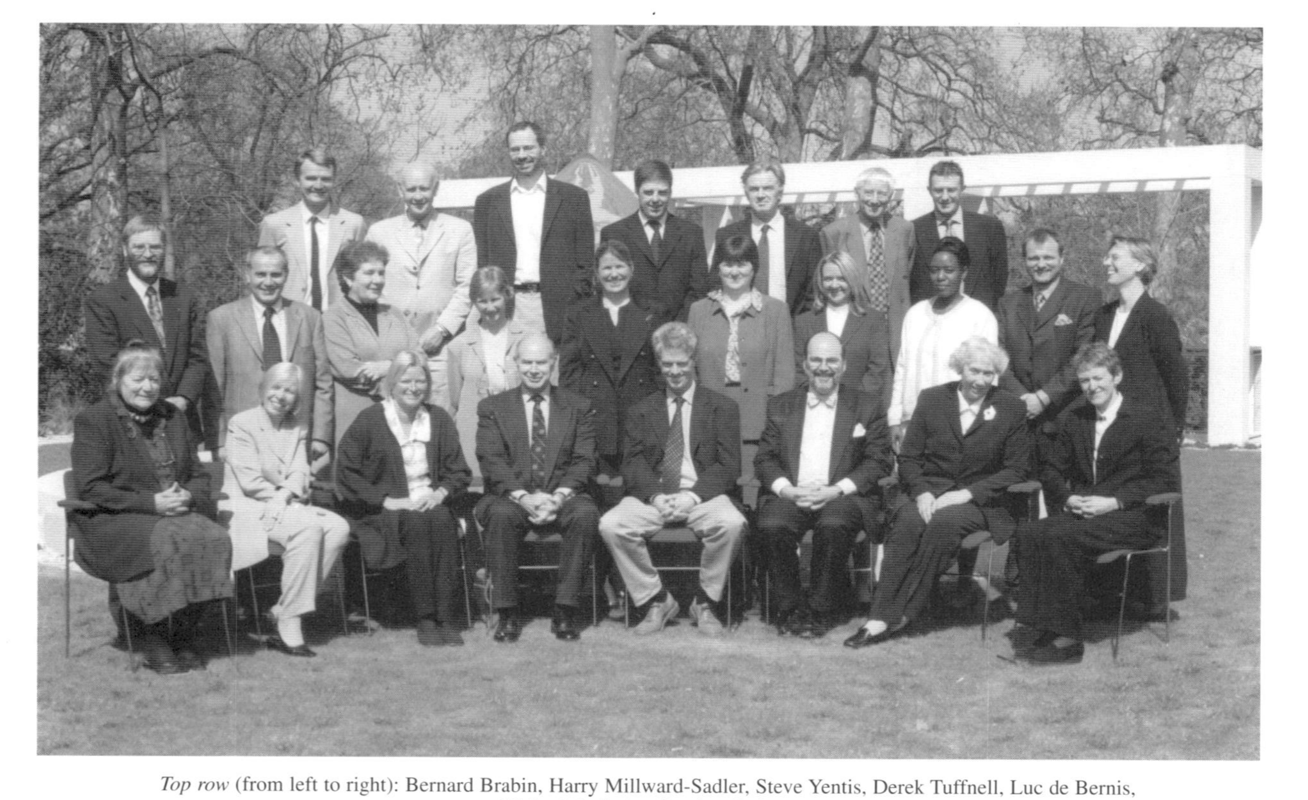

Top row (from left to right): Bernard Brabin, Harry Millward-Sadler, Steve Yentis, Derek Tuffnell, Luc de Bernis, Michael de Swiet, Stephen Robson
Middle row (from left to right): Robert Pattinson, A Metin Gülmezoglu, Margaret Oates, Griselda Cooper, Catherine Nelson-Piercy, Susan Bewley, Tina Lavender, Evelyn Mubiru, Ian Greer, Nynke van den Broek
Bottom row (from left to right): Marion Hall, Wendy Graham, Gwyneth Lewis, Allan MacLean, James Neilson, James Drife, Jean Robinson, Theresa Marteau

Participants

Professor Allan B MacLean
Professor of Obstetrics and Gynaecology, Royal Free and University College Medical School, Royal Free Campus, Hampstead, London NW3 2PT, UK and Convenor of Study Groups, Royal College of Obstetricians and Gynaecologists, UK

Professor James Neilson
Professor of Obstetrics and Gynaecology, University of Liverpool, Liverpool Women's Hospital, Crown Street, Liverpool L8 7SS, UK

Dr Luc de Bernis
Technical Support Unit Head, Making Pregnancy Safer, Reproductive Health and Research, World Health Organization, Avenue Appia 20, CH-1211, Geneva 27, Switzerland

Dr Susan Bewley
Clinical Director, Women's Health Directorate, 9th Floor, New Guy's House, Guy's Hospital, St Thomas's Street, London SE1 9RT, UK

Professor Bernard J Brabin
Professor of Tropical Medicine, Liverpool School of Tropical Medicine, Pembroke Place, Liverpool L3 5QA, UK

Dr Nynke van den Broek
Senior Lecturer in Reproductive Health, Liverpool School of Tropical Medicine, Pembroke Place, Liverpool L3 5QA, UK

Mrs Christine A Carson
National Infant Feeding Advisor and Central Assessor for the Confidential Enquiries into Maternal Deaths, Wellington House, 133–155 Waterloo Road, London SE1 8UG, UK

Dr Griselda Cooper
Senior Lecturer in Anaesthesia, University Department of Anaesthesia and Intensive Care, North 5a, Queen Elizabeth Hospital, Edgbaston, Birmingham B15 2TH, UK

Professor James Drife
Professor of Obstetrics and Gynaecology, Department of Obstetrics and Gynaecology, Clarendon Wing, Belmont Grove, Leeds LS2 9NS, UK

Professor Wendy J Graham
Professor of Obstetric Epidemiology and Director of Dugald Baird Centre for Research in Women's Health, Department of Obstetrics and Gynaecology, University of Aberdeen, Aberdeen Maternity Hospital, Aberdeen AB25 2ZL, UK

Professor Ian Greer
Professor of Obstetrics and Gynaecology, Department of Obstetrics and Gynaecology, Glasgow Royal Infirmary, Queen Elizabeth Building, 10 Alexandra Parade, Glasgow G31 2ER, UK

Dr A Metin Gülmezoglu
Scientist, Department of Reproductive Health and Research, World Health Organization, Avenue Appia 20, Geneva 27, CH-1211, Switzerland

Professor Marion H Hall
Consultant Obstetrician and Gynaecologist, Aberdeen Maternity Hospital, Cornhill Road, Aberdeen AB25 2ZL, UK

Dr Tina Lavender
Reader in Midwifery, University of Central Lancashire, Preston PR1 2HE, UK

Dr Gwyneth Lewis
Director of UK Confidential Enquiries into Maternal Deaths, Wellington House, 133–155 Waterloo Road, London SE1 8UG, UK

Professor Theresa M Marteau
Professor of Health Psychology, Psychology and Genetics Research Group, King's College London, Thomas Guy House, Guy's Campus, London SE1 9RT, UK

Dr Harry Millward-Sadler
Consultant Pathologist and Honorary Senior Lecturer, Department of Pathology, General Hospital, Tremona Road, Southampton SO16 6YD, UK

Dr Evelyn Mubiru
Specialist Obstetrician and Gynaecologist, Mulago Hospital, PO Box 7051, Kampala, Uganda

Dr Catherine Nelson-Piercy
Consultant Obstetric Physician, 9th Floor Directorate Office, New Guy's House, Guy's Hospital, St Thomas's Street, London SE1 9RT, UK

Dr Margaret Oates
Senior Lecturer in Psychiatry and Consultant Perinatal Psychiatrist, Division of Psychiatry, University of Nottingham, University Hospital, Nottingham NG7 2UH, UK

Professor Robert C Pattinson
Director, MRC Unit for Maternal and Infant Health Care Strategies, University of Pretoria, Klinikala Building, Kalafong Hospital, Private Bag X396, Pretoria 0001, South Africa

Ms Jean Robinson
Honorary Research Officer, Association for Improvements in Maternity Services, 56 Lonsdale Road, Oxford OX2 7EP, UK

Professor Stephen Robson
Professor of Fetal Medicine, Department of Obstetrics and Gynaecology, 4th Floor, Leazes Wing, Royal Victoria Infirmary, Newcastle NE1 4LP, UK

Professor Michael de Swiet
Emeritus Professor of Obstetric Medicine and Consultant Physician, Queen Charlotte's Hospital, Hammersmith Campus, Du Cane Road, London W12 0NN, UK

Mr Derek J Tuffnell
Consultant Obstetrician and Gynaecologist, Bradford Royal Infirmary, Duckworth Lane, Bradford BD9 6RJ, UK

Dr Steve Yentis
Consultant Anaesthetist and Honorary Senior Lecturer, Department of Anaesthesia, Chelsea and Westminster Hospital and Faculty of Medicine, Imperial College, 369 Fulham Road, London SW10 9NH, UK

Additional contributors

Dr G Justus Hofmeyer
Director, Effective Care Research Unit, Cecilia Makiwane and Frere Hospitals, Private Bag X9047, East London, South Africa

Ms Esther Maissi
Research Assistant, Psychology and Genetics Research Group, King's College London, Thomas Guy House, Guy's Campus, London SE1 9RT, UK

Professor Florence Mirembe
Head of Obstetrics and Gynaecology Department, Makerere Medical School, PO Box 7062, Kampala, Uganda

Professor Jack Moodley
Chief Specialist, Department of Obstetrics and Gynaecology, Nelson R Mandela School of Medicine, Private Bag 7, Congella 4013, South Africa

Dr Francine Verhoeff
Clinical Research Fellow, Liverpool School of Tropical Medicine, Pembroke Place, Liverpool, L3 5QA, UK

Dr Prabhath Wagaarachchi
Clinical Lecturer in Obstetrics and Gynaecology, Aberdeen Maternity Hospital, Cornhill Road, Aberdeen, AB25 2ZL, UK

Dr Mark Waterstone
Consultant Obstetrician and Gynaecologist, Queen Mary's Hospital, Frognal Avenue, Sidcup, Kent DA14 6LT, UK

Dr Anthony Wilkey
Consultant Anaesthetist, Featherstone Department of Anaesthesia, North 5a, Queen Elizabeth Hospital, Edgbaston, Birmingham B15 2TH, UK

Dr Charles Wolfe
Reader in Public Health Medicine and Director of Research and Development, Division of Primary Care and Public Health Sciences, Capital House, 42 Weston Street, London SE1 3QD, UK

Preface

Fortunately, in the developed world maternal deaths are rare, but each is a tragedy for the woman, her family and for those healthcare professionals who cared for her. Each maternal death tells a story and leaves clues as to whether it might have been prevented. Sometimes individual cases will have such an impact that they will alter the way we practise for the rest of our professional lives. Learning lessons from these deaths has been a crucial part of the Confidential Enquiry into Maternal Deaths (CEMD), first introduced in England and Wales 50 years ago, and whose methodology has subsequently been adapted for use in many other countries. The CEMD is possibly the world's longest-running and most outstanding example of clinical self-audit. The actions taken on the many recommendations made in the reports over the years have made a real contribution to saving women's lives.

So why have a Study Group to examine the subject? First, the process of the Confidential Enquiry only continues because of the ongoing dedication and determination of a few, and the Royal College of Obstetricians and Gynaecologists and the Department of Health must continue to provide support. Second, since the scope of the Confidential Enquiry has widened to include key public health issues, much more needs to be done. It is shocking that in the twenty-first century the most vulnerable women in our society have up to a 20-times-greater risk of dying during or after pregnancy. Many women who die fail to access services. These findings point to the need to rethink how maternity care is provided and to a recognition that each woman requires a flexible package of care tailored to her own particular circumstances. The finding that the leading cause of maternal death is suicide is equally stark and requires serious consideration by those who plan for and provide perinatal mental health services. Thus, the Enquiry remains an extremely important tool in advocating change, which should lead to improvements in clinical management and health service delivery. Without it, we do not have the evidence to push for change. Third, there is a need to address morbidity as well as mortality.

Although deaths in developed countries are rare, each year in developing countries approximately eight million women suffer pregnancy-related complications and over half a million die. Each death or long-term complication represents an individual tragedy for the woman, her children and wider family. More tragically, most deaths are avoidable. More than 80% of maternal deaths could probably be prevented by actions that are proven to be effective and affordable, even in the poorer countries of the world. In the twenty-first century, this represents a potentially remediable cause of human suffering of unimaginable proportions. The College is pleased to be working with the World Health Organization and through the Confidential Enquiry to provide advice and assistance where possible to help overcome one of the worst examples of health inequality in the world today.

This book makes available the contributions of the members of the Study Group to provide a current and relevant record of the continuing challenge of maternal mortality and morbidity, nationally and globally. We hope you find it stimulating.

Allan B MacLean
James Neilson

SECTION 1

MATERNAL MORTALITY: GLOBAL OVERVIEW I

Chapter 1

The global problem of maternal mortality: inequalities and inequities

Wendy J Graham

'All . . . are equal. But some . . . are more equal than others.'

George Orwell, *Animal Farm,* 1945.

Introduction

Over 200 years ago in Aberdeen, Alexander Gordon identified the contagious nature of puerperal fever as it was carried by birth attendants to 'lying-in' women of all social classes.[1,2] This historical association provides a rare example of high maternal mortality alongside higher social class. Almost 100 years ago in Aberdeen, the first enquiry into maternal deaths was conducted, leading the way for national investigations and ultimately for the Confidential Enquiries into Maternal Deaths in the United Kingdom 1997–1999 (CEMD).[3] These early reviews went beyond 'a limited study of clinical factors'[4] by taking account of the mother's social conditions and highlighted a greater risk of maternal death among poor women. In 1952 in Aberdeen, Sir Dugald Baird wrote of the importance of social research in obstetrics and of the inability of even 'the highest standard of obstetric art and skill' to overcome significant social gradients in adverse pregnancy outcomes.[5] Today in Aberdeen, our collaboration is not only with the CEMD report but also with governments and international agencies seeking to reduce the extremely high levels of maternal mortality that still prevail in developing countries.

Two hundred years of research on maternal mortality is indeed a long track record, and one that coincides with a dramatic fall in the obstetric and lifetime risk of maternal death for at least some of the world's women. But the problem of maternal mortality in 2002 remains truly global – as relevant in the UK as in the Kingdom of Nepal – owing to a long-standing and dominant theme: not all women face an equal risk of maternal death within the same society. In itself, this is neither a new nor a surprising statement. Rather, its value lies in illuminating one of the continuing challenges of the modern world – health inequalities and inequities.[6] There are many fine overviews of national levels and trends in maternal mortality, both historical[7,8] and contemporary,[9,10] which I make no attempt to replicate. My intention here is to promote renewed interest in the study of differences in maternal mortality within populations and to provoke debate on the relative importance of geographical, biological and socio-economic determinants – asking whether maternal death in 2002 is not so much a question of where or what you are but who you are.

Of course, dissecting mortality patterns is not a recent field of study or one peculiar to obstetrics. Demographers have long regarded the study of mortality differentials as the very core of their discipline, as witnessed in the work of Malthus in 1798.[11] There is work dating back to the 1800s in Sweden indicating the higher risks of maternal death from puerperal sepsis in the presence of unmarried civil status, poverty and malnutrition.[12] It is now well known that anaemia, one of the main diseases of poverty, complicates sepsis – increasing the risk of maternal death 25–30-fold.[13] In recent years, however, maternal mortality has rarely formed part of the serious international debates on inequality and inequity[14] and differentials have not been a common focus for obstetric research. This situation partly reflects the data constraints of 'small numbers' in developed countries and 'poor numbers' in developing countries, as discussed further below. The comparative neglect of differentials in maternal mortality within populations also reflects the current international agenda, which focuses on levels and trends on a global scale – between major world regions and particularly between the richest and poorest countries. This 'globalisation' of maternal mortality has certainly been a powerful advocacy tool for safe motherhood in the developing world. But the emphasis on these macroscopic differences has often entailed a neglect of common and crucial microscopic inequalities.

Given this neglect, what can be said about differentials in maternal mortality and how confident can we be in relation to any observed patterns? This chapter seeks to answer these questions and is necessarily exploratory. I have drawn on literature in the English language, identified using specific search terms* and the electronic databases Medline, CINAHL, Embase, BIDS, and Popline, and also grey literature accessible through international agencies such as the World Health Organization and the Inter-Agency Group for Safe Motherhood. The chapter comprises four main sections: the first two consider the issues of definitions and data sources, the third highlights the key themes emerging from the current knowledge base and the final section proposes some recommendations for further work.

Defining the problem

There are many examples of how changes in the definition of maternal death have led to a reappraisal – generally upwards – not only of the true magnitude of the problem, but also of the importance of social as opposed to biological factors. Early studies in developed countries, for example, focused on the direct causes of maternal death and the roles of the obstetrician and midwife.[15] It was the later incorporation of indirect causes, many of which were communicable and poverty-related diseases, that stimulated stronger public health interest in maternal mortality,[8] with family doctors and general physicians becoming more involved.[16]

* Search terms: maternal mortality or maternal death or pregnancy-related death and socio-economic factors or differentials or poverty or risk factors or socio-economic gradients, or inequalities or inequities.

A recent example of the influence of definitions is provided by the International Classification of Diseases and Related Health Problems, revision 10 (ICD-10) and the introduction of the categories 'pregnancy-related' and 'late maternal' deaths.* One effect seen in several developed countries is an increase in the proportion of indirect and coincidental deaths. In the UK, for example, the latest CEMD report (1997–99) shows that when late and maternal (direct and indirect) deaths are combined, suicide was the main cause. It also indicated marked social class differences between this and other causes.[17] These definitional changes also have repercussions for developing countries in terms of identifying causes that are socially patterned. HIV/AIDS-related deaths, for example, between 42 days and one year postpartum should now be included in the 'late maternal' category, although the routine information systems in many of these countries still fail to capture many events. Similarly, deaths owing to violence and suicide, both of which have often been regarded as coincidental causes in the past, should now be captured under the 'pregnancy-related' definition.[18]

Just as definitions of maternal death can illuminate or disguise the relative importance of different factors, so can the meanings applied to terms like 'differentials', 'inequalities' and 'inequities'. The first of these can be applied loosely to refer to any characteristic, such as height, place of residence or social class, which can be used to describe (differentiate) a population or health outcome. So, for example, age is a biologically related differential that is well known to influence the risk of maternal mortality; the two other major categories of differentials are geographical and societal (or socio-economic). Although the word 'inequalities' can be used synonymously with differentials, in recent years it has tended to have a 'political' overtone, referring to health differences specifically between geographical areas and/or between socio-economic groups.[19] The distinction between inequality and inequity is more complex, but essentially relates to the concept of avoidability and to principles of fairness and justice. For example, while levels or causes of maternal mortality can vary between population subgroups, some of these differences or inequalities are essentially unavoidable and therefore generally not considered unfair.[20] Deaths from postpartum haemorrhage (PPH), for instance, are generally more common among women of high rather than low parity, but this difference partly reflects the underlying biological risk of haemorrhage, which is not avoidable *per se*. However, deaths from PPH are also more common among women who do not have access to emergency obstetric care, regardless of parity, but this difference partly reflects geographical and/or socio-economic inequalities that are avoidable and thus inequitable. From this perspective, it can be seen that health inequalities and inequities are ultimately ethical and political issues[14] that also touch on the complex matter of human rights.[21,22]

Clearly, what is regarded as 'fair and just' is influenced by the way in which a health problem is perceived in terms of priority and feasible solutions and thus varies widely according to ideology and country.[14,19] This variability begs the crucial question of whose perception matters – those suffering from the problem or those charged with addressing it, be they policy-makers, practitioners or self-proclaimed activists. Varying definitions of avoidability, fairness and justice reflect different perspectives on causality and opportunities for intervention and make international comparisons of health inequalities and inequities problematic. In both developing and developed countries, where services involve user payments, health differentials have been seen primarily as a consequence

---

* Pregnancy-related death: death of a woman while pregnant or within 42 days of termination of pregnancy, irrespective of cause. Late maternal death: death of a woman from direct or indirect obstetric causes more than 42 days but less than one year after termination of pregnancy.

of inequitable access owing to geographical and socio-economic factors, and particularly poverty. The concern in these circumstances has thus been to devise a more equitable supply of services.[20] By contrast, in the UK and other parts of Europe, where health services are essentially free at the point of demand, equitable access has been assumed and thus the focus has been on the aetiology (biology) of poor health and disease with a view to primary prevention. The simplistic distinction between biological, geographical and socio-economic differentials in health outcomes obviously disguises what are invariably multiple and overlapping causal pathways, with some factors being true determinants and others risk factors. For maternal death, however, the crucial mediating effect of access to health services is obvious. The implications for intervention then become a matter of tackling inequities – of ensuring timely access to appropriate care regardless of where a woman is or indeed who she is.

Measuring the problem

How a health problem is perceived and defined influences not only how it is measured but also the importance attached to the accuracy of the findings.[23] The inadequacies in the data sources and collection methods both for maternal mortality and for many socio-economic factors make it hard to distinguish true relationships from measurement artefacts.[24]

The constraints on capturing maternal deaths accurately are well-known.[9,23] An estimated two-thirds of the world's population resides where vital registration and health services data are lacking or highly biased.[18] These are also likely to be populations where maternal mortality is highest and disadvantage most ignored,[25] since these conditions tend to coincide with poor information systems. The lack of reliable routine data sources means that reliance is often placed on modelling methods, survey-based approaches or demographic surveillance.[9] Modelling methods can give only indications of the national level of maternal mortality and thus no insight into differences by area, cause or socio-economic factors. Surveys and surveillance systems have serious logistical implications if population coverage is to be large enough to yield stable estimates. The most common survey-based sources of maternal mortality estimates in developing countries, the Demographic and Health Surveys,[26] do not currently gather any information about the characteristics of the maternal deaths themselves and may miss the very poorest groups owing to the sampling methodology.[27] Demographic surveillance systems can provide information about individual and household-level socio-economic characteristics before and after a maternal death, and thus are also able to look at the adverse consequences for families.[28] However, such population-based sources need to rely on verbal autopsy methods to establish cause of death and these techniques are well known to be unreliable.[29,30] Verbal autopsies could, nevertheless, be a valuable source of information on socio-economic factors as well as on the availability and uptake of health services.

It is primarily errors in reporting causes of death that confound routine statistics on maternal mortality in developed countries. Failure to mention pregnancy status in adult female deaths and misclassification of deaths are the two principal problems,[18] with estimates of the magnitude of under-reporting varying between 17% and 63%.[31] Classification errors are often compounded by analytical obstacles to handling multiple causes of death. Although hierarchies for assigning such causes can be helpful, the inevitable emphasis on a single cause not only masks the multifactorial nature of any death, but also can undermine the importance of associated conditions that are known to be socially related, such as anaemia. Indeed, this and other indirect causes of maternal death tend to be under-reported in developed and developing countries, both in official statistics and in health-facility registers. AbouZahr,[18] for example, noted that more than 50% of the 60 countries reporting vital registration statistics to the WHO for 1990–92 failed to report a single indirect maternal death. These causes are estimated to represent at least 25% of all maternal deaths in developing countries.[10] Interestingly, in the most recent CEMD report,[17] this was the first time in its history that the maternal mortality ratio (MMR) was higher for indirect (6.4/100 000 maternities) than for direct causes (5.0/100 000 maternities), with cardiac problems the single most common medical condition. For much of the developing world, the main indirect causes of maternal death remain the communicable diseases that are also regarded as the 'diseases of poverty' – malaria, tuberculosis and HIV/AIDS. Underestimation of the importance of these indirect causes in health information systems and in international prioritisation exercises, such as the Global Burden of Disease,[32] clearly has major implications for the study of inequalities and inequities in maternal mortality.

Socio-economic factors are also problematic to measure, and typically include a variety of individual or household-level characteristics, such as occupation, wealth or income, absolute or relative poverty, gender, education, social class, ethnicity and marital status. As well as these single indicators, there are various composite measures, such as the Carstairs Deprivation Index,[33] based on postal address, and Poverty Quintiles based primarily on assets.[34] There is an extensive literature[24,35] on the measurement problems – problems that are further complicated in the event of death. In addition to the issue of whether the woman's own characteristics or those of her partner or household should be measured, there are temporal considerations, since circumstances often change as a consequence of the woman's death or prior illness. Many routine health information systems gather only a very narrow range of socio-economic data, much of it based on crude and often gender-insensitive classification schemes.[36] In some settings, privacy and confidentiality laws preclude the recording of information on such potentially relevant factors as home circumstances, sources of income, partners, nationality or birthplace. In the event of an obstetric emergency, where the woman cannot provide information, it obviously falls to those individuals accompanying her to act as proxy respondents.

After death, follow-up data collection raises a number of challenges, even in special studies. There are sensitive issues about the most reliable respondent, particularly owing to culpability bias, as in the case of domestic violence or where there has been neglect in seeking treatment. Issues of privacy and confidentiality are again raised when posing questions on, for example, wantedness of pregnancy, use of contraception, sources of income or partnership status, and, depending on the time period since the death, there may be cultural taboos on mentioning the deceased. Where unpaid hospital fees are involved, a 'wall of silence' may be encountered, including denial of the woman's existence. There may also be significant biases in the reporting by relatives of the timing and use of services, especially where there is migration around the time of delivery. For example, in many cultures women often return to their parents' household to deliver, having received antenatal care elsewhere. In the event of an intrapartum complication, these women may thus appear as 'unbooked' cases if they present at local health facilities, confounding the frequently observed link[37] between booking status and maternal mortality.

Inequalities in maternal mortality – what may we know?

Location is but part of the problem

As mentioned previously, geography or location is one of the main factors used to consider health inequalities. The spatial or geographical mapping of such inequalities dates back to the origins of public health. Today it involves sophisticated data-capture techniques, such as Geographic Information Systems,[38] and complex analytical methods.[39] However, these recent developments have largely escaped the field of maternal mortality, in which the exploration of geographical inequalities still tends to be in terms of international differences and patterns of service uptake.

Historical comparisons of national levels of maternal mortality are numerous. Loudon,[7] for example, highlights the enormous difference in 1930 between the Netherlands, with an MMR of 250 per 100 000 live births, and the USA with 700 – a difference that was essentially eliminated by 1960. Although these international contrasts, themselves fraught with problems of data comparability, clearly cannot reveal subnational variations, they continue to be a focus of attention. Table 1.1 illustrates some common examples of these geographical inequalities. The contrast, for example, between the average lifetime risk of maternal mortality between developed and developing countries is frequently cited as the 'largest discrepancy of all public health statistics' and was used as one of the first rallying calls for the Safe Motherhood Initiative.[40]

The inclusion of two other variables in Table 1.1 – the total fertility rate and female life expectancy at birth – introduces the long-standing reliance in maternal mortality research on correlational analysis. This partly reflects the lack of accurate subnational or individual-level data. The dangers and limitations of such an approach, however, are not always well appreciated. The ecological fallacy, for example, is often ignored and so causality presumed between dependent and independent variables, such as the level of maternal mortality and the proportion of skilled attendants at delivery.[41] To extrapolate from crude geographical comparisons across diverse countries, often without controlling for confounding factors, and derive priorities for programme action within countries is obviously inappropriate. Today, however, there are influential international development targets[42] that not only assume that the proportion of deliveries with a doctor or midwife can be used as a benchmark indicator for progress in reducing maternal mortality, but also that such national levels are indicative of development itself.[43]

There are many examples of the geographical correlational approach to inequalities in maternal mortality at the international level. These are undoubtedly useful as descriptive devices but not as a basis for policy formulation. They do, however, provide pointers to the importance of subnational variations. Shen and Williamson's[44] recent analysis, for example, suggests that the status of women is associated with levels of maternal mortality after controlling for *per capita* gross domestic product and economic group. The status markers that were used – women's education, contraceptive prevalence, age at first marriage and total fertility rate – also showed clear subnational variations. In other words, geographical inequalities in maternal mortality are likely to coincide with (but not necessarily be caused by) geographical inequalities in these societal variables. A recent illustration of this is seen in Hoyert *et al.*'s[45] analysis of US data, showing that regional differences in maternal mortality were totally removed after adjusting for racial status.

Table 1.1. Estimates of maternal mortality, fertility and female life expectancy for selected world regions and countries, 1995–99

Selected regions or countries[a]	Estimated annual maternal deaths[65] (*n*)	MMR[65] (per 100 000 live births)	Lifetime risk of maternal death[65] (ratio)	Total fertility rate[66]	Female life expectancy at birth[66]
World	515 000	400	75	2.8	69
Developed countries	2 800	21	2 500	1.6	79
Developing countries	512 000	440	60	3.2	66
Poorest countries	230 000	1 000	16	3.6	64
Northern America	490	11	3 500	2.0	80
USA	470	12	3 500	2.1	80
Europe	2 200	28	2 000	1.4	78
France	150	20	2 500	1.9	83
Germany	90	12	5 300	1.3	81
Romania	150	60	1 000	1.3	74
UK	75	10	4 600	1.7	80
Africa	273 000	1 000	16	5.2	55
Ethiopia	46 000	1 800	7	5.9	53
Libya	170	120	180	3.9	77
Rwanda	6 300	2 300	6	5.8	40
South Africa	3 600	70	340	2.9	54
Asia	217 000	280	110	3.2	66
Japan	140	12	4 600	1.3	84
India	110 000	440	55	3.2	61
Singapore	5	9	5 400	1.6	80
Yemen	6 100	850	13	7.2	61
Latin America and the Caribbean	22 000	190	160	2.8	74
Bolivia	1 400	550	33	4.2	64
Brazil	8 800	260	130	2.4	72
Chile	90	33	1 000	2.3	78
Haiti	2 800	1 100	16	4.7	51

[a] UN classification of world regions; MMR = maternal mortality ratio

The extent to which geographical inequalities in maternal mortality are essentially mediated by access to health services can be hard to disentangle. Socio-economic inequalities are also likely to coincide with service inequalities, as illustrated by comparisons between rural and urban areas in developing countries. Indeed, rural–urban differences in the risk of maternal death can be seen in historical data; Dugald Baird, for example, noted the cancelling-out of the benefits of good nutrition among rural women in Scotland in the 1950s by poor access to emergency services.[46] Today, geographical inequalities in maternal mortality in developed countries are less apparent, possibly through improved physical supply of services, but perhaps also being masked by small numbers. What is striking, however, in the literature is that after controlling for geography or location and thus the physical availability of services, there are clear differentials in use or uptake. In other words, it is realised access rather than potential access that is crucial.[47] This demand side of the service equation has been comparatively ignored in studies of maternal mortality. One extreme illustration of the influence of uptake can be seen in a religious group in the USA for whom the use of health professionals and emergency obstetric care is prohibited. This group apparently experiences a 100-fold higher level of maternal mortality than the general population, albeit based on small numbers.[48] In developing countries, some evidence of the non-geographical barriers to use can be seen in maternal mortality studies conducted among urban populations. These reveal significant delays in presentation by some women, who experience case fatality rates and causes, such as obstetric haemorrhage, that would be expected among rural populations with poor physical availability of care.[49] Such findings are suggestive of socio-economic inequities and thus of the importance of 'who you are'.

Poverty is a key contributory factor

Foremost among the socio-economic factors in current debates on development and health is poverty. Simply stated, poverty is a term used to describe the condition of an individual or a group for which there is a lack of resources, usually taken to include money and material possessions, significantly affecting health and wellbeing.[19] Whereas today lack of resources is often measured by asset possession and/or household income, in the past other surrogates for wealth or poverty, such as occupation, social class and education, were used. Table 1.2 illustrates the inequalities in maternal mortality for different populations and time periods using such factors. Although based on individual level comparisons rather than correlations of aggregate measures, there are still significant limitations to such bivariate analysis and more powerful multivariate techniques should preferably be used.

The link between poverty and health, both absolute and relative, has in fact been clear for well over a century and is backed up by an extensive literature. There is, however, renewed interest now in tackling poverty among governments in developed and developing countries and among international agencies.[19,20] This has been stimulated by the suggested potential for improved health to contribute to the reduction of poverty and thus to development.[50] The correlation between economic growth and health is constantly being revisited, but only confirms what older studies revealed – that variations in crude measures of health, such as life expectancy, are not 'explained' by variations in crude economic measures, such as *per capita* health expenditure.[20] Figure 1.1 repeats this correlation specifically using maternal mortality and points to a similar conclusion: for countries with *per capita* health expenditure below US$500 there is an enormous range in maternal mortality, while above this figure there is an enormous range in health expenditure but little difference in maternal mortality. Such a simple correlation must obviously be interpreted cautiously. There is a clear need for more refined data and sophisticated approaches that reveal the distribution within countries – be this for wealth or poverty[51,52] or for service use.

For developing countries, it is often assumed that the primary mechanism through which poverty affects maternal mortality is uptake of services, with poor women facing significant barriers to the timely use of appropriate quality care. Indeed, service use is often the primary type of information relating to maternal health available in these countries, and is presumed to be a reliable proxy for poor health outcomes.[10,53] There is, however, a lack of rigorous demonstrations of the link between process measures of service use and improved maternal outcomes at the population level. This gap provides one rationale for a major new research endeavour – the Initiative for Maternal

Table 1.2. Selected studies reporting poverty-related inequalities in maternal mortality

Country[a]	Period	Differential	Total deaths (n)	MMR per 100 000 live births (95% CI)	Adapted from reference
England and Wales	1930–32	Social class:[b]			7 (Table 2)
		I and II (professional, middle and upper classes)		444.00	
		III		411.00	
		IV		416.00	
		V (unskilled labourer)		389.00	
UK	1997–99	Social class	378[c]		17 (Table 1.16)
		1 (Professional)		7.65[d] (4.07–13.08)	
		2 (Managerial)		8.37 (6.21–11.04)	
		3 (Skilled, non-manual)		24.53 (18.21–32.34)	
		4 (Skilled, manual)		8.06 (5.99–10.63)	
		5 (Partly skilled)		15.01 (11.03–19.96)	
		6 (Unskilled)		15.14 (8.65–24.58)	
		7 (Armed forces)		27.21 (11.75–53.61)	
		8 (Inadequately described)		46.75 (17.16, 101.75)	
		9 (Housewife, student, carer, sick, private income, no occupation, not stated)		191.33 (159.32, 233.33)	
USA	1997	Education	298[e]		45 (Table 1)
	< 12 years			9.5 (95% CI: 8.1, 10.9)	
	> 12 years			6.3 (95% CI: 5.3, 7.8)	
Nigeria (Zaria: Ahmedu Bello University Hospital)	1976–79	Education[f]	238[e]		67 (Table 12.1)
		Some (unbooked cases)		0.00	
		Some (booked cases)		261.00	
		None (unbooked cases)		2926.00	
		None (booked cases)		104.00	

[a] National figures unless indicated otherwise; [b] direct maternal deaths only; [c] direct, indirect, coincidental and late maternal deaths; [d] maternal deaths per 100 000 maternities (deliveries after 24 weeks of gestation; [e] direct and indirect maternal deaths; [f] booked/unbooked cases are defined on the basis of whether the woman had booked for antenatal care and received at least two visits, the last no more than two weeks before delivery;[68] CI = confidence interval; MMR = maternal mortality ratio

Mortality Programme Assessment (IMMPACT) to build an evidence base on effective and cost-effective intervention strategies for reducing maternal mortality in developing countries.[54]

Increasing service use overall cannot be assumed to produce health gain, precisely because of the inequalities and inequities between population subgroups. These differentials are disguised by such national statistics as the proportion of deliveries with health professionals. Recent work has revealed major discrepancies between the rich and the poor as regards uptake of maternal health services – discrepancies that are often greater within countries than between them.[51,52] Moreover, there is a growing concern that the health sector reforms under way in many of these countries may in fact increase rather than decrease the inequities specific to maternal health.[55] Figure 1.2, for example, shows significant gradients between the poorest and richest groups but also indicates a steeper trend for the service indicator for maternal rather than child health.

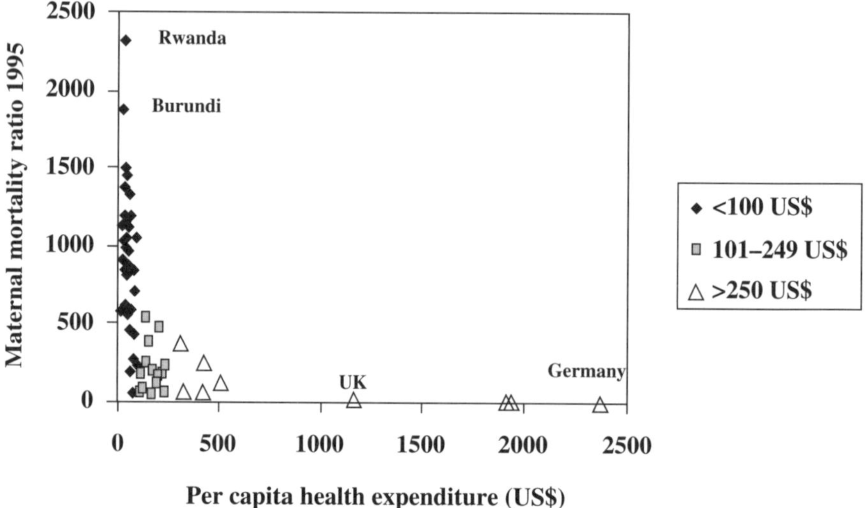

Figure 1.1. Maternal mortality ratio (MMR)[65] per 100 000 births (1995) by per capita health expenditure[74] (1997) for 66 developed and developing countries

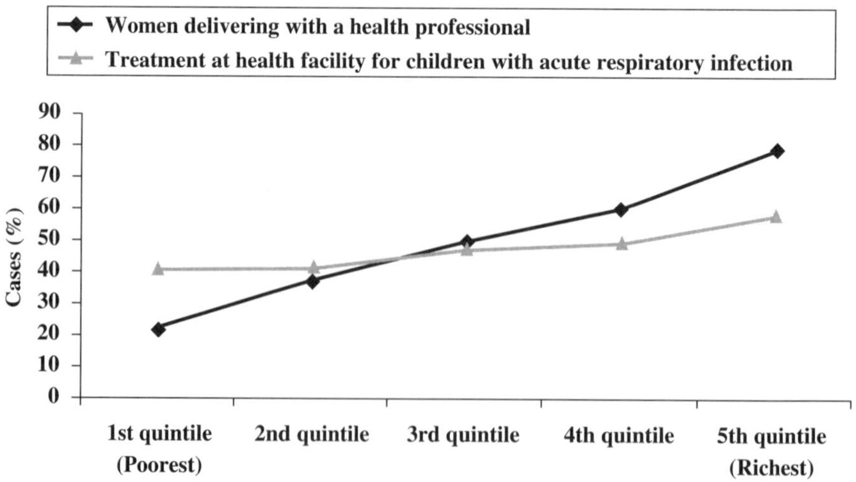

Figure 1.2. Poor–rich inequalities[51] in access to different types of health care (unweighted average from ten developing countries); reproduced with permission from the World Bank

The disadvantage that women face is also reflected in gender-specific analyses of mortality risk, with the apparent biological advantages that women are born with in terms of life expectancy often being reversed in the reproductive years.[36] This has also been linked with poverty, and it is now estimated that women constitute 70% of the world's poor.[56]

The use of services is, however, itself confounded with clinical need. For example, an extremely low proportion of deliveries with doctors is not necessarily a sign of huge unmet need, since these may in fact be the very women requiring obstetric intervention. Crude indicators of deliveries with health professionals are thus hard to interpret, since they encompass both women who need professional care and those who have the resources to choose such care. Although service use is undoubtedly linked in many countries with levels of poverty and economic disadvantage, obviously underlying biological factors should also be acknowledged. A topical illustration of this is provided by the prediction that levels of maternal mortality will increase in the near future in several European countries owing to increasing age at first birth.[57] This demographic trend is predominantly found in higher socio-economic groups, who also tend to use services more often, confounding the relationship with maternal mortality risks – risks that are well known to rise with age regardless of income.

Health inequalities are not just economically determined

Clearly it would be simplistic to assume that economic factors are the only determinants of inequalities in maternal mortality. Both historical and contemporary research shows a number of aspects to disadvantage that operate through subtle and indirect pathways to influence outcomes. Some of these 'who you are' societal factors are group characteristics such as ethnicity, caste or race, while others, such as marital status, social standing, self-esteem or psycho-social stress, are specific to individuals (Table 1.3). These differentials may of course be masking underlying biological or economic factors, although this does not appear to be the case. In the USA, for example, the four-fold increase in the risk of maternal death in black women versus white women for every cause contrasts with only a two-fold increase in the risk of complications. Moreover, economic factors cannot explain the higher risks of maternal death among black versus Hispanic women, since they have comparable poverty status.[45] Indeed, Ibison *et al.*[58] found that the immigrant women in England and Wales who died of maternal causes were more likely to come from high-income groups compared with non-immigrant women. Razum *et al.*,[59] on the other hand, suggest that the higher risks of maternal death among unmarried women observed in Germany transcend nationality, and are in fact the reflection of economic disadvantage among single mothers.

These examples raise one of the major difficulties in studying the determinants of health inequalities – the temporal dimension. Socio-economic status can change dramatically for individuals and families not only in one generation, but also across generations. This is now well recognised to complicate studies of the early origins of health inequalities,[24] possibly including some of the indirect causes of maternal deaths in developed countries. Thus, measures of disadvantage, social or economic, close to the time of death may conceal the influence of familial or early environment factors. This is also relevant to developing country populations, where education can make a dramatic difference to income levels within one generation, and yet may not be able to

Table 1.3. Selected studies reporting socially related inequalities in maternal mortality

Country[a]	Period	Differential	Total deaths (*n*)	Measure of maternal mortality	MMR per 100 000 live births (95% CI)	Adapted from reference
USA	1925–37	Race:		MMR per 100 000 live births		7 (Table 1)
		White			510–630	
		Non-white			900–1200	
USA	1997	Race:	303[b]	MMR per 100 000 live births		45 (Table 1)
		White (non-Hispanic)			5.2 (4.3–6.1)	
		Black			20.8 (17.2–24.5)	
		Hispanic			8.0 (6.1–10.4)	
		Marital status:	327[b]	MMR per 100 000 live births		
		Married			7.1 (6.1–8.1)	
		Unmarried			11.2 (9.4–13.1)	
Guatemala	1986	Ethnic group:	419[b]	MMR per 100 000 live births		68 (Table 3)
		Indigenous			165	
		Non-indigenous			94	
England	1997–99	Ethnic group:	213[b]	MMR per 100 000 live births		17 (Table 1.15)
		White			11.0	
		Pakistani/Indian/Bangladeshi			32.4	
		Black African/Caribbean/mixed/other			16.4	
		Asian/other			13.9	
West Germany	1989–96	Nationality:	334[b]	MMR per 100 000 live births		59 (Table 2, Table 4)
		German			5.8	
		Non-German			7.6	
		Marital status:		Age-adjusted relative risk		
		Unmarried versus married			1.85	
		Married non-German versus married German			1.73	
		Unmarried non-German versus married German			0.92	
Former East Germany (after reunification)	1991–96	Marital status:	45[b]	Relative risk		69
		Unmarried versus married (crude)			1.91 (1.06–3.45)	
		Unmarried versus married (age-adjusted)			2.56 (1.41–4.63)	

[a] National figures unless indicated otherwise; [b] direct and indirect maternal deaths; CI = confidence interval; MMR = maternal mortality ratio

counteract relevant childhood factors, such as poor nutrition. The application of life-course approaches[24] to inequalities in maternal mortality therefore deserves further consideration.

Avoidable maternal deaths are, by definition, inequities

The concept of avoidable maternal deaths has long been used in obstetric research. If all inequities are acknowledged as avoidable or preventable differences in health outcomes that are unjust or unfair, from this perspective it could be argued that all avoidable maternal deaths are inequities. As proposed in the European Atlas of Avoidable Mortality,[60] for those conditions or diseases where deaths are substantially avoidable by adequate and timely health care, variations in the incidence or prevalence of these conditions may help to explain but rarely to justify differences in mortality. Thus factors that increase the risks of pregnancy-related complications rarely justify the varying risks of maternal death within the same population. Avoidable maternal deaths are therefore injustices to all women regardless of where, what or who they are.

It is estimated that 88–98% of maternal deaths in the world are avoidable with timely and effective care.[61] Table 1.4 presents empirical data on the lack of such care across a wide variety of settings. At all levels of maternal mortality, there are some service-related avoidable factors that are essentially a function of the health system and others that appear to be driven by the interaction between the provider and the patient. This interaction seems to be mediated by who the patient is. In the USA, for example, the quality of care received has been shown to have a direct relationship with the socio-economic status of the individual.[45] Similarly, in the CEMD report it is acknowledged in the discussion on avoidable factors that 'health professionals who work with disadvantaged clients need to be able to understand a woman's social and cultural background'.[17] In developing countries, poor-quality care is well known to be a serious deterrent to women seeking care, as well as a direct cause of maternal deaths.[62] This poor-quality care, in turn, is influenced by the woman's socio-economic position and often aggravated by the huge divide between her status and perspectives and those of the provider. This is clearly illustrated in the case of unwanted pregnancy and abortion-related mortality. The providers' willingness to deliver an appropriate, timely and high-quality termination or post-abortion service can be the determinant of a woman's life or death in many developed and developing countries.[63] In the USA, for example, the case–fatality rate from abortion is over four-times greater in black than in white women.[45] The mortality rate from abortion in developing countries is estimated at almost 700 per 100 000 terminations, versus 0.2–1.2 in developed countries[63] – a stark geographical inequality that is undoubtedly masking a bigger inequity between women.

Conclusion and recommendations

The global problem of maternal mortality persists despite significant technological progress and greater understanding, and despite economic advance for the rich minority of the world. The focus on the size of the problem – on the MMR and, where information systems permit, on time trends, has deflected attention away from the question of differentials within populations or countries. The extent to which these

Table 1.4. Selected studies reporting avoidable factors in maternal deaths

Country[a]	Period	Avoidable deaths (%)	Avoidable deaths (n)	Comment	Adapted from reference
Japan	1991–92	37 (preventable) 16 (possibly preventable)	72/197 32/197	Direct and indirect maternal deaths; mistake or error constituting substandard care must have occurred for death to qualify as preventable	70
West Africa[b]	1994–96	74 (avoidable) 69 (received substandard or no care)	38/55 32/43	Direct obstetric deaths Direct, indirect and late	49
Afghanistan[c]	1999–2000	67 (preventable)	18/27	Direct and indirect deaths among refugee population; authors do not define preventable	71
Egypt	1992–93	47 (substandard care from the obstetric team)	334/718	92% of direct and indirect deaths had one or more factors contributing to death, including for example patient delay and no/lack of antenatal care	72 (Table 8)
Sri Lanka[d]	1985–87, 1990–97	73 (preventable) 79 (received substandard care) 66 (received poor institutional care) 60 (mismanaged)	97/133 105/133 88/133 80/133	Pregnancy-related deaths	73
UK	1997–99	Direct deaths: 60 (some substandard care) 50 (major substandard care)	 64/106 53/106		17 (Table 1.4)
		Indirect deaths: 22 (some substandard care) 13 (major substandard care)	 46/205 26/205		17 (Table 1.5)
		Late and coincidental deaths: 10 (some substandard care) 7 (major substandard care)	 12/123 9/123		

[a] National figures unless indicated otherwise; [b] death identified among women living in specified areas of Abidjan (Côte d'Ivoire), Bamako (Mali), Niamey (Niger), Nouakchott (Mauritania), Ougadougou (Burkina Faso), Saint-Louis, Kafrine, Fatik (Senegal); [c] deaths in 12 Afghan refugee settlements in Pakistan; [d] maternal deaths at Castle Street Hospital, Colombo, Sri Lanka

differences can be regarded as inequalities or inequities involves value-judgements about fairness and justice. These values obviously vary between societies and over time but the avoidability of the majority of maternal deaths in all countries remains a universal violation of human rights.

Health inequalities and inequities are not static or inevitable phenomena, but rather have a dynamic driven by the interaction of geography, biology and society that is mediated by the health system. This implies that they are amenable to change and so gives some grounds for optimism.[14] After more than 200 years of research on maternal mortality, much of it focusing on clinical or biological risk factors, it is time to promote a stronger societal perspective. This will help to throw light on crucial barriers both to the demand from women for care and to the supply of effective, cost-effective and equitable services. Such a perspective can usefully be labelled 'social obstetrics' in honour of one of the first social obstetricians – Sir Dugald Baird.

With this perspective come four responsibilities and recommendations for action.

1. Concerted efforts are needed to improve routine data sources and enquiry methods for determining inequalities in maternal health. Outcomes need to be broadened beyond maternal mortality to include severe maternal morbidity (near-misses), addressing the constraints of small numbers of deaths and of reliance on proxy respondents. The range and nature of socially relevant data routinely gathered for case management need to be reviewed. In the context of weak information systems, the role of verbal autopsy techniques should be reassessed specifically for collecting socio-economic information. The potential for follow-up of maternal deaths or near-misses requires further consideration in order to supplement routine sources, particularly as regards social circumstances. Maternal health research should learn lessons and benefit from developments in other relevant fields. These include the use of multilevel modelling to overcome problems of small numbers and of individual versus aggregate data, the use of Geographic Information Systems to map outcomes against service provision and other covariates, and the use of small-areas statistics and analytical methods, for example, from the 2001 UK Census.[14]

2. There needs to be a renewed call for multidisciplinary teamwork. Reflecting on a similar observation by Sir Dugald Baird[64] over three decades ago, the call must go beyond obstetricians, midwives, sociologists, statisticians, nutritionists and psychologists. It should now include health economists who can inform our understanding of poverty, cost-effectiveness and equity, and demographers and epidemiologists who can bring to maternal mortality more sophisticated approaches to studying differentials.

3. Greater attention is needed to the indirect causes of maternal mortality. These represent a growing proportion of the total in developed and developing countries and may reflect different socio-economic inequalities from those linked with direct causes. In poor countries, the old challenge of communicable diseases such as malaria and tuberculosis now needs to be tackled together with the new onslaught from HIV/AIDS. These are indeed the diseases of poverty, and their inclusion in the global burden of maternal mortality will further emphasise the inequalities and inequities within rather than between developing countries. Indirect causes also highlight a possible role for life-course approaches to the study of maternal mortality, both for medical conditions such as heart disease and for mental illness and suicide.

4. Finally, in judging the success of intervention strategies in reducing maternal mortality it is crucial that not only clinical effectiveness and cost-effectiveness are considered, but also the implications for equity goals. The health-sector reforms under way in many developed and developing countries may indeed decrease the gap between advantaged and disadvantaged groups for some health outcomes. But they may also inadvertently increase inequities for others, and thus require mechanisms and advocates for monitoring positive and negative effects. 'Social obstetrics' must recognise these political dimensions to maternal health and acknowledge that safe motherhood should be the equal right of all women.

Acknowledgements

Thanks are given to my colleagues in Aberdeen for helpful comments on an earlier version of this paper, particularly Professor Marion Hall, Dr Colin Bullough, Dr Gillian Penney, Dr Julia Hussein, Julie Bruce, Dr Janet Tucker and Dr Edwin van Teijlingen. This paper is dedicated to the lasting memory of the late Dr Paul Arthur, Director of the Kintampo Health Research Centre, who died suddenly on 9 March 2002. Paul's contribution to safe motherhood, both in his home country of Ghana and internationally, lives on through the standards he set for rigorous research and for multidisciplinary collaboration.

References

1. Lowis GW. Epidemiology of puerperal fever: the contributions of Alexander Gordon. *Med Hist*1993;37:399–410.
2. Louden I. *Death in Childbirth: An International Study of Maternal Care and Maternal Mortality 1800–1950.* Oxford: Clarendon Press; 1992.
3. Macfarlane A. Enquiries into maternal deaths during the 20th century. In: *Why Mothers Die 1997–1999. The Confidential Enquiries into Maternal Deaths in the United Kingdom.* London: RCOG Press; 2001. p. 346–57.
4. Godber G. The Confidential Enquiry into Maternal Deaths. A limited study of clinical results. In: McGlachan G, editor. *A Question of Quality.* London: Nuffield Provincial Hospitals Trust; 1976. p. 25–33.
5. Baird D. Preventive medicine in obstetrics. *N Engl J Med* 1952;246:561–8.
6. Feachem RGA. Poverty and inequity: a proper focus for the new century. *Bull World Health Organ*2000;78:1–3.
7. Loudon I. Maternal mortality in the past and its relevance to developing countries today. *Am J Clin Nutr* 2000;72:241S–246S.
8. van Lerberghe W, de Brouwere V. Of blind alleys and things that have worked: history's lessons on reducing maternal mortality. *Studies in Health Service Organisation and Policy* 2001;17:7–33.
9. AbouZahr C, Wardlaw T. Maternal mortality at the end of the decade: signs of progress? *Bull World Health Organ* 2001;79:561–73.
10. Liljestrand J. Strategies to reduce maternal mortality worldwide. *Curr Opin Obstet Gynaecol* 2000;12:513–17.
11. Malthus TR. *An Essay on the Principle of Population as it Affects the Future of Society.* London: Johnson; 1798.
12. Hogberg U, Wall S, Brostrom G. The impact of early medical technology on maternal mortality in late 19th century Sweden. *Int J Gynaecol Obstet* 1986;24:251–61.
13. Harrison KA. Anaemia, malaria and sickle cell disease. *Clin Obstet Gynaecol* 1982;9:445–77.
14. Leon DA, Walt G. Poverty, inequality, and health in international perspective: a divided world? In: Leon DA, Walt G, editors. *Poverty, Inequality and Health.* Oxford: Oxford University Press; 2001. p. 1–16.
15. Fathalla MF. When medicine rediscovered its social roots. *Bull World Health Organ* 2000;78:677–8.
16. de Brouwere V, Tonglet R, Van Lerberghe W. Strategies for reducing maternal mortality in developing countries: what can we learn from the history of the industrialized West? *Trop Med Int Health* 1998;3:771–82.
17. Drife J, Lewis G, editors. *Why Mothers Die 1997–1999. The Confidential Enquiries into Maternal Deaths in the United Kingdom.* London: RCOG Press; 2001.
18. AbouZahr C. Maternal mortality overview. In: Murray CJL, Lopez, AD, editors. *Health Dimensions of Sex and Reproduction. Global Burden of Disease and Injury Series. Volume III.* Geneva: WHO; 1998. p. 111–64.
19. Calman KC. Equity, poverty and health for all. *BMJ* 1997;314:1187–91.
20. Leon DA, Walt G, Gilson L. Recent advances: international perspectives on health inequalities and policy. *BMJ* 2001;322:591–4.
21. Cook RJ, Dickens BM. Ethics, justice and women's health. *Int J Gynaecol Obstet* 1999;64:81–5.

22. Freedman LP. Using human rights in maternal mortality programs: from analysis to strategy. *Int J Gynaecol Obstet* 2001;75:51–60.
23. Graham WJ, Campbell OMR. The measurement trap. *Soc Sci Med* 1992;35:967–76.
24. Davey-Smith G, Gunnell D, Ben-Sholomo Y. Life-course approaches to socio-economic differentials in cause-specific adult mortality. In: Leon DA, Walt G, editors. *Poverty, Inequality and Health.* Oxford: Oxford University Press; 2001. p. 88–124.
25. Braveman P, Krieger N, Lynch J. Health inequalities and social inequalities in health. *Bull World Health Organ* 2000;78:232–5.
26. Stanton C, Abderrahim N, Hill K. An assessment of DHS maternal mortality indicators. *Stud Fam Plann* 2000;21:111–23.
27. Diamond I, Matthews Z, Stephenson R. *Assessing the Health of the Poor: Towards a Pro-poor Measurement Strategy.* London: DFID Health Systems Resource Centre; 2001.
28. Sankoh OA, Ngom P, Nyarko P, Mwageni E, Kahn K, editors. INDEPTH Network. *Population and Health in Developing Countries. Volume 1: Population, Health and Survival at INDEPTH Sites.* Ottawa: International Development Research Centre; 2002.
29. Sloan NL, Langer A, Hernandez B, Romero M, Winikoff B. The etiology of maternal mortality in developing countries: what do verbal autopsies tell us? *Bull World Health Organ* 2001;79:805–10.
30. Chandramohan D, Rodrigues LC, Maude GH, Hayes RJ. Verbal autopsies for adult deaths: their development and validation in a multicentre study. *Trop Med Int Health* 1998;3:436–46.
31. Bouvier-Colle MH, Varnoux N, Costes P, Hatton F. Reasons for the underreporting of maternal mortality in France, as indicated by a survey of all deaths among women of childbearing age. *Int J Epidemiol* 1991;20:717–21.
32. Abou Zahr C, Vaughan JP. Assessing the burden of sexual and reproductive ill-health: questions regarding the use of disability-adjusted life years. *Bull World Health Organ* 2000;78:655–66.
33. Carstairs V, Morris R. *Deprivation and Health in Scotland.* Aberdeen: Aberdeen University Press; 1991.
34. Gwatkin DR. Health inequalities and the health of the poor: what do we know? What can we do? *Bull World Health Organ* 2000;78:3–18.
35. Valkonen T. Problems in the measurement and international comparisons of socio-economic differences in mortality. *Soc Sci Med* 1993;36:409–18.
36. Oakley A. Who cares for health? Social relations, gender, and the public health. *J Epidemiol Community Health* 1994;48:427–34.
37. Harrison KA. Maternal mortality in Nigeria: the real issues. *Afr J Reprod Health* 1997;1:7–13.
38. Loslier L. Geographic information systems (GIS) from a health perspective. In: de Savigny D, Wijeyaratne P, editors. *GIS for Health and the Environment. Proceedings of an International Workshop*, 5–10 September 1994, Colombo, Sri Lanka; 1995. p. 13–20. Colombo: Colombo University Press.
39. Kaufman L, Rousseeuw PJ. *Finding Groups in Data: An Introduction to Cluster Analysis.* New York: Wiley; 1990.
40. Mahler H. The Safe Motherhood Initiative: a call to action. *Lancet* 1987;i:668–70.
41. Graham WJ, Bell J, Bullough CHW. Can skilled attendance at delivery reduce maternal mortality in developing countries. *Studies in Health Service Organisation and Policy* 2001;17:97–130.
42. United Nations. *Key Actions for the Further Implementation of the Programme of Action for the International Conference on Population and Development.* New York: UN; 1999.
43. World Health Organization. *Reduction of Maternal Mortality. A Joint WHO/UNFPA/UNICEF/World Bank Statement.* Geneva: WHO; 1999.
44. Shen C, Williamson JB. Maternal mortality, women's status, and economic dependency in less developed countries: a cross-national analysis. *Soc Sci Med* 1999;49:197–214.
45. Hoyert DL, Danel I, Tully P. Maternal mortality, United States and Canada, 1982–1997. *Birth* 2000;27:4–11.
46. Baird D. The evolution of modern obstetrics. *Lancet* 1960;2:557–64.
47. Goddard M, Smith P. Equity of access to health care services: theory and evidence from the United Kingdom. *Soc Sci Med* 2001;53:1149–62.
48. Kaunitz AM, Spence C, Danielson TS, Rochat RW, Grimes DA. Perinatal and maternal mortality in a religious group avoiding obstetric care. *Am J Obstet Gynecol* 1984;150:826–31.
49. Bouvier-Colle MH, Ouedraogo C, Dumont A, Vangeenderhuysen C, Salanave B, Decam C, for the MOMA Group. Maternal mortality in West Africa: rates, causes and substandard care from a prospective survey. *Acta Obstet Gynecol Scand* 2001;80:113–19.
50. World Health Organization. *Macroeconomics and Health. Investing in Health for Economic Development.* Geneva: WHO; 2001.

51. World Bank. *Safe Motherhood and the World Bank. Lessons from 10 years of experience. Human Development Network.* Washington DC: The World Bank; 1999.
52. Kunst AE, Houweling T. A global picture of poor-rich differences in the utilisation of delivery care. *Studies in Health Service Organisation and Policy* 2001;17:297–315.
53. Wardlaw T, Maine D. Process indicators for maternal mortality programmes. In: Berer M, Ravindran TKS, editors. *Reproductive Health Matters. Safe Motherhood Initiatives: Critical Issues.* London: Blackwell Science; 1999. p. 24–30.
54. Graham WJ. Now or never: the case for measuring maternal mortality. *Lancet* 2002;359:701–4.
55. McDonagh M, Goodburn E. Maternal health and health sector reform: opportunities and challenges. *Studies in Health Service Organisation and Policy* 2001;17:317–85.
56. Department for International Development. *Breaking the Barriers: Women and the Elimination of World Poverty*. London: DFID; 1999.
57. Salanave B, Bouvier-Colle MH. The likely increase in maternal mortality in the UK and France until 2005. *Paediatr Perinat Epidemiol* 1996;10:418–22.
58. Ibison JM, Swerdlow AJ, Head JA, Marmot M. Maternal mortality in England and Wales 1970–1985: an analysis by country of birth. *Br J Obstet Gynaecol* 1996;103:973–80.
59. Razum O, Jahn A, Blettner A, Reitmaier P. Trends in maternal mortality ratio among women of German and non-German nationality in West Germany, 1980–1996. *Int J Epidemiol* 1999;28:919–24.
60. Holland WW. *European Community Atlas of Avoidable Death*. 2nd ed. Oxford: Oxford Medical Publications; 1993.
61. World Health Organization. *Prevention of Maternal Mortality: report of WHO Inter-Regional Meeting, Geneva November 11–15, 1985*. Geneva: WHO; 1986.
62. Koblinsky M, Conroy C, Kureshy N, Stanton ME. *Issues in Programming for Safe Motherhood.* Washington DC: MotherCare; 2000.
63. Berer M. Making abortions safe: a matter of good public health policy and practice. *Bull World Health Organ* 2000;78:580–91.
64. Baird D. Social research and obstetric practice. *Question* 1969:3–13.
65. World Health Organization. *Maternal Mortality in 1995*. Estimates developed by WHO, UNICEF, UNFPA. WHO/RHR/01.9. Geneva: WHO; 2001 [http://www.who.int/reproductive-health/publications/RHR_01_9_maternal_mortality_estimates/index.en.html].
66. Population Reference Bureau. *2001 World Population Data Sheet*. Washington: PRB; 2001.
67. Harrison KA. Child-bearing, health and social priorities: a survey of 22,774 consecutive births in Zaria, northern Nigeria. *Br J Obstet Gynaecol* 1985;92 Suppl 5.
68. Kestler E. Guatemala: maternal mortality in Guatemala: assessing the gap, beginning to bridge it. *World Health Stat Q* 1995;48:28–33.
69. Razum O, Jahn A, Snow R. Maternal mortality in the former East Germany before and after reunification: changes in risk by marital status. *BMJ* 1999;319:1104–5.
70. Nagaya K, Fetters MD, Ishikawa M, Kubo T, Koyanagi T, Saito Y, *et al*. Causes of maternal mortality in Japan. *JAMA* 2000;283:2661–7.
71. Bartlett LA, Jamieson DJ, Kahm T, Sultana M, Wilson HG, Duerr A. Maternal mortality among Afghan refugees in Pakistan, 1999–2000. *Lancet* 2002;359:643–9.
72. Egypt Ministry of Health. *National Maternal Mortality Study: Findings and conclusions.* Cairo: Child Survival Project. Egypt Ministry of Health; 1994.
73. Wagaarachchi P, Fernando L. Trends in maternal mortality and assessment of substandard care in a tertiary care hospital. *Eur J Obstet Gynecol Reprod Biol* 2002;101:36–40.
74. World Health Organization. *World Health Report 2000.* Geneva: WHO; 2000.

Chapter 2

Contributing to making a difference: the World Health Organization's 'Making Pregnancy Safer' strategy

Luc de Bernis

Introduction

Each year more than 20 million women experience ill health as a result of pregnancy; for some the suffering is permanent. The lives of eight million are threatened, and over half a million women[1] die from causes related to pregnancy and childbirth. In addition, about 3.9 million newborn infants die within the first week of life, and another three million babies are born dead.[2] Although the term 'newborn' is used here, it is recognised that some interventions during pregnancy and delivery will also have an impact on risk of stillbirth and, thus, perinatal statistics.

Estimates recently published[1] show that, despite all efforts conducted for more than ten years under the Safe Motherhood Initiative (SMI), trends are not tending to decrease in the poorest countries.

The reasons why these maternal mortality ratios (MMRs) are not decreasing are complex and include lack of a clear internationally agreed strategy, lack of governmental commitment and lack of coordination and funding. Experience over the past decade has also shown that the challenge of maternal and newborn illnesses and deaths is highly dependent upon a functioning healthcare system that responds to pregnant women's needs by improving access to quality maternal health services, especially among the poor and vulnerable populations. Access to maternal health services has been seriously lacking in all of the countries with high MMRs.

Burden of disease

Maternal and newborn ill-health are substantial contributors to the global burden of disease, together accounting for some 8% of the total burden globally and much higher proportions in the developing world. Maternal and newborn health services, therefore, need to be given due attention and need to be complementary to other core cost-effective public and private health interventions (HIV/AIDS, tuberculosis, malaria, etc.). Increased efforts are needed to measure the maternal and newborn health-related burden of disease: information about maternal and newborn morbidity and the consequences for the family and household of maternal deaths is not widely available. Measurement of maternal and newborn morbidity is facing enormous problems related to the lack of agreed definitions, relevant data and research funding. For example, we do not yet know the prevalence of critical problems such as vesicovaginal fistula, which are creating the worst life we can imagine for thousands of women, mostly poor and adolescent. Equally, the social and economic costs of such maternal and newborn conditions needs to be calculated and analysed.

Determinants of maternal deaths are complex and relate to many factors including:

- women's status
- poverty
- illiteracy
- low economic development
- weakness of health systems
- barriers caused by regulations and laws.

However, the majority of the causes of death are preventable or treatable. There is evidence that the five main direct obstetric causes of deaths account for nearly 80% of maternal deaths. These deaths can be prevented by actions that are effective and affordable in developing country contexts (Tables 2.1 and 2.2).

Effective interventions

Effective interventions to reduce morbidity and mortality exist and have for the past few decades been used in developed countries. Although research is needed to adapt technologies and protocols to poor settings, the need to implement these cost-effective interventions is clearly established. Addressing the complex challenge of maternal and newborn morbidity and mortality depends upon an enabling environment that includes human resources management, equipment, drugs, supplies, transport and the necessary community mobilisation. Effective interventions include preventive measures such as the 'Plan for Birth'[3,4] (antenatal care), family planning to prevent unwanted pregnancies, management of normal birth to prevent infections and detect early complications, iron and folic acid supplementation and malaria prophylaxis during pregnancy.

Gender and reproductive rights

Maternal mortality is symptomatic of gender inequality. Preventing maternal death and illness is an issue of social justice and women's human rights. Redefining maternal mortality from a 'health disadvantage' to a 'social injustice' provides the legal and political basis for governments to ensure maternal health care for all women.[5]

'If hundreds of thousands of men were suffering and dying every year, alone in fear

Table 2.1. Maternal and newborn deaths and stillbirths: causes and main interventions

Causes of death	%	Proven interventions
Maternal		
Bleeding after delivery (postpartum haemorrhage)	25	Treating anaemia in pregnancy Skilled attendant at birth to prevent/treat bleeding with correct drugs and replace fluid loss by intravenous drip/transfusion if severe
Infection after delivery	15	Skilled attendant at birth: clean practices, antibiotics if infection arises
Unsafe abortion	13	Skilled attendant to give antibiotics, empty uterus, replace fluids if needed, counsel and provide family planning; access to safe abortion where legal
High blood pressure (hypertension) during pregnancy: most dangerous when severe (eclampsia)	12	Detection in pregnancy Referral to doctor or hospital Treating eclampsia with appropriate anticonvulsive (magnesium sulphate) Referring unconscious woman for expert urgent assistance
Obstructed labour	8	Detection in time and referral for operative delivery
Other direct obstetric causes	8	Refer ectopic pregnancy for operation
Indirect causes	19	Disease-specific interventions (malaria, HIV etc.)
Newborn		
Infections (sepsis, meningitis, pneumonia, neonatal tetanus, congenital syphilis)	33	Maternal tetanus toxoid immunisation Syphilis screening and treatment Clean delivery Warmth Support for early and exclusive breastfeeding Early recognition and management of infections
Birth asphyxia and trauma	28	Skilled attendant at birth Effective management of maternal obstetric complications
Preterm birth and/or low birthweight	24	Antimalarials for women at risk during pregnancy, more attention to warmth Breastfeeding counselling and support Infection control and early detection and management of complications Treatment of sexually transmitted diseases Smoking cessation
Stillbirths		
Birth asphyxia and trauma	40	Skilled attendant at birth Effective management of obstetric complications
Other known causes (pregnancy complications, maternal diseases, malaria, malformations)	25	Pregnancy care Presumptive treatment for endemic diseases Effective management of pregnancy complications
Congenital syphilis	8	Maternal syphilis screening and treatment of positive cases
Cause unknown	27	

and agony, or if millions upon millions of men were being injured and disabled and humiliated, [some] sustaining massive and untreated injuries and wounds to their genitalia, leaving them in constant pain, infertile and incontinent, and in dread of having sex, then we would have heard about this issue long ago, and something would have been done'.[6]

Several human-rights treaties, including the Convention on the Elimination of all Forms of Discrimination against Women (the Women's Convention, ratified by more

Table 2.2. Major maternal complications

Complication	Actions
Postpartum haemorrhage	Plan for birth, active management of third stage of labour (UNIJECT) Manual removal of the placenta
Complicated abortion	Prevention, manual vacuum aspiration, antibiotics
Postpartum sepsis	Prevention (universal precautions, antibiotic prophylaxis for caesarean section), antibiotics
Obstructed labour	Early detection (partograph), caesarean section, vaginal extraction
Severe pre-eclampsia, eclampsia	Magnesium sulphate (Mg SO_4), antihypertensives
Anaemia	Screening, prevention and treatment, blood transfusion
Essential drugs	First-line: oxytocic (UNIJECT), Mg SO_4, antibiotics, iron/folic acid, tetanus toxoid vaccine Second-line: intravenous fluids, hydralazine, blood, anaesthetics
Laboratory tests	Syphilis, HIV, haemoglobin, blood group

than 160 countries) make specific mention of states' obligations relating to the prevention of maternal mortality and provision of appropriate services for pregnant women.

Inequality

This is one of the biggest inequalities between rich and poor communities. Women from the world's poorest households (income of less than US$1 per day) are at least 300 times more likely to suffer in this way than those who are more prosperous. In developing countries where populations have high levels of fertility, such as Eastern Africa, one woman in 11 may die of pregnancy-related causes during her lifetime, compared with one in 5000 in developed, low-fertility settings such as Southern Europe.[1]

Poverty-related maternal deaths are a reality that rich countries, such as the UK, are also facing. 'Women from the most disadvantaged groups of society were about 20 times more likely to die than women in the highest two social classes.'[7] Internationally agreed targets for reducing inequality include:

- a reduction of MMR by 50% between 1990 and 2000 and a further 50% reduction by 2015, i.e. an overall reduction of 75% between 1990 and 2015
- a reduction of infant mortality to below 35/1000 live births by 2015
- provision of access to all those who need reproductive health services by 2015.[8]

Where the maternal mortality rate is very high, at least 40% of all births should be assisted by skilled attendants by 2005. By 2010, this figure should be at least 50% and, by 2015, at least 60%. Globally, by 2005, 80% of all births should be assisted by skilled attendants, by 2010, 85%, and by 2015, 90%.[9]

Other international development goals, including the reduction of extreme poverty, gender equity and the education of girls and women should, if met, also contribute to the improvement of maternal and newborn health.

Building on the lessons learned after ten years of the Safe Motherhood Initiative (1997, Colombo meeting), the WHO/UNICEF/UNFPA/World Bank Joint Statement on Reduction of Maternal Mortality was developed in 1999,[10] which formed the basis for consensus on:

- prevention and management of unwanted pregnancy and unsafe abortion
- skilled care during pregnancy and childbirth
- access to referral care when complications arise.

Making pregnancy safer

In order to respond to this challenge and for the World Health Organization (WHO) to fulfil its mandate, the Making Pregnancy Safer (MPR) initiative has recently been established as one of the 11 high priorities that the organisation pledges to focus on.

The WHO MPR strategy is a next step in the operationalisation of the Joint Statement on Maternal Mortality Reduction. This initiative represents the WHO's strengthened contribution to the global Safe Motherhood Initiative, aiming to reduce maternal and newborn morbidity and mortality worldwide.

MPR is a health-sector strategy that focuses on a systematic and integrated planning approach to address the key clinical and health-systems interventions necessary to reduce maternal and newborn morbidity and mortality. The strategy places particular emphasis on skilled attendance and the provision of appropriate and effective continuum of care.

The objectives of the MPR initiative are therefore to provide guidance on how to:

- improve equitable access, use and quality of maternal and newborn services
- improve family and community practices for maternal and newborn health.

Making Pregnancy Safer initiative's added value

The initiative is focusing on evidence-based and cost-effective interventions that are intended to achieve international targets. These interventions cover pregnancy, childbirth and postpartum care, including family planning, abortion (where abortion is legal) and post-abortion care.

Experience increasingly calls for professionalisation of birth care in the form of skilled attendants. Professionals (obstetricians, gynaecologists and midwives) know that the reduction of MMR depends to a large extent on the access to quality skilled care for all pregnant women and their newborn. The international definition of a 'skilled attendant' has therefore been developed.[9]

The impact of implementation of skilled attendants has never been measured because such interventions are complex and multifactored. It is hoped, however, that the Initiative for Maternal Mortality Programme Assessment Project at the Dugald Baird Centre for Research on Women's Health (Aberdeen University) will be able to provide useful findings on this issue. However, many experiences from countries in the North and South, such as the recently studied examples of Sri Lanka and Malaysia,[11] clearly show the importance of establishing a strong human-resources strategy based on midwives accompanied by investments in a functioning health system in the dramatic reduction of MMR. In Thailand, to give another example, the maternal mortality reduction by three-quarters in the 1960s and 1970s has been obtained mainly by quadrupling the number of new midwifes. It is important to add that although the number of professionals is important, the question is also how professional staff perform and behave. Delivery structures need to be adequately equipped and staffed by well-trained and well-motivated health workers.

Traditional birth attendants

Traditional birth attendants are not skilled attendants. Strategies will need to be put in place to accelerate the production of skilled attendants. However, the two roles need to be clearly defined, as traditional birth attendants continue to be necessary pending the availability of skilled attendants. Traditional birth attendants will continue to play a role as a crucial link between the communities and formal health-service delivery system.

Assessing the Safe Motherhood Initiative from a human rights perspective

MPR is using a rights-based approach to help countries with assessing regulations and laws that may have an impact on maternal and newborn health. An assessment tool has been developed to assist a national stakeholder team to review laws, policies and health-systems considerations against the major health outcome indicators. It will be field-tested in Mozambique.

Poverty focus

MPR focuses especially on poor and marginalised women, especially adolescents, in developing countries, as the burden of disease associated with maternal morbidity and mortality is highest among this group of women.

Entry point

MPR focuses on maternal and newborn health services that provide an entry-point for other health interventions, such as prevention and management of HIV, sexually transmitted infections, tuberculosis and malaria. What is the best way to implement mother-to-child transmission prevention programmes if pregnant women are not using antenatal care services? MPR is working with other programmes in order to give guidance in integrated care and ensuring provision of necessary care.

Health systems requirements

In order to create an enabling environment for the skilled attendant, MPR addresses the health systems requirements focusing on the key functions of the health system such as stewardship (overall system design, performance assessment, priority setting, intersectoral advocacy, regulation and consumer protection), financing (revenue collection, fund pooling and purchasing), resource generation (human resources, physical resources and knowledge) and service provision (combination of inputs into a production process that takes place in a particular organisational setting and leads to the provision of a series of interventions).[12] Maternal and newborn care services, including first and referral levels to provide essential and comprehensive obstetric care, require a functioning health system. MPR will address these needs in focusing mainly on the health service provision function that addresses the health-systems requirements that are necessary to ensure the provision of the key clinical interventions (Figure 2.1).

In other words, MPR will not take on entire health systems but will focus on areas that are crucial and pertinent to the provision of evidence-based maternal and newborn healthcare interventions. Skilled attendants, human-resource policy and strategies are key to MPR and need to be addressed accordingly. Strengthening midwifery services, addressing the respective and complementary roles of midwives and doctors, the professional status, the professional behaviour, in order to improve accessibility and quality of care will be crucial.

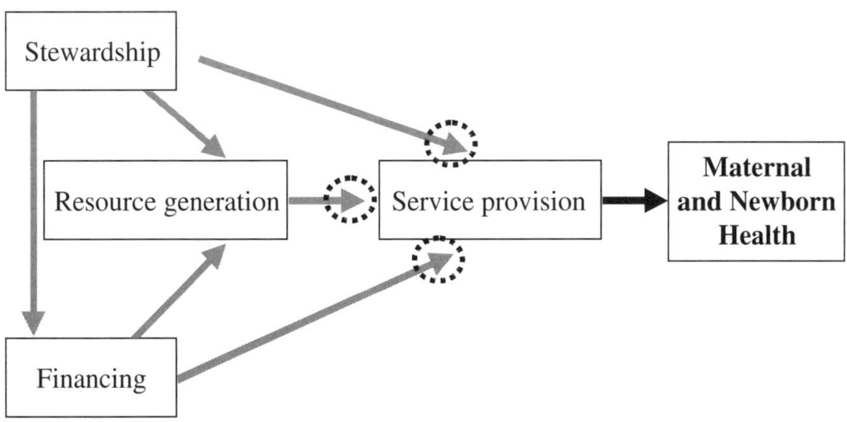

Figure 2.1. The WHO framework for health system performance assessment

Health system and sector reform gains

MPR seeks to highlight and integrate effective evidence-based interventions and activities into national health-planning processes such as health-sector reforms and health-development plans that have a profound impact on the development and delivery of services, including those that contribute to making pregnancy safer. Strengthening health systems to ensure the availability of skilled attendants for delivery and provision of an effective continuum of care, including emergency referral, will not only have a positive impact on maternal and newborn health but also on other services.

Expected outputs

MPR focuses on health outcomes and the importance of improving health systems in order to attain long-term, sustainable and affordable results in terms of safe motherhood. More specifically, the MPR expected process/output indicators (Table 2.2) include:

- increased maternal and newborn health services provided by a skilled attendant backed up by a functioning referral system properly equipped to manage complications
- increased best practices in the care of pregnant women and newborns
- increased healthy behaviour among women, including seeking timely maternal and newborn care
- availability of an environment conducive to the implementation of MPR activities.

Only strong governmental commitment, with adequate funding and strong support from donors, will achieve these ambitious but realistic objectives. The WHO's Commission on Macroeconomics and Health has recently estimated the necessary funds to achieve the Millennium Development Goal of reducing MMR by 75%, between 1990 and 2015, in the 83 worst-off countries. In order to increase the coverage to 90% in 2015, with refocused antenatal care and skilled birth attendance, the annual incremental cost is estimated as US$2.8–4.5 billion until 2007 and as US$4.3–6.7 billion until 2015. This represents 13.0% of the cost of expanding coverage of the 49 priority interventions needed in these countries to address the primary causes of the avoidable mortality (US$8–11 per capita or US$40–52 billion by 2015). The US$27 billion by 2007 would represent around one-tenth of 1% of the gross national product of the donor countries.[13]

'Making Pregnancy Safer' objectives

To achieve the MPR objectives, the WHO will focus on six areas of work:

1. providing technical support to countries
2. advocacy

3. partnership building
4. establishing norms and standards, and developing tools
5. promoting and coordinating research and disseminating findings
6. monitoring and evaluation.

Under each of these areas of work, a number of activities are developed to be undertaken at global, regional and national levels.

Technical country support

MPR is initially working in ten spotlight countries (Bolivia, Ethiopia, Indonesia, Laos PDR, Mauritania, Moldova, Mozambique, Nigeria, Sudan, Uganda), providing technical and policy support for national coordination and developing national capacities to plan, design and implement evidence-based medical and health-systems interventions, including policies, regulations and laws relating to maternal and newborn health services. MPR is carefully documenting lessons learned with a view to applying the experience gained in other countries in the future.

In providing technical support at the country level, MPR:

- supports the development of a comprehensive national reproductive health/Safe Motherhood Initiative/MPR strategy and plan (Indonesia, Nigeria etc.);
- supports the establishment of supportive policies, regulations and laws related to MPR and the Safe Motherhood Initiative (Mozambique, Mauritania)
- supports the development and adoption of evidence-based national norms, standards and tools related to maternal and newborn care (all ten countries)
- helps to identify and apply cost-effective maternal and newborn interventions (all ten countries)
- helps to coordinate MPR and Safe Motherhood Initiative plans and activities (all ten countries)
- supports activities that aim to maximise resources available for the Safe Motherhood Initiative (all ten countries).
- links with other programmes that are involved in areas of work relevant to safe motherhood, such as HIV/AIDS, malaria and blood safety (all ten countries)
- integrates into sector-wide approach and intersectoral efforts, including national poverty-reduction efforts (Indonesia, Uganda, Mozambique, Bolivia), national development plans (Ethiopia, Indonesia, Moldova, Bolivia, Nigeria, Mauritania) the UN Development Assistance Framework (Mozambique, Nigeria, Mauritania).

Norms, standards and tools

Currently MPR is developing a comprehensive package of norms, standards and tools (IMPAC), which includes standards for maternal and newborn care, training modules (midwifery modules), manuals (*Managing Complications of Pregnancy and*

Childbirth: A Manual for Midwives and Doctors – MCPC)[14] and decision-making tools for health providers, as well as managerial tools for policy-makers and district managers (the MPR planning guide, midwifery services, costing spreadsheets, planning workshop tools, etc.). Regularly updated and expanded, including useful comments from developing countries health providers, the Reproductive Health Library, available as a CD and on the web (www.who.int/reproductive-health) provides the evidence on interventions for maternal and newborn mortality reduction.

With the MCPC, the professionals have for the first time in obstetric history a generic compilation of the internationally agreed key interventions. This manual is under worldwide dissemination and has been already translated into French, Spanish, Russian, Laotian, Indonesian and is being translated into other languages, e.g. Chinese. This manual has been adopted as national standards by Bolivia. A second revised version is planned to be produced at the end of 2003. Normative work in MPR during the biennium will thus focus on further development of clinical guides (*Essential Care Practice Guide*),[15] guides and materials designed to strengthen midwifery services, managerial tools, including development of an MPR planning guide (and human-resources planning materials and developing the skills of health workers and health services for linking with the community. MPR is publishing a guide[14] to implement the New WHO antenatal care model promoting evidence-based and cost-effective interventions during pregnancy

The WHO is working with individual countries to establish medium- and long-term human-resources strategies in order to fill the enormous gap that they are facing in this respect. The normative role of MPR in developing generic materials at the global level and supporting adaptation, development and implementation of national norms, standards and tools is essential to support this strategy.

Advocacy

There is evidence that expanding the coverage of maternal and newborn health services, including a relatively small number of key interventions, to women in poverty could save a great number of lives each year, reduce poverty levels, spur economic development and promote global security. Governments, aid agencies and international agencies need to be convinced that investments in maternal and newborn mortality, as human-rights, public-health and human-development issues, need to be promoted by the Global Fund, in order to implement proven evidence-based cost-effective interventions.

Advocacy will be carried out at both a global level, to ensure that safe motherhood is kept high on the health and development agenda, and at a national level, to promote consistent, ethical and evidence-based policies, as well as to ensure that use of current resources is maximised and additional resources are secured for maternal and newborn health services.

MPR is developing efficient messages to partners, governments and policy-makers, based on the evidence-based cost-effective interventions and lessons learned from implementation activities. MPR will develop an advocacy strategies/tool (REDUCE model/RHCS – Mozambique, Nigeria, and Uganda) to support countries with their advocacy activities. MPR will develop a user-friendly website and continue publication of the *Safe Motherhood Newsletter*, targeted at all healthcare providers.

Table 2.3. Process and output indicators

Indicator	Definition
Process	Indicator of the manner in which the services are provided and often are reflected by quality of care, efficiency of the services and its management; a measure of the extent, efficiency or quality of service provided
Output	Indicator of the immediate results of the services targeted to achieve specific improvements in health (e.g. proportion of mothers educated, proportion of women immunised)

Partnership

Partnerships are being fostered and developed to strengthen involvement and coordination between governments, multilateral and bilateral donors, non-governmental organisations and other partners in the implementation of focused maternal and newborn plans and efforts (Ethiopia, Nigeria, Uganda – MPR/RH collaboration).

- MPR participates actively in Safe Motherhood Initiative interagency groups at global, regional and national levels.
- MPR is planning a global summit for Making Pregnancy Safer.
- MPR is promoting donors' collaboration at a national level (Ethiopia donor group for MPR, Indonesia).
- MPR is establishing collaborative work with professional organisations (International Federation of Obstetrics and Gynecology, International Confederation of Midwives) and wishes to support a professional consortium to reduce maternal and newborn mortality.
- MPR is promoting collaborative and coordinated activities between programmes to maximise the investments and increase the efficiency of the interventions.

Monitoring and evaluation

MPR continues to pay particular attention both to programme monitoring and evaluation and to global monitoring in order to maintain sustained interest in and attention to the issue of maternal and neonatal mortality. MPR will support the improvement of national and sub-national information systems and the use of agreed process and output indicators.[16] MPR will collaborate with the Initiative for Maternal Mortality Programme Assessment Project (Aberdeen University) designed to measure the outcomes of the key interventions (skilled attendants).

Conclusion

We know which interventions are needed to correct the unacceptable inequality of maternal and newborn illnesses and death. WHO/MPR is trying to find the path, giving guidance to partners, to implement these interventions with policy-makers and professionals in a sustainable way in poor countries. WHO/MPR will measure the process and the impact of these cost-effective evidence-based interventions and share lessons learned. The success will be the access to and use of the quality care provided by the pregnant women and their newborns, fully supported by their communities. A long-term effort in terms of commitment, funding and support is needed.

Professionals have a central role to play, in the developing countries in being highly active for changes, and in rich countries in advocating adequate aid and effective support.

- measuring morbidity and mortality
- disseminating the use of audits to improve quality of care
- conducting research and adapting technologies
- improving efforts on training
- advocating maternal and newborn health services, including accessible and well-equipped services within a functioning referral system.

The MPR initiative intends to build solid, effective and long-term partnerships for addressing the scandal of persistent high maternal and newborn mortality ratios.

References

1. World Health Organization. *Maternal Mortality in 1995. Estimates Developed by WHO, UNICEF and UNFPA*. Geneva: WHO; 2001 [www.who.int/reproductive-health/index].
2. WHO/EIP database 2001.
3. World Health Organization. *Essential Care Practice Guide for Pregnancy, Childbirth and Newborn Care*. Geneva: WHO; 2002.
4. WHO Antenatal Care Randomized Trial. *Manual for the Implementation of the New Model*. Geneva: WHO; 2002 WHO/RHR/01.30.
5. Safe Motherhood Inter-Agency Group (IAG), 1998.
6. Sister Anne Thompson, quoted in: *Birth Rights, New Approaches for Safe Motherhood*. PANOS Institute. 2001.
7. Drife J, Lewis G. *Why Mothers Die 1997–1999. The Confidential Enquiries into Maternal Deaths in the UK*. London: RCOG Press; 2001.
8. United Nations. *Population and Development*. Volume I: Programme of Action adopted at the International Conference on Population and Development, Cairo, 5–13 September 1994, Chapter VIII Health, Morbidity and Mortality, paragraph 8.1. New York: United Nations; 1995.
9. United Nations General Assembly. *Report of the Ad Hoc Committee of the Whole of the Twenty-first Special Session of the General Assembly. Key actions for the further implementation of the Programme of Action of the International Conference on Population and Development*, paragraph 64. New York: UN; 1999.
10. World Health Organization. *Reduction of Maternal Mortality. A Joint WHO/UNFPA/UNICEF/World Bank Statement*. Geneva: WHO; 1999.
11. World Bank. Determinants for MMR reduction in these two countries. 2002. In press.
12. Murray, C, Frenk, J. *A WHO Framework for Health System Performance Assessment. GPE Discussion Paper No. 6*. Geneva: WHO; 1999.

13. Jha P, Mills A, Hanson K, Kumayanarake L, Conteh L, Kurowski C, *et al*. Improving the health of the global poor. *Science* 2002;295:2036–9.
14. World Health Organization. *Managing Complications of Pregnancy and Childbirth: A Manual for Midwives and Doctors*. Geneva: WHO; 2000, WHOI/RHR/00.07
15. UNICEF, WHO, UNFPA. *Guidelines for Monitoring the Availability and Use of Obstetric Services*. Geneva: UNICEF, WHO, UNFPA; 1997.
16. World Health Organization. *Essential Care Practice Guide for Pregnancy, Childbirth and Newborn Care*. Geneva: WHO; 2002.

Chapter 3

Confidential enquiry into maternal deaths in South Africa

Robert C Pattinson and Jack Moodley

Introduction

In 1952, the first year of the modern Confidential Enquiry for England and Wales, the maternal mortality ratio (MMR), excluding early pregnancy deaths, was 54/100 000 births. After almost 50 years of the Confidential Enquiry, the MMR in the 1997–1999 triennium for the UK was 11.4/100 000 maternities.[1] In 1994, the MMR for South Africa was unknown.

The post-apartheid government in South Africa made maternal and child health a priority issue for the new administration. To fulfil this objective, the new administration recognised the need to gather information concerning all aspects of maternal deaths. The government decided to establish a confidential enquiry system similar to that practised in the UK. A confidential enquiry system allows for determining the MMR, but also the factors associated with maternal deaths and this in turn allows for remedial action. To achieve this, deaths during pregnancy, childbirth and the puerperium were made notifiable events on 1 October 1997, in terms of the National Policy Health Act, Number 116 of 1990. The Minister of Health also appointed a National Committee on Confidential Enquiries into Maternal Deaths (NCCEMD) to manage the process.

The NCCEMD is responsible for the confidential enquiry into maternal mortality in South Africa and is tasked with 'making recommendations, based on the confidential study of maternal deaths to the Department of Health such that the implementation of the recommendations should result in a decrease in the maternal mortality'.[2] The NCCEMD comprises experts from the medical and midwifery professions throughout South Africa who are appointed for three years and representatives from the Maternal, Child and Women's Health, Health Information Systems and Epidemiology and Research Departments of the National Department of Health.

Methodology

After each maternal death in a facility, a defined process is followed. First, the facility completes a Maternal Death Notification Form that is sent to their provincial office within seven days of the maternal death along with a photocopy of the patient's case records. The province forwards all documentation to a provincial assessing team and informs the NCCEMD that the maternal death has occurred. The NCCEMD secretariat issues the case a unique file number. The provincial assessing team, comprising an obstetrician and a midwife appointed by the province, is responsible for completion of an assessor's form that provides information on the primary, final and contributory causes of death and establishes whether there were avoidable factors, missed opportunities or any other aspects of substandard care present in the maternal death. No assessor team assesses deaths that occurred in their health district and each province has a least two teams. The assessor team completes and returns all documentation to the province within 30 days. In some provinces, with cases where an anaesthetic may have played a role in a maternal death, all documentation is also sent for an anaesthetic evaluation. The NCCEMD performs quality assurances by reassessing a random sample of maternal deaths and comparing its findings to those of the provincial assessor team. In this way, standards can be maintained and weak assessor teams identified. The documentation is anonymised except for the unique NCCEMD file number at the provincial level. All documentation is then forwarded to the NCCEMD for collation and analysis. The NCCEMD uses these data to compile a report on maternal deaths and make recommendations for reducing the number of deaths.

An annual provincial assessors' workshop is held to inform the assessors of the previous year's results and discuss problems. The reports are discussed at the workshop and consensus is obtained for recommendations of the NCCEMD. Once the report is accepted, all case files are destroyed and work begins on the next report. Detailed reports are produced every three years, but there are annual interim reports that document changing patterns in disease and mortality rates. Details of the process and method of assessment are shown in Figure 3.1.

Following the report's publication, the provincial maternal children's and women's health units are responsible for disseminating the information it contains. Workshops are held in the health districts throughout South Africa and usually the provincial assessor teams provide the feedback to the health workers of the various health districts.

This system has a number of advantages. The first is that an obstetrician and midwife evaluate each case. The case is discussed between them and a joint assessment is made. This means that the report and recommendations have the support of both the medical and nursing fraternities. The second is that each province appoints its own assessors, so that the system is inclusive. Bringing the assessors to annual workshops allows for maintenance of standards and discussion of results. The assessors are then in an excellent position to distribute the information back to their provinces.

The major disadvantage of the system is the worry that confidentiality may be breached. Confidentiality is stressed at each opportunity. The Maternal Death Notification Form and the assessors' report belong to the state and are not case records, which according to South African law belong to the patient. Hence the information given by the assessors is not available to the family; however, the family may access

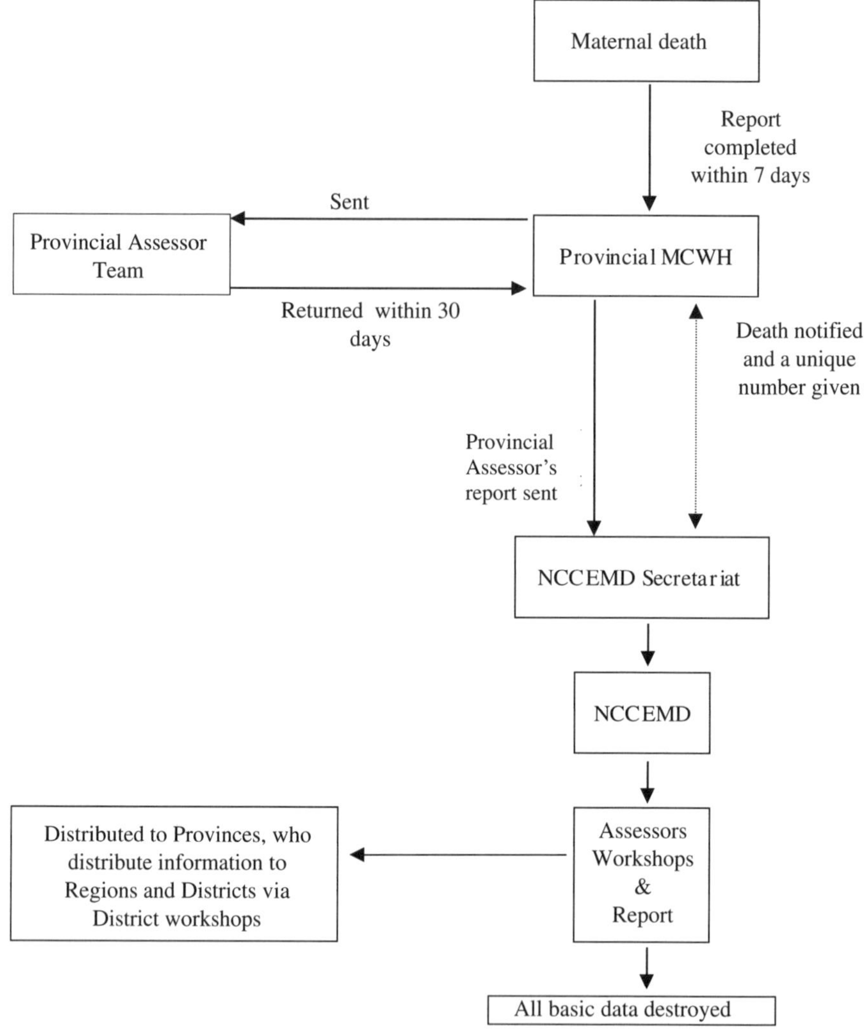

Figure 3.1. The process of confidential enquiry into maternal deaths; MCWH = Maternal, Child and Women's Health Units; NCCEMD = National Committee for the Confidential Enquiries into Maternal Deaths

the case records and these may be assessed independently. The family is thus in no way compromised. The cases are anonymised and later destroyed, so that the provincial assessors or NCCEMD members cannot be subpoenaed in a court case. To give the health profession confidence that no assessor can influence any medico-legal case in any way, no assessor is permitted to be involved in any medico-legal case involving a maternal death.

Another disadvantage is the large number of people involved, which can make the system inefficient. South Africa has nine provinces and, throughout the country, over a hundred health districts. Currently the NCCEMD receives more than 1000 maternal death notifications a year. To improve on this, a new computer programme has been devised to allow for electronic transfer of data and more rapid turnaround and analysis of the cases.

It can rightly be questioned whether establishing such a system in a developing country is putting scarce health resources to the most appropriate use. In monetary terms, the system is not expensive, as the assessors are not financially rewarded. The provinces often allocate one call shift per month to the assessor for this purpose. The major cost involves the holding of meetings and workshops and the production of the report. An unmeasured cost is the sometimes considerable time spent analysing the cases, which arguably could be spent treating patients. The counter-argument is that reducing maternal mortality is a priority for obstetricians, midwives and health administrators alike and the time spent identifying the problems in the health system is well spent. How can improvements be made without proper appreciation of the situation? Lack of data leads to lack of understanding of the problem and consequently lack of priority given to it by decision-makers and politicians and hence to lack of resources to address the problem.[3]

The actual process of performing the confidential enquiry follows five clear steps.

Step 1. Identification of maternal deaths and their demographics.

Step 2. Allocation of the primary and final cause of death.

Step 3. Identification of avoidable factors, missed opportunities and substandard care.

Step 4. Recommendation of solutions to the problems identified.

Step 5. Feedback of the findings to all stakeholders.

Step 1: Identification of maternal deaths and their demographics

The International Classification of Diseases, Injuries and Causes of Death Revision 10 defines a maternal death as 'the death of a woman while pregnant or within 42 days of termination of pregnancy, from any cause related to, or aggravated by the pregnancy or its management, but not from accidental or incidental causes'.

The maternal death notification process requires that all deaths of women occurring in pregnancy or within 42 days of being pregnant be reported. These deaths are then subdivided into 'direct', 'indirect' and 'fortuitous' deaths. The NCCEMD does not report on *late* deaths, that is deaths occurring between 42 days and one year after abortion or delivery that are due to direct or indirect maternal causes. Only *direct* and *indirect* deaths are counted for statistical purposes.

Coincidental (fortuitous) deaths are included in the recording of maternal deaths in South Africa, to identify the magnitude of the problem of violence against women and to identify the number of suicides in pregnancy.

Estimating maternal mortality ratio in South Africa

The number of births per year is not known for the whole of South Africa, hence no MMR can be calculated. However, it was possible to calculate the MMRs for three provinces in 1998 as they have an accurate method for recording the number of births, and this varied from 50/100 000 births in the Western Cape, to 67/100 000 births in Gauteng and 135/100 000 births in the Free State.[3] These provinces have the best infrastructure and the MMR in the poorer provinces will be higher.

The estimated MMR for the country as a whole has been independently calculated in the South African Demographic and Health Survey (SADHS) report and was estimated at 150/100 000 live births.[4] This is compatible with the findings of the NCCEMD.

Obtaining accurate numbers for births and maternal deaths is difficult in developing countries because the vast majority of home births and deaths are not recorded. This is clearly a weakness in the system. The confidential enquiry system is health-institution-based, and deaths at home are not systematically collected. In the more rural provinces it is estimated that up to 25% of births occur at home, compared with 3–5% in the mainly urban provinces.[4] An awareness campaign has been run to inform traditional healers, state mortuaries, church leaders and community leaders of the confidential enquiry system and these people have been requested to notify their closest institution if they identify a maternal death. This approach has not had much success to date. The death certificate has been altered to document whether the person was pregnant or not, but at present this system is not efficient enough to allow for cross-checking to ascertain whether all maternal deaths have been collected.

Since its inception in October 1997, the number of maternal deaths being reported to the NCCEMD has been steadily rising.[5] It is not known whether this is due entirely to improved reporting or to an actual increase in maternal deaths. Comparisons made between provinces of similar background show wide variations in numbers of deaths reported. By using the last census, an estimated number of maternal deaths can be calculated and using these data it is probable that some provinces are significantly underreporting and should probably be recording double the number reported. There are probably at least 200 maternal deaths that have not been reported in 2000. Overall, it would appear that the number of maternal deaths is, in reality, rising.[5]

Step 2: Allocation of the primary and final cause of death

The causes of death are classified using two systems. Each death is classified according to a primary (underlying) cause, namely the disease process that initiated the events that led to the woman's death. Each death is also classified as to final and contributory causes of death. For example, if a woman died from an intracerebral haemorrhage resulting from severe hypertension following pre-eclampsia, pre-eclampsia would be allocated as the primary cause and the final cause would be intracerebral haemorrhage. Postmortems are not readily available in South Africa and in the majority of cases the cause is allocated after assessing the case records. Non-pregnancy-related infections belong to a group of infections that are incidental to the pregnancy, hence an indirect cause of maternal death. The most common cause of non-pregnancy-related infections is AIDS. AIDS is only allocated as a primary cause if a positive HIV test has been recorded and a CD4+ T-lymphocyte count of less than 200/μl or if an AIDS-defining disease such as tuberculosis or cryptococcal meningitis was present. In women who are HIV-infected but do not have AIDS and subsequently die, the primary cause is not classified as AIDS. In many cases the HIV status is unknown; the impact of the HIV/AIDS epidemic on maternal deaths is therefore obviously being underestimated.

Primary obstetric causes of maternal death

The primary obstetric causes of reported maternal deaths for 1998–2000 are shown in Table 3.1.[5] There has been a significant reduction in the proportion of direct causes of maternal death (1998 – 63.3%, down to 1999 – 59.1% and 2000 – 58.5%), with a concomitant increase in the proportion of indirect causes of death (1998 – 33.6%, up to 1999 – 37.5% and 2000 – 38.6%). This is largely due to the increased proportion of deaths due to non-pregnancy-related sepsis, mainly AIDS.

The 'big five' causes of maternal death in 2000 were non-pregnancy-related infections (29.7%, mainly deaths due to AIDS), complications of hypertension in pregnancy (22.7%), obstetric haemorrhage (13.5%), pregnancy-related sepsis (12.4%, including septic abortions and puerperal sepsis) and pre-existing maternal disease (8.9%, mainly cardiac disease). These five account for 87.2% of maternal deaths. These data are consistent with those of 1998 and 1999, with the only difference being a real increase in deaths due to AIDS (Table 3.1 and Figure 3.2).

In 2000, HIV-testing was reported in only 38% of maternal deaths and 78% of these were HIV-infected. In the category of non-pregnancy-related infections, 22% of these maternal deaths, including those with pneumonia, tuberculosis and meningitis, did not have HIV-testing performed. Thus, the number of women reported to have died due to AIDS is an underestimate. All women dying from septic abortion whose HIV status was tested were HIV-infected, as were 73% of women dying from puerperal sepsis.

Table 3.1. Primary obstetric causes of reported maternal deaths: 1998–2000; data derived from the Maternal Death Notification Form received by the NCCEMD by 15 March 2001

Primary cause of maternal death	1998		1999		2000	
	(*n*)	%	(*n*)	%	(*n*)	%
Direct deaths	358	63.4	418	59.2	402	58.5
Hypertension in pregnancy	131	23.2	149	21.1	155	22.7
Postpartum haemorrhage	48	8.5	65	9.2	71	10.4
Antepartum haemorrhage	27	4.8	29	4.1	21	3.1
Abortion	32	5.7	37	5.2	26	3.9
Ectopic pregnancies	11	1.9	9	1.3	6	0.9
Pregnancy-related sepsis	41	7.3	62	8.8	55	8.5
Anaesthetic accidents	27	4.8	24	3.4	27	3.9
Acute collapse and embolism	41	7.3	43	6.1	41	6.0
Indirect deaths	190	33.6	258	36.5	264	38.6
Non-pregnancy-related infections	130	23.0	202	28.6	203	29.7
AIDS	82	14.5	110	15.6	131	19.2
Pre-existing maternal disease	59	10.4	56	7.9	61	8.9
Cardiacs	28	5.0	26	3.7	22	3.2
Not classifiable (unknown)	18	3.2	30	4.2	18	2.6
Total maternal deaths	565	100.0	706	100.0	684	100.0
Fortuitous deaths	20		15		18	

Reported deaths due to AIDS rose from 82 in 1998 to 110 in 1999 and 131 in 2000. However, in 2000 a further 45 women who, if they had been tested for HIV and had been found to be infected, would have been classified as dying of AIDS. The HIV epidemic is having a major impact on maternal deaths in South Africa. Non-pregnancy-related infections have become the major cause of maternal deaths at all levels of care, superseding complications of hypertension in pregnancy.

In 2000, there appears to have been a decline in the number of women dying as a result of complications of an abortion (1998 – 32 cases, 5.7% of all maternal deaths; 1999 – 37 cases, 5.2% and 2000 – 26 cases, 3.9%). This may be due to the effect of the Choice of Termination of Pregnancy Act of 1996. Further evidence has been obtained by studying the severe acute maternal mortality in the Pretoria Region of Gauteng.[6] Here, a significant decline in maternal deaths and severe acute maternal mortality in Pretoria has coincided with a doubling of terminations, especially in the second trimester.

All hospitals are classified as level 1, 2 or 3, with level 1 being primary-level hospitals, with no specialists but often performing caesarean sections, level 2 being secondary-level care with general specialists being available and level 3 being tertiary-level care with subspecialists available. The pattern of the causes of maternal deaths varies according to the level of care and analysing this gives valuable information concerning the functioning of the tiered healthcare system. In level-1 institutions, obstetric haemorrhage remains the most important direct cause of death, but anaesthetic-related causes are the third most common cause. Anaesthetic-related causes that are classified in this category are women who were well and who developed a problem that was specifically due to the anaesthetic. Examples are a woman who had

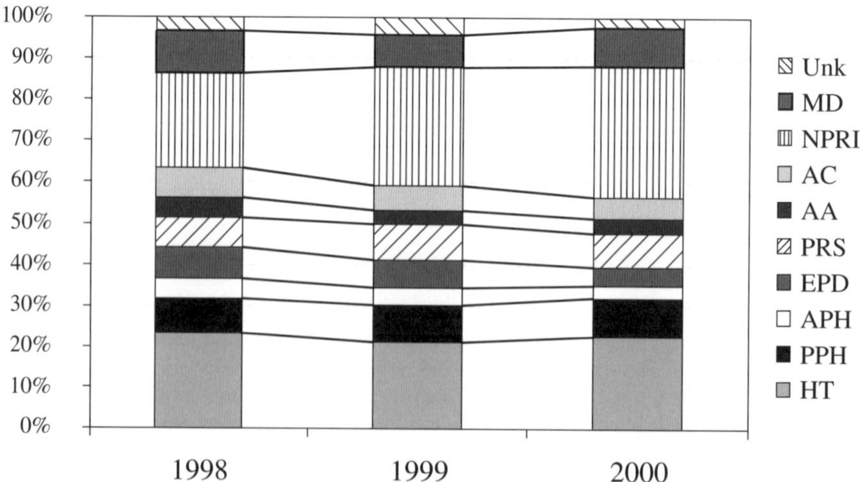

Figure 3.2. Primary obstetric cause of reported maternal deaths 1998–2000; Unk = unknown, MD = pre-existing medical disease, NPRI = non-pregnancy-related infections, AC = acute collapse and embolism, AA = anaesthetic-related, PRS = pregnancy-related sepsis, EPD = early pregnancy death, APH = antepartum haemorrhage, PPH = postpartum haemorrhage, HT = hypertension

general anaesthetic for an elective caesarean section for a previous caesarean section and there was a failed intubation or a healthy woman who had a spinal anaesthetic for a caesarean section for the indication cephalopelvic disproportion and who had a cardiac arrest due to a high spinal anaesthesia. These deaths at level-1 institutions clearly indicate a problem in administering anaesthetics to pregnant women at this level. Complications of hypertension in pregnancy are the most common direct causes of death in level-2 and -3 institutions (Table 3.2).

Step 3: Identification of avoidable factors, missed opportunities and substandard care

Substandard care

The NCCEMD adopted the definition of substandard care that is used by the UK. The term 'substandard care' has been used in this report to take into account not only failure in clinical care but also some of the underlying factors that may have produced a low standard of care for the patient. This includes situations produced by the actions of the woman herself, or her relatives, which may be outside the control of the clinicians. It also takes into account shortage of resources for staffing facilities and administrative failure in the maternity services and the back-up facilities, such as anaesthetic, radiological and pathology services. It is used in preference to the term 'avoidable factors' that was used previously in the England and Wales reports until 1979 and has also been used in the Scottish and Northern Ireland reports. This was sometimes misinterpreted in the past and taken to mean that avoiding these factors would necessarily have prevented the death. 'Substandard' in the context of the report means that the care that the patient received, or that was made available to her, fell below the standard that the authors considered should have been offered to her in this triennium.[7]

It is important to understand that in assessing the case, the assessors look at the care in totality, which includes the functioning of the healthcare system. The basic guidelines that the assessor employs are those commonly used in the country and those that are applicable to the level of care. The Maternal Manual of the Perinatal Education Programme[8] is used as a basis for assessing care at a primary level, and the standard

Table 3.2. Comparison of the relative importance of direct primary causes of maternal death per level of care: 1998–2000

Cause	Level 1			Level 2			Level 3		
	1998	1999	2000	1998	1999	2000	1998	1999	2000
Deaths (n)	110	115	118	116	137	148	103	143	114
Hypertension in pregnancy (%)	27.3	24.3	21.2	34.5	34.3	44.6	47.6	47.6	46.5
Obstetric haemorrhage (%)	28.2	31.3	29.7	22.4	19.7	20.2	9.7	16.8	18.4
Early pregnancy deaths (%)	10.9	7.0	4.2	12.1	11.7	8.8	15.5	14.7	12.3
Pregnancy-related sepsis (%)	9.1	16.5	12.7	12.1	15.3	11.5	16.5	14.0	19.3
Anaesthetic-related (%)	13.6	11.3	16.9	7.8	4.4	3.4	1.0	2.8	1.8
Acute collapse (%)	10.9	9.6	15.3	11.2	14.6	11.5	9.7	4.2	1.8

textbooks used in medical schools for undergraduates for secondary-level and local protocols are used for tertiary-level care.

The assessment of care system used in the Confidential Enquiry

The basic structure of the care assessment system devised for the Confidential Enquiry is to analyse (1) the woman and her environment; (2) the administrative circumstances surrounding the care and (3) the standard of health care, each individually. Analysis in these three categories has the obvious advantage that information gained in these areas can be fed back immediately to the relevant sectors for action.

Patient-related problems (the woman and her environment)

Assessment of avoidable factors or missed opportunities related to the woman and her environment is divided into three sections:

1. Issues relating to the woman herself; for example, a woman may delay reporting to a clinic that her membranes have ruptured and this delay may result in chorioamnionitis that ultimately leads to her death. This delay may have been due to lack of knowledge.
2. The influence the family has on the woman's behaviour; for example, the woman may decline a hysterectomy for severe puerperal sepsis until she has consulted with her family, and this delay may contribute to her death.
3. The effect of the environment (community) in which the woman lives on her behaviour; for example, the lack of a telephone to call the ambulance service in a community or the attitude of the community towards the health services may influence the outcome.

When collecting and interpreting the information on patient-related factors, it is important not to 'blame the victim'. The full story tends to be complicated and it is often circumstances rather than neglect or desire to do damage on the part of the woman that dictate the behaviour.

Administrative problems

Administrative problems are easier to classify and the information is easier to obtain. The problems are classified as:

- transport, e.g. lack of transport from the clinic to hospital or hospital to hospital
- barriers to access to healthcare facilities, e.g. hostile reception at clinics or hospitals
- inaccessibility, e.g. lack of termination of pregnancy services
- lack of healthcare facilities, e.g. intensive-care beds
- lack of personnel or of appropriately trained staff
- communication problems, such as breakdown in communication between patients and healthcare workers or between healthcare workers.

Standard of health care

The assessment of the standard of care given to the woman by the health workers is divided into distinct periods (antenatal, intrapartum and postpartum, emergency event, resuscitation and anaesthesia) and the care is assessed in each period where applicable.

The assessment of each section is based on how the following were performed in each case:

- initial assessment, i.e. history, examination and special investigations
- problem identification or diagnosis
- adherence to management plan or management protocol
- follow-up monitoring.

Cases where a death might not be assessable because of missing or incomplete notes are also recorded. Valuable information is obtained here. An absence of notes itself suggests substandard care and missing files indicate a major administrative problem.

The assessors have a checklist that covers the aspects of the case as described above. The checklist is used to ensure a uniform approach to case-assessment. The areas where substandard care is thought to occur are recorded and all the information is then computerised. The cause of each death is recorded and the assessment of care in each case is linked. In this way, disease-specific information is obtained and the problems related to a particular disease are identified. Consequently, it is easier to formulate specific solutions.

Table 3.3 summarises the magnitude of the problems in care experienced in 1998.[2] In almost half of the maternal deaths, there was a missed opportunity for preventing death related to the behaviour of the woman herself or her community. The most

Table 3.3. Avoidable factors, missed opportunities and substandard care for 1998; 559 maternal deaths were analysed with respect to avoidable factors as some information was available on them

Category	Assessable cases (*n*)	Incidence of avoidable factors in assessable cases (%)
Patient-orientated problems	410	48.8
Administrative factors	485	33.2
Level 1	NA	37.2
Level 2	NA	30.5
Level 3	NA	33.1
Medical personnel orientated:		
Routine care:		
Antenatal	234	38.9
Intrapartum	199	31.2
Postpartum	99	34.3
Emergency event	463	56.8
Level 1	NA	74.2
Level 2	NA	56.8
Level 3	NA	43.6
Resuscitation	295	28.8
Anaesthetic care	170	25.3
Unprofessional conduct	559	12.5

NA = not available

common factors were not attending antenatal care and delay in seeking help (Table 3.4). It is not known what the specific reasons for non-attendance at antenatal clinics or the reasons for delay in seeking help were. More attention will need to be placed on establishing these reasons, so that interventions can be introduced. Self-induced termination of pregnancy occurred in 30% of women dying from complications of abortion.

Problems with the administration were evenly distributed throughout the levels of care. However, delay in transporting patients between institutions was seen in 13.6% of cases requiring transport (Table 3.4). The problem varied considerably between provinces, with the lowest being 5% in the mainly urban provinces to the highest of 38% in rural provinces. The problem of transport is probably even greater than this because the delays in transporting women from their homes to health institutions could not be estimated due to lack of information.

A lack of intensive-care facilities, beds, equipment and personnel was found to be a factor in 15.6% of cases where mothers died in tertiary institutions. This is also probably an underestimate of the magnitude of the problem because it is not known in how many cases doctors from level-1 and -2 hospitals wanted to refer patients but were informed that there was no intensive-care bed available and to try other hospitals. Blood transfusion facilities were unavailable in 11.7% of cases that required urgent blood transfusions.

Lack of personnel was rarely mentioned as an avoidable factor. This may be due to health workers at the institution not thinking of inadequate staffing because they have become so used to the shortages that they regard it as normal – or to lack of information available to the assessors for them to allocate it as an avoidable factor.

Management of the emergency event revealed problems of care in more than half the cases (Table 3.5). The major problems in the management related to non-adherence to the standard protocols for the management of the conditions (39% of cases) and misdiagnosis (13% of cases). It is not known whether this is due to ignorance or 'laziness' on the part of the staff. In 18.4% of cases either there was a delay in referring patients or they were managed at an inappropriate level of care. This may represent

Table 3.4. Avoidable factors, missed opportunities and substandard care for 1998

Category	Major problems	%
Patient-orientated problems (*n* = 349)	Non-attendance antenatal care	21.2
	Infrequent attendance	8.9
	Delay in seeking help	18.6
	Self-induced termination[a]	30.0
	Self-discharge from hospital	2.9
Administrative factors (*n* = 485)	Delay in transport from home to institution	4.1
	Delay transport between institutions[b]	13.6
	Delay in admissions area	1.9
	Insufficient intensive-care beds[c]	15.6
	Lack of laboratory facilities	2.2
	Lack of availability of blood transfusion[d]	11.7
	Lack of appropriately trained medical officers	2.9
	Lack of communication between health workers	3.7

[a] denominator for self-induced termination is 30; [b] denominator 235 (total number of maternal deaths who were transported within the health services; [c] denominator 273 (total number of maternal deaths who died in tertiary institutions); [d] denominator for lack of availability of blood transfusion is 94

Table 3.5. Medical personnel orientated problems: emergency event and resuscitation

Emergency event (n = 462)	Major problems	Incidence (%)
Initial assessment	No notes	4.5
	Done incompletely at any level	28.4
Problem recognition	No notes	4.8
	Done incompletely at any level	30.7
Management plan/ protocol followed	More senior assistance not called	8.0
	More senior assistance not available	3.5
	Delay referral to secondary/tertiary centre	9.1
	Patient managed at inappropriate institution	9.3
	Wrong diagnosis	13.0
	Standard protocol not followed	39.0
	Delays in getting treatment performed	5.2
	Technical skill not adequate or available	2.2
Continued monitoring	Not done/no notes	6.5
	Failure to get special investigation results	4.5
	Observations done infrequently/incompletely	19.5
	Prolonged abnormal observations without action	5.8
Resuscitation (n = 295)	Airway not secured	3.7
	Breathing not supported	7.1
	Circulation not supported	11.2
	Drugs not given	4.4
	Investigations not done	3.1
	Special monitoring not performed	4.4
	Central venous pressure line not inserted	5.4
	Ongoing monitoring not performed	5.4
	Subsequent management not planned	9.8

transport problems, difficulty in appreciating the severity of the condition or lack of an identified referral hospital that will accept the patient. In 25.3% of cases, either observations after the emergency event were made infrequently or incompletely or there were prolonged abnormal observations without any action. It is not known what the reason for this is. It could be due to lack of staff or to laziness on their part. Almost one-third of cases had an anaesthetic at some point in the course of their management, and it was found that there was some form of substandard care in anaesthesia in 25.3% of these cases.

Unprofessional conduct occurred on a few occasions. The most common problems were not attending patients when called and not performing observations when prescribed.

Step 4: Recommendation of solutions to the problems identified

Complete analysis of the data usually identifies the major problems. Producing the recommendations is not so easy. In a developing country, there are many deficiencies in the healthcare system and there are also severe budget constraints. The NCCEMD decided that to have a major impact the recommendations must involve diseases or conditions that made a major contribution to maternal deaths and that their implementation must be feasible within the South African context. 'Feasible' in the context of this report means that they must be affordable and practical. They also stated that implementation must occur within the next triennium, and that the impact should be measurable for the next triennial report. The recommendations also had to be specific so that health authorities could measure the progress of their implementation. Furthermore, the recommendations had to be based on the data contained in the report and there had to be clear evidence from the literature that implementation of such a recommendation would reduce the problem. Within these constraints, the NCCEMD made the following ten key recommendations for the 1998 report:[3]

1. Guidelines on managing conditions that commonly result in maternal death to be developed, distributed and implemented throughout the country by 2002.
2. Referral routes and criteria for referral to be established and implemented by 2001.
3. Staffing and equipment norms per level of care to be established in every health institution concerned with the care of pregnant women by 2001.
4. The distribution of the termination of pregnancy services (especially with respect to second-trimester termination) to be expanded and the sites must be advertised to the public.
5. The partogram to be used for monitoring labour in every pregnant woman and problems detected on the partogram to be managed accordingly.
6. Blood to be available at every institution where caesarean sections are performed.
7. Medical obstetric clinics to be established to ensure the optimal management of women with pre-existing medical conditions, especially women with heart disease and diabetes mellitus.
8. Regional anaesthesia should be promoted in all sites performing caesarean sections.
9. Family planning services must intensively educate women 30 years and older or with five or more children about the dangers of pregnancy. Contraceptive use should be actively promoted in this group of women.
10. A national HIV/AIDS policy geared towards managing these women and dealing with the ethical considerations to be available by 2001.

Several of these recommendations have been implemented and their effect will be measured in the next triennial report due in October 2002.

Step 5: Feedback of the findings to all stakeholders

No system of audit or quality assurance is complete without feeding back the information obtained to the relevant stakeholders. The stakeholders are the public, the government and the health workers. The structure the NCCEMD developed had this as one of its main priorities. The system of devolution of the data collection to the provinces means that the provincial administrators are directly involved. The national

Department of Health's involvement with the NCCEMD has enabled it to budget for the various meetings and to put progress in the implementation of the ten key recommendations as a permanent agenda item for the regular meetings of the provincial ministers of health with the national minister of health. This demonstrates that the political commitment is there. This commitment is essential to implement the necessary changes. The devolution of assessment to the provinces also means that the health professionals, namely the obstetricians and midwives, are directly involved and take ownership of the process. Regular provincial meetings are held to discuss problems and progress with data collection and the implementation of the recommendations.

However, changing practice in the institutions is the hardest nut to crack and innovative methods will need to be introduced to achieve this. Programmes aimed directly at the public to change some of their health behaviours are also required, most notably in the prevention of HIV infection.

Conclusion

It is highly unlikely that the MMR in South Africa – approximately twelve times higher than in the UK – is due to a global lack of knowledge of how to manage severely ill pregnant women; it is more likely to be due to maternity services in South Africa not implementing available knowledge. This is borne out by the findings of the *Saving Mothers* report.[2] This knowledge is essential for planning the packages of care or strategies to be implemented in South Africa.[3]

It is possible to set up a confidential enquiry system into maternal deaths in a developing country first to describe the current position, then to monitor the effect of the introduction of new programmes. This is the essential first step in starting quality assurance in maternal care. To be successful, the system should have the confidence of the public, the profession and the Department of Health.

De Brouwere *et al.*[9] described a few essential ingredients for effecting a reduction in maternal mortality. The first phase is to identify the magnitude of the problem and to realise that it is feasible to improve significantly on the current state of affairs. The second phase is to obtain the knowledge to improve the situation, to persuade health workers to use that knowledge and to make the knowledge and facilities available to the vast majority of the population. Political will is a prerequisite for implementation of the necessary changes.

The South African government is at the point where it can realistically give a reasonably accurate estimate of the MMR; it knows the common causes of maternal mortality and that there are many avoidable factors, missed opportunities and substandard kinds of care surrounding maternal deaths. Most importantly, it knows that the problem is manageable because it knows what the factors are and that they are remediable. This fulfils the first phase necessary for a reduction in maternal deaths.[9]

Furthermore, the medical knowledge is available to prevent these maternal deaths and the health system is in place to make this knowledge available to the vast majority of pregnant women. Thus, all the ingredients are in place to reduce maternal mortality in South Africa, except for persuading the population, the health workers and the administrators to use the knowledge available. This is the next main challenge.

References

1. Drife J, Lewis G. *Why Mothers Die 1997–1999: The Confidential Enquiries into Maternal Deaths in the United Kingdom*. London: RCOG Press; 2001.
2. Pattinson R, editor. *Saving Mothers. Report on Confidential Enquiries into Maternal Deaths in South Africa, 1998*. Pretoria/Cape Town: Government Printers; 1999.
3. Graham WJ. Now or never: the case for measuring maternal mortality. *Lancet* 2002;359:701–4.
4. Department of Health, South Africa. *South African Demographic and Health Survey: 1998*. Pretoria/Cape Town: Government Printers; 1999.
5. Department of Health, South Africa. *Third Interim Report on Confidential Enquiries into Maternal Deaths in South Africa 2000*. Pretoria/Cape Town: Government Printers.
6. Vandecruys H, Pattinson RC, Macdonald AP, Mantel GD. Severe acute maternal morbidity and mortality in the Pretoria academic complex: changing patterns over 4 years. *Eur J Obstet Gynecol Reprod Biol* 2002;102:6–10.
7. Department of Health, Welsh Office, Scottish Home and Health Department, Department of Health and Social Services, Northern Ireland. *Report on Confidential Enquiries into Maternal Death in the United Kingdom, 1985–87*. London: HMSO; 1991.
8. Theron GB, editor. *Perinatal Education Programme, Manual I, Maternal Care*. Cape Town: Perinatal Education Trust; 1993.
9. De Brouwere V, Tonglet R, van Lerberghe W. Strategies for reducing maternal mortality in developing countries: what can we learn from the history of the industrialised west? *Trop Med Int Health* 1998;3:771–82.

Chapter 4

Maternal mortality: global overview I

Discussion

Discussion following the papers by Professor Graham, Dr de Bernis and Professor Pattinson

Drife: Linking one of Professor Pattinson's final remarks with the thrust of Professor Graham's paper, I made a note at the end that Dugald Baird was not just a researcher – he had an agenda. He did not have to study poverty in Glasgow for ten years to know that it was a bad thing; he knew before he started. One of Professor Pattinson's final remarks was that the problems and the solutions have been identified; the problem is in the implementation of that knowledge.

I wonder if, in terms of the research that formed the basis of Professor Graham's recommendation, there is an endpoint. The classic process in academic research is to answer one question, find ten more and answer them and so on, so that we are all continuing our research. However, to take the example of the L-shaped curve that you showed relating mortality to the number of doctors, is it naïve to say that you can simply make a recommendation that a certain number of doctors are required to reduce maternal mortality, or does further work remain to be done? I am asking what the endpoint of the research is because the two presentations give different messages as to whether further research is required or not.

Graham: The issue is the level at which we need proof of effectiveness and cost-effectiveness. The Initiative for Maternal Mortality Programme Assessment is focusing on assessing strategies for reducing maternal mortality and morbidity – in other words, on composite interventions rather than individual clinical interventions. It may be, at the level of effective and cost-effective strategies that impact at the population level, that the current evidence base is weakest. In very poor countries, decisions need to be made on what to prioritise and actions must be taken based on the best advice available at the time. This need to act should not, however, eclipse the concurrent need to improve the evidence-base for decision-making, particularly around implementation barriers but also around the methods and tools to demonstrate health gain from alternative strategies. In other words, we cannot simply assume that improving processes of care will necessarily produce a health gain, i.e. a reduction of maternal mortality and morbidity; we must reliably demonstrate a gain at the population level.

If you look at a range of developing countries, the various international recommendations on action for safe motherhood have not necessarily been followed. There are many reasons for this but, as Professor Pattinson mentioned with De Brouwere's historical work,[1] the first priority was to demonstrate the magnitude of the problem and also to convince governments that something can be changed – that progress can be made and demonstrated. Today in developing countries we need to show that link between implementation of services and direct health gain.

In some countries, there are hard decisions to be made. For example, let us take a particular controversy in safe motherhood between the focus on emergency obstetric, i.e. facility-based care, and a package of activities that involve community outreach. There is a major debate about this. There is one school of thought that stresses the importance of improving the hospital rather than community outreach. On the other hand, there are situations where it is clear that if you simply get the 'house in order', people do not come.

The point is that we need stronger evidence of the health gains at a population level and in terms of effective health care. The countries I am talking about are somewhat different from South Africa, situations that have seriously malfunctioning health systems, where the choices of where they concentrate their services and what is most cost-effective at that point in history are very important. It is quite a complex question, but when we say 'we know what needs to be done', we need to distinguish between knowing what to do at a clinical level and knowing what to do for very large populations and poor countries, which is another matter.

De Swiet: Professor Graham, when you were talking about inadequate data, I imagine you meant with regard to pregnancy. In fact, the data regarding causes of cardiac maternal mortality outside of pregnancy are also inadequate, and that is not confined to developing countries; it is strongly apparent in developed countries. It is desperately important to have these data because it is only then that we can look at the true impact of pregnancy on maternal health.

Graham: My main area of work is the measurement problems in maternal mortality. It is true to say that when we look at a lot of data sets it is hard to know if what we are seeing is an artefact of the measurement process or the true pattern. This is very serious and it is so hard to know if these proportional mortality ratios are fact or fiction. As you were saying, any proportion is greatly affected by a component that happens to be missing.

I have a major problem when we start to examine this, particularly with this balance between the direct and the indirect causes of mortality. International statistics suggest that 25% of the deaths are indirect but the question is: 'what is the unknown fraction?' We have to be extremely cautious in all of those percentage distributions, where the measurement barriers are so severe that we might be looking at the measurement artefacts. That is particularly true for the indirect causes.

Brabin: Dr de Bernis, I was interested in your comment on maternal education and the important association that was identified between a low level of maternal education and maternal mortality. In children, we know that maternal education is the most important predictor of child survival. My question is whether you can expand on that at all. Is this just an association, or can you tell us something about mechanisms? In particular, how does this relate to female literacy, which is different from maternal education?

De Bernis: This is a very difficult question for me because to my knowledge, as I have said, we have no evidence of any direct link between maternal education and the maternal mortality ratio – and I agree with you that it may be more a question of literacy than education. There are no studies that clarify this, only broad ones that discuss health improvement and educational access in general.

For maternal mortality reduction itself, I have no recollection of any specific useful study, but scientifically this can be debated. If educational access is right for the child, it could also be important from the viewpoint of the woman's health . There is an obvious link between general degree of awareness, access to information and ability to understand and to discuss issues with professionals and the readiness and capacity to seek out health care.

In the community side of maternal health we do not have much evidence and we recently organised a meeting simply to map the evidence in order to establish which interventions are critical for improving maternal health. Ultimately there is no evidence; we have many experiences that are specific to different countries and contexts. Improving the status of women and creating more opportunities for advancement and for financial autonomy within the family, for example, are certainly all very important. Many non-governmental and partner organisations are working in these areas.

To answer your question, I cannot state that there is a proven link between maternal education and literacy and maternal death.

Brabin: My second question is: 'what is your strategy on adolescent health in terms of preparing the mother for pregnancy?'

De Bernis: This is a very important question. When I discuss poverty and vulnerable groups, I do need to discuss adolescents. This point is a very important one for us and, as you probably know, there are now several teams working on adolescent issues. Regarding pregnancy, we do not think that adolescent pregnancy is an especially important topic. The pregnancy itself from a purely medical viewpoint is not the fact; the fact is the context, and the socio-economic context is very important in addressing questions concerning adolescence.

This context is very difficult to address and, as you probably know, a lot of research is now being conducted into this. There are many proposals for creating special services for adolescents because we know that adolescents do not seek care without clear guarantees of confidentiality and increased respect. Much research shows that there is a lot of work to be done with the providers to improve quality of care, recognition of the specific problems of adolescents and, again, respect and confidentiality.

Regarding the care itself, there is no study that indicates a specific area to be managed. I would say that there is no specific management for the care, but the problem is more how to address adolescents within the delivery services.

Drife: A comment and a question: sadly, this country is one of those that are buying skilled attendants from countries that need them more than we do, and it is deeply embarrassing for some of us. It is sad to think that we do not know what to do about it – just to apologise to you for that.

The question is: can you sum up what happened in the islands of the south-west Pacific? There was a spectacular improvement in maternal mortality between those two columns in the table that you showed. Although these are small numbers of people, were there any lessons to be learned from what they did there?

De Bernis: Unfortunately I cannot answer your question, and I do not really know. There are two studies soon to be published by the World Bank about Malaysia and Sri Lanka. It is very important to see that at the end of the analysis of all the determinants and the data from these two countries for 40 years, the main determinant remains midwifery – the establishment of a clear system based on midwives who are well supported by the health system and well recognised by the community, which means strong political commitment and community recognition. I remind you of this fact because it could be interesting for the discussion.

Drife: It was not a rhetorical question by any means, but I know there has been a lot of partnership between Australia and other parts of Oceania and it may be that this is an example of co-operation between a developed country and a developing area that would repay study.

Hall: I wanted to comment on your point that maternal mortality in women having terminations of pregnancy was declining. That is certainly a cause for congratulation to the service because in Britain it took a long time after legalisation of terminations before maternal mortality did improve. In Britain it was probably about 20 years after legalisation before the service really took stock of the fact that they ought to be providing a good service that actually met women's needs. The fact that many of the women are still not using the service is not at all surprising at such an early stage after legalisation.

I wanted to ask whether most of the self-induced terminations were among young schoolgirls or adolescents or whether they were mostly in grande multiparae.

Pattinson: We only have specific data for the Gauteng region on that question. The majority of our deaths are in the older women, those having a parity of three and above and aged 30 years and above, not in teenagers.

Graham: It is very interesting and you have some information that I was not aware of on inequalities and inequities. I have a question about the increase in postpartum haemorrhage (PPH) that you were suggesting. There is some evidence in parts of West Africa – those countries that have particularly high rates of HIV – that the problem is basically one of blood supply. You mentioned that there is increasing difficulty in obtaining blood. This is always difficult, but there are also stigmatising issues and the beliefs about people being tested as a consequence of providing blood. In many countries there is evidence of an increasing reluctance to provide blood and this has started to impact on PPH cases.

Pattinson: The availability of blood at all sites performing caesarean sections is one of the points on which the provinces have to report back to their ministers of health – it is one of those ten recommendations. It appears that the availability of blood is not our major problem. It is more of a problem of poor management. However, we might be seeing more PPH because women who are HIV-infected are at a greater risk of haemorrhage due to the HIV-associated thrombocytopenia.

Neilson: Professor Pattinson, I was very impressed by the ambitious nature of your programme and I was particularly intrigued by the difficulties of trying to measure impact when clearly there are anxieties in some regions about the underascertainment of deaths. If there were a way of measuring impact, this might have major global relevance. Are there ways of measuring impact on a regional basis, where you think you have higher-quality and more complete data, rather than on a national basis?

Pattinson: The aim is to do a random sample from various hospitals around the country to look at the specific issues, such as whether they have protocols in place because that is one of the recommendations. It has been done fairly well for terminations of pregnancy, where there have been six-monthly progress audits. The ultimate impact on maternal death will take longer to assess. In the interim, we are looking at measurable endpoints derived from the ten recommendations. We want to see that what we recommend is being done. The onus is however on us to make certain that what we recommend is appropriate and will make an impact.

MacLean: One of the things that did not appear in your list of interventions was symphysiotomy. Does this mean that the last one has been done? Is it something that you no longer recommend?

Pattinson: An article has just been published in *BJOG* on this topic.[2] We do not see much of obstructed labour as primary cause of death. It is not recorded as a primary cause. We record it under 'sepsis' and under 'haemorrhage' and it accounts for about 3% of the deaths in our institutions – I must stress that this is an institution-based audit. Our transport system between institutions is sufficiently good that our ambulance service can get patients to hospitals performing caesarean sections before major catastrophes occur.

The other endpoint would be looking at vesicovaginal fistulae, which are not common, because we are able to see the patients in time. They are only common in the Free State Province and most of those patients are referred from Lesotho. The very few obstetric vesicovaginal fistulae we see is a measure of the infrastructure that we have in South Africa. I am sure that there is a place for symphysiotomy in specific circumstances, but our problem will be teaching people how to do it.

Brabin: I have a comment and a question. First, I was also interested in the rise in PPH that you documented. It has been shown recently in Papua New Guinea that there was an greater increase in PPH in areas with high malaria exposure. I wonder whether this might relate in any way to the emergence of drug-resistance malaria. My question is: 'what does this confidential enquiry framework cost?'

Pattinson: The costs are essentially hidden. Most assessors are given a session, which means a call off, in which to carry out their assessment. The midwives ask their matrons if they can have the time off and the only direct costs are organising the publications and the workshops, which have been sponsored by the World Health Organization recently. So I cannot tell you the actual costs but a workshop will cost about 80,000 South African rand to bring the 60 people up from around the country, which is about £5000.

Gülmezoglu: I wanted to ask a question because this exercise has clearly been very useful and you have generated a huge amount of information. You said that now we have to act on our findings and Professor Graham referred to the composite interventions; this whole area of knowing what to do and putting it into practice, as you know, is a very complex matter. I know that you have an interest in this area as well, and I want to ask how you want to go about transferring this knowledge into practice.

Pattinson: It is one of the important points that I have tried to make, which is the difference between guidelines and protocols. Work by Grimshaw and Russell[3] suggests that the greatest chance for successful implementation of a protocol depends on various factors; it must be home-grown (i.e. developed within the institution), facilitation is best with face-to-face, one-to-one contact and specific issues must be addressed, not a whole lot at one time. That is our approach. We have produced policy guidelines for the common causes of maternal deaths in South Africa, and the maternal child and women's health coordinators have to go to each institution and facilitate the change from those policy guidelines to their institutional protocols. For example, the policy guideline says that magnesium sulphate should be used for eclampsia but the institutional protocol specifies where it is kept, the dosage and what the indications are for its use in that institution. Also, specific local information such as the telephone number of the site to which the patient should be referred would be in the protocol. That is the level of detail at which institutional protocols should be written and we anticipate that home-growing the protocol at the institution will give better results, but we will have to wait and see. We will be looking at the establishment of protocols by taking a random sample of 80 hospitals to see whether they have the protocols in place. However, this is only an interim measure. The impact of this method of implementation of the protocols on maternal deaths will be measured only in years to come.

References

1. De Brouwere V, Tonglet R, van Lerberghe W. Strategies for reducing maternal mortality in developing countries: what can we learn from the history of the industrialised west? *Trop Med Int Health* 1998;3:771–82.
2. Bjorklund K. Minimally invasive surgery of obstructed labour: a review of symphysiotomy during the twentieth century (including 5000 cases). *BJOG* 2002;109:236–48.
3. Grimshaw JM, Russell IT. Effect of clinical guidelines on medical practice: a systematic review of rigorous evaluations. *Lancet* 1993;342:1317–22.

SECTION 2

MATERNAL MORBIDITY AND MORTALITY: GLOBAL OVERVIEW II

Chapter 5

The effects of the HIV/AIDS pandemic on maternal morbidity and mortality

Florence M Mirembe and Evelyn Mubiru

Introduction

While the 1980s ushered in a period of unprecedented expectations in the history of medicine following the eradication of major diseases such as smallpox, in the same decade we witnessed the emergence of yet another formidable and baffling opponent in the form of the HIV/AIDS pandemic. This new and fearsome enemy did not respect the same science and technology that had eradicated smallpox and the disease has spread all over the world, sparing no colour, age or ethnicity. It continues to tax all human brains, science and technology, and has sent the world back to the drawing board, into the laboratories and into communities in the effort to generate new knowledge, skills and strategies for its control.

The disease has caused global concern ever since its appearance in the mid-1980s. It remains a great challenge to the development efforts of many countries, especially the developing world and in particular sub-Saharan Africa, where poverty and preventable endemic diseases remain a menace.

The uniqueness of its modes of transmission – in as much as they are natural, social, biological and physiological, i.e. through whatever form of sexual relationship, through the placenta, mother-to-child transmission and breastfeeding – makes HIV/AIDS a real challenge. Furthermore, other routes such as drug injections, blood transfusions and contamination by infected instruments also play a part.

The disease particularly affects young and middle-aged people, 'the productive and reproductive', especially in the developing world, where poverty, low status, human-rights violations, poor decision making and gender inequities are commonplace. Women are particularly afflicted by HIV by virtue of their biological make-up and the low sociocultural and economic status in which they find themselves entangled.

Vulnerability to HIV/AIDS hinges heavily on individuals' lack of power over their immediate circumstances. This is more so among women who succumb to the circumstances through traditional/cultural, socio-economic and political factors; being poorer and of lower social status, many are rendered powerless to negotiate for their rights.

Social pressures and cultures force women to continue having children even when they are aware of their serological status and know that the next pregnancy will be life-threatening. Men are also under pressure to demonstrate their virility by having children. These and many other factors make women highly vulnerable to HIV/AIDS. The dangers that it poses to women have been described as a triple jeopardy to woman, mother and baby.

Status of the HIV/AIDS pandemic

Currently an estimated 33 million people are believed to be living with the virus, with more than two-thirds of these living in Africa, especially in the sub-Saharan region. In addition, more women than men are known to be infected.[1] In particular, HIV infection is acquired by women during adolescence and young adulthood, with the peak infection age between 20 and 29 years, while male infection peaks much later. Due to early acquisition of HIV infection, women in reproductive age will die from AIDS at an earlier age than the men.[2] The HIV/AIDS pandemic in the sub-Saharan region is described as a 'roaring lion', with rates of 30–50% in some areas. In Uganda, the infection rate seems to be declining from 30% in the early 1990s to an estimated new infection rate of 6.1% (4.3% in rural and about 8.0% in urban areas). However, in antenatal mothers in the urban areas the rate remains 12–13% (Figure 5.1).

Maternal mortality

The definition used is death during pregnancy, labour or childbirth and within 42 days of termination of pregnancy regardless of the site or duration of pregnancy from any cause related to the pregnancy or its management.[3] Maternal deaths remain a tragedy – a silent one in most countries. Worldwide, an estimated 600 000 women die annually as a result of complications resulting or arising from pregnancy and childbirth.

It is also a well-known fact that maternal mortality is a rare occurrence in the developed world but an everyday encounter in labour wards and homesteads in developing countries, mainly due to global inequities in income distribution and access to health services (Table 5.1).[4] The fact that the maternal mortality ratio (MMR) averages 27 deaths/100 000 live births in the developed world and 480–>1000 deaths/100 000 live births in the developing world makes the problem of maternal death a much more severe one for the developing world. Globally it is estimated that around 80% of all maternal deaths are the direct result of complications arising during pregnancy, childbirth or puerperium (Figure 5.2).

HIV/AIDS is a new cause of maternal mortality. HIV infection is prevalent in young people who are productive and reproductive. Looking at East Africa in the mid-1990s, in Kenya 20–30% of women attending antenatal clinics tested positive, in Uganda 28–30% and in Tanzania 25–30%. This shows that HIV/AIDS places a disproportionate burden on women,[5] causing morbidity and subsequent mortality among women of reproductive age.

The high rate of HIV infection is compounded for women by poverty, low social status, poor health services and endemic infectious diseases such as malaria and tuberculosis, making its impact more severe.

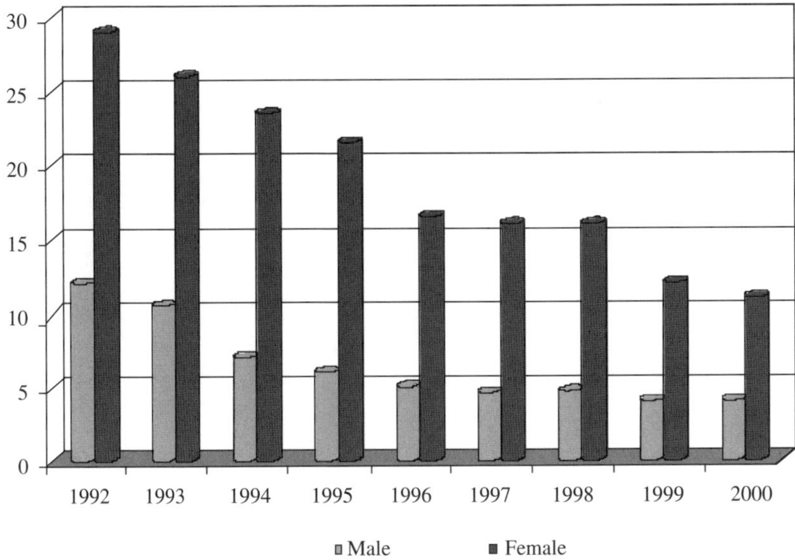

Figure 5.1. HIV rates for 15–24-year-olds by sex among first-time testers; source: AIDS Information Centre, Kampala

The effect of HIV infection on the causal pattern of maternal deaths

HIV/AIDS appears to have undone all the efforts towards the reduction of maternal death. Despite the 50% reduction target for maternal mortality by 2000, the total global figure is progressively rising, especially in the developing world and particularly in sub-Saharan Africa.

Table 5.1. Adults and children estimated to be living with HIV/AIDS as of end 1997

Region	Incidence (n)
North America	860 000
Western Europe	530 000
Eastern Europe and Central Asia	150 000
Caribbean	1.3 million
North Africa and Middle East	210 000
South and South-East Asia	6 million
Latin America	310 000
Sub-Saharan Africa	20.8 million
Australia and New Zealand	12 000
Total	30.6 million

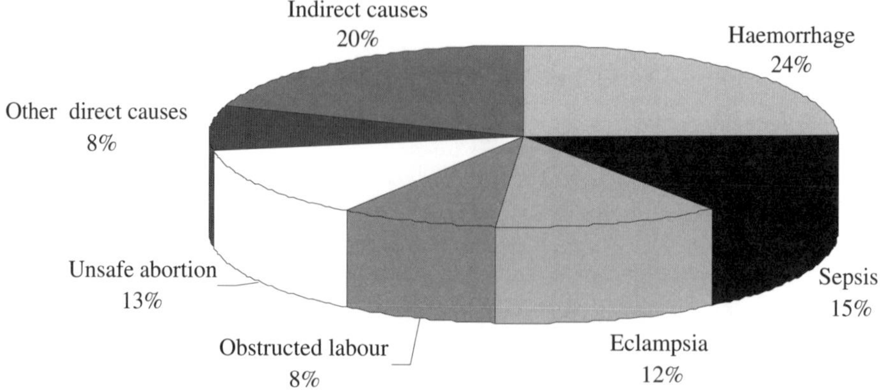

Figure 5.2. Causes of maternal deaths: global estimates that vary in different settings; source: WHO, Geneva 2000

In addition, the causes of death seem to be changing in pattern, especially in the developing world. In Uganda and in many countries such as India,[6–9] although not everybody is screened for HIV serological status, almost 40% of maternal deaths have a strong base of possible HIV infection. This has been supported in Ugandan study by Okong where it was found that 80–90% of all deaths were from HIV/AIDS-related diseases.[10]

Non-traditional conditions are now prevalent and lead to death in pregnancy puerperium and soon after a current pregnancy. These include:

- meningitis
- tuberculosis
- kaposi sarcoma and other malignancies
- severe malaria (exacerbated by HIV infection)
- severe anaemia (exacerbated by HIV infection)
- sepsis.

Although these conditions seemed to be under control through definitive efforts and strategies, especially in the developing world, they have since made a comeback and particularly affect pregnant mothers, leading to death. Efforts have been made within the Safe Motherhood Initiative to address these aetiological factors through integrative approaches, but the toll remains high in extremely poor areas with limited access to medical services.

While formerly most women died in labour and the puerperium, we now see an increasing number of women dying during pregnancy and as a continuation from pregnancy in the puerperium from causes unrelated to pregnancy. In addition, their survival seems to be reduced after delivery.[7]

Scenarios in HIV/AIDS status

In developed countries, the prospects for combating HIV/AIDS have been improved by the discovery of anti-retroviral drugs and easier access to treatment. In the developing world, the picture is bleak; HIV/AIDS infection means death because:

- poverty does not allow access to life-saving anti-retroviral drugs
- intercurrent infections are prevalent and immunosuppression increases morbidity
- nutrition is suboptimal for many, making them vulnerable to infections.

The effect of pregnancy on HIV progression

A meta-analysis that evaluated several studies did not find significant differences in the risk of death and progression to AIDS-related illness or decrease in CD4+ T-lymphocytes. Therefore pregnancy *per se* seems not to be a major underlying factor in the causation of death. It is also well documented that in countries with high HIV-infection rates maternal mortality is also high as a result of other operating risk factors.[9]

However, Berer[7] concluded that pregnancy, delivery and induced abortion complications are more frequent and severe among HIV-seropositive mothers than their counterparts. AIDS was observed to be a key underlying factor in direct and indirect maternal death in those countries where high HIV-infection rates exist. This was also demonstrated in Uganda by Hom *et al.*[11] in a study on the natural history of HIV infection where 30 HIV-positive mothers among 549 followed up died within 50 months.

The impact of HIV/AIDS on maternal mortality

The well-known direct and indirect causes of maternal mortality in the developing world have continued to claim numerous lives of young women. These include:

- haemorrhage
- sepsis
- abortion (unsafe)
- eclampsia
- ruptured uterus and obstructed labour.

These remain major causes, especially during delivery and in early puerperium. The tragedy is that all are preventable with good obstetric care.

Premature death of mothers

There is a progressive increase in the maternal deaths during the antenatal period. These mothers tend to die from diseases such as meningitis, tuberculosis, severe

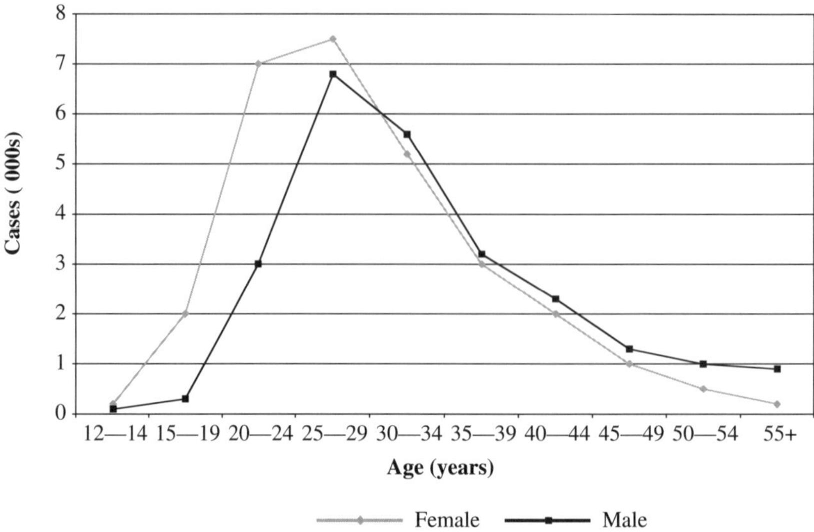

Figure 5.3. Distribution of adult AIDS cases by age and sex; source HIV/AIDS surveillance report, June 2001 Ministry of Health

malaria, unexplained anaemia and toxoplasmosis. This also tends to be at a young age, particularly in the 20–29 years age-group. This age-group happens to be the most actively reproductive. HIV/AIDS brings premature death to the most economically active and productive population groups, imposing an enormous economic and social toll on the afflicted communities. In a study carried out by Urassa *et al.*[12] in a rural district in Tanzania they were able to demonstrate the major cause of adult deaths among the (15–44-year-olds) as being AIDS. The study also demonstrated that more women died of HIV/AIDS than men and that women died younger (aged 25–34 years) than with men (aged 45–54 years) (Figure 5.3).

Reduction of life expectancy

HIV/AIDS has shown and in many areas reversed the gains made in life expectancy in the less developed countries of the sub-Saharan Africa region that has been most affected. In Tanzania mortality rates were 15 times higher among HIV-infected than in HIV-seronegative adults.[12] In Botswana, life expectancy has dropped from 63 years to 54 years of age.

Consequences of maternal death on the children

The death of a productive mother providing support to the children offsets the household economy by removing one of the family's productive pillars. The consequences for the children include:

- death of the young ones – from AIDS acquired from the mother but also from intercurrent infection
- morbidities due to lack of care
- malnutrition leading to stunting
- dissolution of homes
- violence and sexual abuse
- psychological trauma due to stigmatisation
- child labour, unrivalled poverty
- early marriage and repetition of the whole cycle whereby the children could become trapped in the same HIV problems as the mother
- dropping out from school for financial reasons while possibly becoming heads of the household and taking care of the young ones
- early marriage and repetition of the whole cycle whereby the children could become trapped in the same HIV problems as their mothers.

Children's safety and survival is therefore severely threatened, more so as countries continue to experience high death rates resulting from previous infections that are estimated to continue into 2020–2030.[13]

Children orphaned by AIDS – a new challenge

The HIV/AIDS pandemic has tremendously increased the number of orphans. USAID estimates[13] that 13.2 million children under 15 years of age had lost their mothers or both parents; nine out of ten AIDS-orphaned children are in sub-Saharan Africa. There are estimated to be at least one million AIDS-orphaned children in each of Uganda, Ethiopia, Tanzania and Nigeria.

Conclusion

Maternal mortality remains a major problem, a silent one despite the efforts being made, as the ratios in many of the developing countries continue to rise. The emergence of HIV/AIDS on to the world scene has compounded the problem, especially in the developing world, where poverty, intercurrent infections, low status and poor decision making are rampant among women.

HIV/AIDS has brought new dimensions to maternal deaths. While traditionally women died, as they still do, from poor obstetric care, HIV/AIDS is causing death from diseases of poverty that were seemingly being eradicated in the developing world.

The escalating MMR is having an unprecedented effect on child survival and development and there is huge loss of productive life and subsequently of income to households and families as a whole. The burden of orphans has escalated, resulting in children becoming heads of households, caring for their siblings and so on. As a consequence, life expectancy in these countries seems to be declining.

In the context of HIV/AIDS, we need to redouble our efforts to reduce maternal mortality and commitment and investment are required if the trend is to be reversed. We need to treat and offer hope to HIV-seropositive mothers, so that they can survive longer in order to bring up their children and treat the mothers during pregnancy to reduce mother-to-child transmission rates to ensure that children are born unaffected. We also need to support and strongly advocate voluntary confidential counselling and testing and to ensure that pregnant women become aware of their serological status and encourage men to support their wives and to be tested themselves, so that the couples can be assisted in making rational, informed decisions about their reproduction and entire future. We also need to support and strongly advocate voluntary confidential counselling and testing, ensure that pregnant women become aware of their serological status and encourage men to support their wives and to be tested themselves, so that couples can be assisted to make rational, informed decisions about their reproduction and entire future.

In the development paradigm the emphasis is not on individual and risk but on society and vulnerability, targeting the solidarity of communities, ensuring empowerment and working to improve living conditions. We need to address and focus on those areas and interventions in which the investment of time and human resource should have a sustainable and long-term impact.

References

1. Medisone M, Garenne M, Tarautola D, Testa J. Demographic impact of HIV/AIDS in three West African Cities II. Ouagadougou (preliminary report). July 1994.
2. Ugandan Ministry of Health – STD/AIDS Control Programme. *HIV/AIDS Surveillance Report*. Kampala: Ministry of Health, Uganda; 2001.
3. World Health Organization. Reduction of maternal mortality. A joint WHO/UNFPA/UNICEF/World Bank statement. Geneva: WHO; 1999.
4. Rosenfield A, Figdor E. Where is the 'M' in MTCT? The broader issues in mother-to-child transmission of HIV. *Am J Public Health* 2001;91:703–4.
5. Offei Anshah J. African women prepare for Beijing #5. EAC outlines progress since 1995. World conference and challenges ahead. *African Recovery* 2000;14:18.
6. Kumar RM, Rizk EE, Khurrana AK. AIDS in pregnancy among Indian tribal women. *Int J Gynaecol Obstet* 1997;56:59–60.
7. Berer M. HIV/AIDS, pregnancy and maternal mortality and morbidity implications for care. In: Berer M, Sundari Ravindran TK, editors. *Safe Motherhood Initiatives. Critical Issues*. Oxford: Blackwell Science; 1999. p. 198–210.
8. Mirembe FM, Okong P, Nyaphis H, Makoea L. Risk factors for maternal mortality in Lesotho, Malawi, Uganda and Zambia. *Journal of Obstetrics/Gynaecology for East, Central and Southern Africa* 1998;4:1–6.
9. Mirembe F. Clinical report review (unpublished report). Makerere University; 2001.
10. Okong P. Deaths among women of reproductive age (unpublished report); 2000.
11. Hom D, Guay L, Marum L, Svilar A, Ndugwa C, Mmiro F. Mortality among HIV-1 infected mothers in Uganda. *International Conference on AIDS* 1993; 9:695. Abstract no. PO-04-2868.
12. Urassa M, Boerma JT, Isongo R, Ngalula J, Ng'weshean J, Mwaluko G, Zaba B. Impact of HIV/AIDS on mortality and household mobility in rural Tanzania. *AIDS* 2001;15:2017–23.
13. Hunter S, Williamson J. Children on the brink. Updated estimates and recommendations for intervention. Washington DC: United States Agency for International Development; 2000.

Chapter 6

The contribution of malaria

Bernard J Brabin and Francine Verhoeff

Introduction

Pregnant women, especially primigravidae, are more susceptible to malarial infection than non-pregnant women. Malaria prevalence increases from early in gestation in women living in areas of high malaria transmission, and this constitutes a major public health problem in many developing countries. *Plasmodium falciparum* infection during pregnancy increases the risks of abortion, stillbirth, prematurity, intrauterine growth restriction and maternal anaemia.[1] It is associated with increased risk of low birthweight and perinatal, neonatal and infant mortality.[2] Despite the wealth of information on malaria-related maternal morbidity, few studies have attempted to evaluate the contribution of malaria to maternal mortality.

The term 'malaria deaths' can refer either to the deaths ascribed to malaria if every death were correctly assigned to its cause or to the deaths that would be prevented if malaria were removed. There are problems with both these formulations; the first assumes that each death is attributable to a single cause and the second lacks any reference to time.[3] A distinction is also made between 'direct' and 'indirect' maternal malaria deaths. Direct malaria deaths are those of which malaria is a necessary cause and indirect malaria deaths are those of which malaria is a necessary but not a sufficient cause, resulting from a pre-existing condition that is aggravated by malaria. In the former, deaths are prevented by the removal of malaria (through prevention or cure) and, in the latter, deaths are prevented either by the removal of malaria and/or by the removal of the pre-existing condition.[3]

In areas of low malaria endemicity, the risk of direct malaria death following infection (e.g. cerebral malaria) tends to increase, although the proportion of women infected may be low. As endemicity increases, lethal infections such as cerebral malaria become relatively less frequent and severe malarial anaemia relatively more frequent. Malaria in pregnancy in highly endemic areas is extremely common, but is often only mildly symptomatic or asymptomatic. It is plausible that as endemicity increases, the overlap between the risk of lethal malaria and the risk of conditionally lethal other diseases tends to increase, with a corresponding effect on the indirect malaria mortality rate.[3] This notion is shown diagrammatically in Figure 6.1, which illustrates that the ratio between direct and indirect malaria mortality is variable and probably affected by malaria endemicity.

The relationship of malaria as a risk factor for maternal mortality is derived mainly from cross-sectional studies and can be confounded for several reasons. Problems related to the estimation of maternal mortality from such studies have been outlined by Graham.[4] Most report hospital data for moribund women and there is often limited attention to prior treatment, maternal nutritional status or concurrent infections. The accuracy of reported causes is difficult to ascertain and misclassifications occur. Few studies are supported by autopsy data.[5–7] For these reasons, many reports form an inadequate basis for determining the causal connection between malaria and maternal survival and the extrapolation from hospital delivery data must be considered an approximation.

Methods

Published studies on maternal mortality and malaria were identified using Medline, references in published papers, Cochrane reviews and personal communications. Manual searches of predigital data for the major tropical journals were also conducted. The bibliographies of all articles collected were checked for additional references. Studies that included postnatal deaths up to 42 days were included, although in practice few studies reported follow-up data beyond delivery. Studies included cross-sectional,

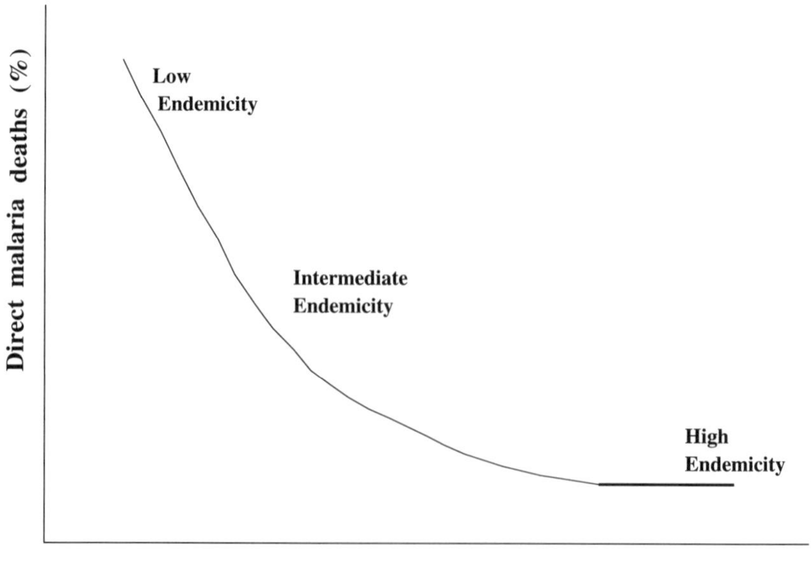

Figure 6.1. A simple model of direct and indirect maternal malaria mortality in relation to levels of malaria transmission; a mathematical formulation of this has been developed by Molineaux[3]

longitudinal, and a small number of randomised controlled trials of malaria chemoprophylaxis in which maternal mortality was reported, although it was not the primary outcome variable. Data from the WHO compilation of maternal mortality were reviewed.[8] All data were categorised by source (hospital or community), direct or indirect malaria deaths, region and sample size.[8] Data were not generally available for classification by parity.

The definition of maternal death used in this review is based on the International Classification of Diseases, revision 10 (ICD-10), which defines it as the death during pregnancy or within 42 days of termination, regardless of the duration and site of the pregnancy.[9] Direct and indirect malaria deaths were as reported in the reviewed studies. The malaria-attributable maternal mortality ratio (MMR) was calculated using the proportion of maternal deaths attributable to malaria, due to indirect and direct causes, and all-cause MMRs as reported by the study authors.

The following methods of estimation were adopted: MMRs were correlated with malaria parasite ratios; the latter is a measure of the intensity of malaria transmission and is the cross-sectional prevalence of infection among asymptomatic children below 15 years of age. These data were available from a recent review of anaemia among pregnant women in sub-Saharan Africa[10] and as far as possible studies were matched by location and date. Malaria-attributable MMR was then calculated from MMR multiplied by the percentage of all deaths attributed to malaria. Case fatality rates from pregnancy malaria, season as an associated risk factor for maternal mortality from malaria and population-attributable risk estimates of MMRs were also used.

Analysis of results

Maternal mortality and malaria endemicity

Cross-sectional reports considered for this review are shown in Table 6.1 for African studies and Table 6.2 for studies outside Africa. Of the 34 reports, only six were community-based. The majority of the hospital-based studies were from the capital city of the country concerned. The malaria-attributable MMRs listed in Tables 6.1 and 6.2 range from one to 9491 in 100 000 births. The levels of malaria endemicity under which these pregnant women were living varies widely between the studies. This is shown for the African reports by the wide range for the malaria parasite ratio (range <2.0–58.5%). Areas for which parasite ratios were not available were classified as low, medium or high endemicity or as an epidemic area.

In areas of low malaria endemicity, many women have low levels of malaria immunity and acute symptomatic malaria would follow infection, which would carry a high mortality rate if due to *P. falciparum* malaria. This was reported during the Ceylon (now Sri Lanka) epidemic in the 1930s, when malaria case fatality during pregnancy ranged from 6.5–24.2% in three different hospitals.[33] Mortality in cerebral malaria cases was 89.5%. In non-immune women in Malaysia, case fatality rates of around 13% were also reported.[44]

There is evidence to suggest that the effectiveness of health services may be limited by the endemicity of malaria and the presence of severe malaria. In Sri Lanka before 1939, there were eleven areas where health units were established to provide intensive maternal and child welfare services; two areas were in the endemic malarious zone and

Table 6.1. Studies reporting malaria as a cause of death in Africa

Country	Years	Sample (*n*)	Deaths (*n*)			Malaria death (%)	MMR	Malaria MMR	Parasite ratio (%)	Reference
			Total	Malaria (direct)	Malaria (indirect)					
Ethiopia (Addis Ababa)	1980–85	Hospital (x 1)	216	–	4	1.8	964	18.0	–	11
Guinea-Bissau (Bofata)	1988–89	Community	31	3 (?)	–	9.7	1490	144.0	–	12
Kenya (Kwale district)	1987	Community	35	1 (?)	–	2.9	657	19.0	–	13
Madagascar	1989	Community	17	3 (?)	–	17.6	3594	634.0	–	14
Malawi	1989	Hospitals (x 12)	214	2 (?)	–	0.9	609	6.0	58.5	15
Mozambique (Maputo)	1984	Hospital (x 1)	40	–	2	5.0	371	19.0	38.5	16
Mozambique (Maputo)	1989–93	Hospital (x 1)	239	37	–	15.5	320	50.0	38.5	6, 17
Nigeria (Ibadan)	1953–54	Hospital (x 1)	76	–	1	1.3	1300	17.0	57.1	18
Nigeria (Benin)	1970–71	Hospital (x 1)	30	–	1	3.3	466	16.0	–	19
Senegal (National)	1988–89	Hospitals (x 5)	100	–	23	23.0	933	215.0	–	20
Sierra Leone (Freetown)	1976	Hospital (x 1)	48	–	2	4.2	589	25.0	–	21
Sudan (Omdurman)	1980–85	Hospital (x 1)	102	–	1	1.0	306	3.0	–	22
Tanzania (Dar es Salaam)	1974–77	Hospital (x 1)	188	1[a]	–	0.5	213	1.0	20.3	23
Tanzania (Moshi)	1971–77	Hospital (x 1)	80	2[a]	4	7.5	329	24.6	32.8	24
Tanzania (Bagamayo)	1993	Community	76	4	–	–	961	51.0	–	24
Uganda (Kampala)	1980–86	Hospitals (x 5)	372	–	3	0.8	347	3.0	–	25
Zimbabwe (Harare)	1972–73	Hospital (x 1)	73	3	–	4.1	170	7.0	< 2.0	26
Zimbabwe (Harare)	1983	Hospital (x 1)	51	1	–	1.2	–	–	–	27, 28
Zimbabwe (Harare)	1989–90	Hospital (x 1)	61	0	1	1.6	85	1.0	–	29
Zambia (Masringo)	1989–90	Community	105	0	8	7.6	168	13.0	–	29
Zambia	1983–88	Hospitals (x 6)	145	–	11	7.6	105	8.0	–	30
Zambia (Lusaka)	1982–83	Hospital (x 1)	60	3[a]	1[b]	6.6	118	5.9	< 5.0	31
Zambia (Lusaka)	1996–97	Hospital (x 1)	251	17	–	6.8	921	62.0	–	32

[a] cerebral malaria; [b] tropical malaria splenomegaly; MMR = maternal mortality ratio/100 000 births; (?) = probable direct malaria death

Table 6.2. Studies reporting malaria as a cause of maternal death outside Africa

Country	Years	Sample (*n*)	Deaths (*n*)			Malaria[a] deaths (%)	MMR	Malaria MMR	Malaria endemicity	Reference
			Total	Malaria (direct)	Malaria (indirect)					
Sri Lanka (Colombo)	1934–35	Hospital (x1)	47[b]	7[c]	27	72.3	13128	9491	Epidemic	33
Guyana	1937–4	Community	1152	128	–	11.1	4729	525	High	34
(sugar estates)	1947–50	Community	232	7	–	3.0	1727	52	Intermediate	
	1951–60	Community	363	0	–	0.0	630	0	Eradicated	
El-Salvador (National)	1983–87	Hospital (x 23)	315	–	2	0.6	148	1	Low	35
Hong Kong	1945–83	Hospital (x 1)	118	1	–		–		Non-endemic	36
Myanmar (Rangoon)	1983–87	Hospital (x 1)	8	1 (?)	–	12.5	197	25	Low	37
Thailand (Bangkok)	1973–77	Hospital (x 3)	212	–	2	0.9	80	1	Low	38
Yemen (Aden)	1977–86	Hospital (x 1)	60	–	2	3.3	330	11	Low	40
Papua New Guinea (National)	1984–86	Hospitals and health centres	304	–	15	4.9	700	34	High	41
Papua New Guinea (Goroka)	1964–73	Hospital (x 1)	142	1	–	0.7	1907	13	Low	42
India (Chandigarh)	1984–85	Hospital (x 1)	87	2[d]	–	2.3	–	-	Low	43

[a] proportion of maternal deaths in pregnancy attributable to malaria x all-cause MMR/100 000; [b] malaria parasites not identified in 13 deaths; [c] cerebral malaria; [d] *Plasmodium vivax* (x 1), *P. falciparum* (x 1); MMR = maternal mortality ratio/100 000 live births; (?) = probable direct malaria death

Table 6.3. Infant and maternal mortality in malarious and non-malarious health unit areas in Sri Lanka[45]

Area	Average infant mortality/1000 births	Average maternal mortality /1000 births
Seven malaria non-endemic health unit areas	117.3	10.1
Two malaria-endemic health unit areas	187.5	23.9
Sri Lanka (all areas)	159.5	20.0

nine were in the non-endemic zone.[45] As shown in Table 6.3, the average infant and maternal mortality rates for the health unit areas in the endemic zone were higher than those of the health unit areas of the non-endemic zone and exceeded the rates for Sri Lanka as a whole. Thus, despite the concentrated medical services, mortality among mothers (and children) remained excessive in the malarious areas. Details of malaria parasite prevalence were not reported for the malarious areas.

The relationship between the malaria parasite ratio and malaria-attributable maternal mortality was examined for eight African studies listed in Table 6.1. Two areas with low parasite ratios (<5%) had malaria-attributable mortality below 7/100 000 births. The six areas with high parasite ratios had a wide range for malaria mortality from 1–50/100 000 births. There appears to be no association of maternal mortality with parasite ratio (correlation coefficient R^2 0.1; $P = 0.5$), but the number of studies with matching parasite ratios available was small. Taking only the 18 hospital-based studies in Africa, the median level for malaria-attributable malaria mortality was 16/100 000 births (95% CL: 2.1–54.5). For the five community-based African studies, the median level was higher at 51/100 000 births with wide confidence limits (95% CL: –155–+499).

The data available outside Africa are summarised in Table 6.2. Categories of malaria transmission as described by malaria parasite ratios were not available. The Sri Lankan epidemic illustrates the devastating effects of non-immune pregnant women's exposure to infection.[33] High malaria-related mortality also occurred prior to malaria-control activities in the sugar estates of Guyana. These prospective data show the dramatic decline in malaria as a cause of death in females of reproductive age during successive periods of improved malaria control leading to malaria eradication.[34] This suggests a wide-ranging influence of endemic malaria on maternal mortality.

Figure 6.2 shows the plot between all-cause and malaria-attributable MMRs for the studies listed in Tables 6.1 and 6.2. The association is highly significant, with a best line fit for a linear curve (correlation coefficient R^2 76.2%; $P < 0.001$). The data suggest a dose–response relationship between malaria-attributable and all-cause maternal mortality when the latter is above 400/100 000 births. In the *Global Factbook on Maternal Mortality*,[7] only a few studies from malarious areas specifically reported that no malaria deaths occurred and a large number of others from malarious areas in Africa make no specific mention of malaria (n = 69). In some of these, it may have been classified under 'other' causes of death, although in the detailed analysis of hospital deliveries by Harrison and Rossiter[46] on maternal mortality in northern Nigeria, no mention is made of malaria as a cause and it is not listed among several infections associated with maternal deaths. Also in a prospective community-based study of 672 women in rural Gambia, where malaria is seasonal, maternal mortality was high (2232/100 000 live births) but none of the 15 deaths documented was attributed to malaria.[47] However, in view of the strong association between malaria-attributable and

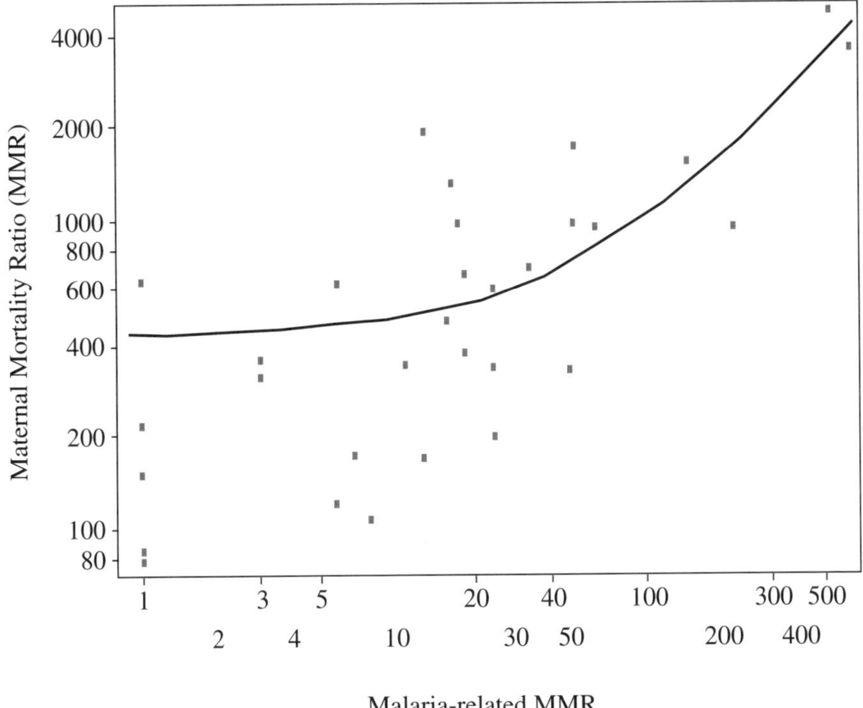

Figure 6.2. Malaria-attributable and all-cause maternal mortality ratios (excluding data for the Sri Lankan epidemic)

all-cause maternal mortality, it seems unlikely that for malarious areas with MMRs above 400 that no malaria deaths occur.

Case fatality rates in areas of low endemicity

Table 6.4 shows malaria case fatality rates for three study areas in India and for the Karen population on the Thai–Burmese border. These areas are endemic for *P. falciparum* and *P. vivax* malaria, and both malaria transmission and maternal prepregnancy immunity were probably low. The case fatality reported for the Indian studies would be equivalent to an MMR of 1832/100 000 births. On the Thai–Burmese border a 1% maternal death rate from malaria in pregnant women was reported during 1985, which was the year before antenatal care was started. The table shows that following the effective introduction of antenatal care case fatality was zero. Few other studies report case fatality data. Adolescent maternal mortality has been reported from urban Mozambique, where a 30% higher institutional mortality ratio in adolescents was observed compared with non-adolescents.[16] Average case fatality during the Sri Lanka epidemic was 13.1%, illustrating the devastating effects of epidemic malaria in women with low malaria immunity. In non-immune pregnant women, the clinical

Table 6.4. Case fatality rates from malaria in pregnancy in India and Thailand

Location	Years	Malaria prevalence at antenatal clinics (%) (%)	(*n*)	Deaths (*n*)	Survivors (*n*)	Case fatality (%)	Reference
India:							
Chandigarh	1984–85	1.40	(14/1000)	3 (1 Pv, 2 Pf)	75	3.85	43
Surat	1987–88	1.16	(104/8900)	4 (all Pf)	99	3.85	57
Jabalpur	1992–95	1.52	(365/24000)[a]	3 (all Pf)	362	0.83	58
Thailand	1986–89	5.86	(888/15147)[b]	0	1 358	0.0	39

[a] estimated average number of deliveries, over five years; [b] 888 positive smears in 15147 antenatal visits; in 1986, incidence of Pf 1.6 and Pv 0.5 / woman / six months (R. McGready, personal communication); Pv = *Plasmodium vivax*; Pf = *Plasmodium falciparum*

features of falciparum malaria develop rapidly and death may occur following the onset of symptoms within two to three days unless correct treatment is given. The details of the pathophysiology and management of malaria in pregnancy have been reviewed in an earlier RCOG Study Group.[48]

Seasonal factors and malaria-related maternal mortality

In pregnant women, malaria-related mortality may be greater in areas with high seasonal transmission. The mechanism to explain this could relate to a reduced likelihood of developing parity-specific malaria immunity due to the less frequent and intermittent exposure to infection that occurs with seasonal transmission. Parity-related mechanisms associated with malaria immunity have been reviewed.[49] Seasonal maternal malaria deaths, confirmed by autopsy, were reported from urban Maputo and Mozambique[6] in a catchment population with an estimated malaria-attributable mortality of 50/100 000 births[16] (Table 6.1). Both severe anaemia and cerebral malaria were common. Delayed hospitalisation and/or treatment, young age, lack of antenatal care and primiparity increased risk of death. This was the highest malaria-related mortality estimate of all hospital-based studies from Africa, except for the national estimate for five hospitals in Senegal, which is also an area with high transmission seasonal malaria.[20] In the Gambia, another area with seasonal malaria, Greenwood *et al.*,[50] in a randomised community-based controlled trial of malaria chemoprophylaxis, also reported maternal mortality data. There were one in 518 deaths in the experimental and three in 631 deaths in the chemoprophylaxis control group, and a further nine women died from the group not reporting for chemoprophylaxis. In South Africa, an increase in malaria-attributable maternal deaths was reported from areas affected by the flooding in Mozambique in 1999. For non-pregnancy-related infections, the percentage of deaths due to malaria increased from five in 130 deaths in 1998 to 20 in 262 deaths in 1999.[51]

Population-attributable risk of maternal mortality due to malaria

Maternal mortality from malarial anaemia has been estimated by attributing the anaemia excess in primigravidae compared with multigravidae in malarious areas as

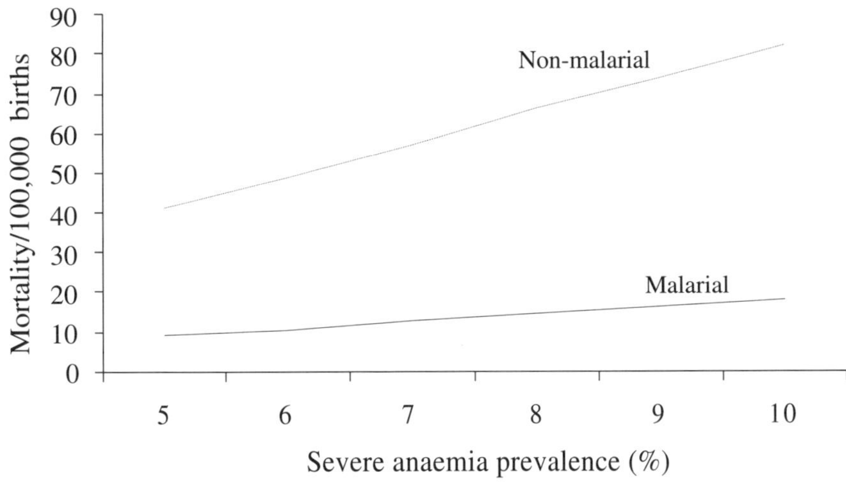

Figure 6.3. Malarial and non-malarial maternal mortality associated with severe anaemia (haemoglobin levels <7 g/l) in primigravidae living in malarious areas (modified from Brabin *et al.*[53])

due to the excess of malaria experienced by primigravidae. This assumption is reasonable because in areas of high transmission a large number of studies have confirmed that *P. falciparum* malaria and anaemia are more frequent in primigravidae.[2,52] Cause-specific malaria mortality in primigravidae can then be estimated if a case fatality rate is assumed.[53] The case fatality estimate for severe anaemia (haemoglobin levels of less than 70 g/l) in developing countries was taken as 1%, which is derived from a recent analysis of anaemia and pregnancy-related maternal mortality for a large number of hospital-based studies in Africa.[52] Using this method, in areas with perennial malaria transmission and a 5% severe anaemia prevalence there would be nine severe malaria anaemia-related deaths per 100 000 births to primigravidae. At a 10% severe anaemia prevalence, there would be 18 severe malaria anaemia-related deaths. Figure 6.3 shows the trend in mortality estimates for malarial and non-malarial anaemia using this approach. The relative risk of mortality associated with extremely severe anaemia (haemoglobin levels of less than 4.7 g/l) was estimated at 3.51 (95% CI 2.05–6.00). Population-attributable estimates can be defended on the basis of the strong association between severe anaemia and maternal mortality. An outline of this methodology for determining malaria-attributable maternal mortality from severe anaemia has been published.[53]

The values in Figure 6.3 are of the same order of magnitude as median values for malaria-attributable mortality (direct and indirect) in hospital studies which were estimated from Tables 6.1 and 6.2 (6/100 000 births). However, the above estimate for primigravidae relates to deaths from severe malarial anaemia and does not include other malaria-related deaths (e.g. cerebral malaria).

Figure 6.4 shows the plot of malaria estimates of maternal mortality by year of study for hospital reports from Africa. The estimates remain low (<20/100 000 births) until the late 1980s, when four studies showed values above 50/100 000 births between 1988

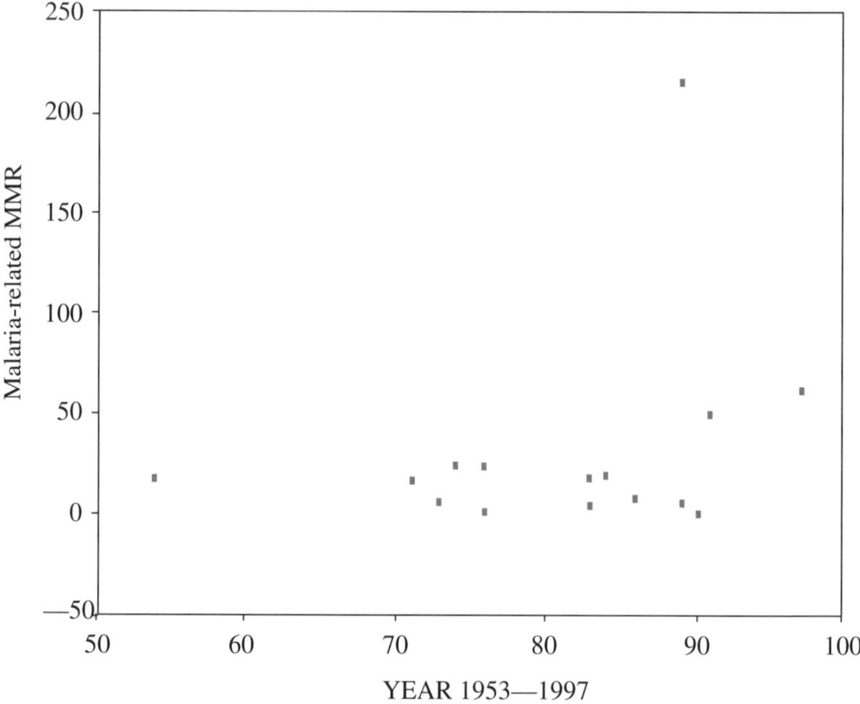

Figure 6.4. Secular trend in malaria-attributable maternal mortality ratios (MMR) in hospital-based studies from Africa, 1953–1997

and 1997. These were from Mozambique, Senegal and two from Zambia. This may relate to the emergence during this period of the HIV epidemic and drug-resistant *P. falciparum* malaria. In Zambia, malaria is considered a major cause of maternal death.[33]

Discussion

The estimation of maternal mortality in countries with defective data is rife with difficulties. There are problems with identifying catchment populations of hospitals in order to calculate rates or to claim that the estimates have any relevance beyond the population of women using a particular hospital.[4] For hospital deliveries, it is not always clear whether only live births are referred to or whether fetal deaths are included. Conversely, hospital deliveries provide higher-quality cause-specific information and may provide a better indicator of the proportion of maternal deaths associated with malaria. The classification of some indirect malaria deaths was probably more affected by the subjective view of the observer. The rate at which the institution's statistics covers births is important and a high coverage of births equates with a high coverage of maternal deaths. No single source is satisfactory and multiple sources are essential for this type of analysis.

The extent to which large differences in the estimates of malaria-related maternal mortality in this analysis reflect the pattern of risk rather than the pattern of data deficiencies is uncertain. The data provide little information on when mothers' deaths occur: in which trimester, at delivery or in the postpartum period. Maternal complications related to malaria in early pregnancy may be underestimated. In the study from Maputo, Mozambique, malaria was considered one of the reasons why adolescents died more often than older women in the second trimester.[6,16] Authors' definitions of malaria deaths were frequently not provided and in only a few reports was cerebral malaria specifically mentioned. The cause of death was often assigned from a clinical diagnosis generally made by the obstetrician researcher. This was based on verbal autopsy and clinical case notes by health workers who attended the patient. Postmortems to confirm diagnosis were conducted in only a minority of studies. In an early study from Ibadan in Nigeria, with postmortem examination in 111/114 maternal deaths, anaemia was the most common obstetric cause listed but malaria was not mentioned specifically.[5] Conversely, in the Maputo study maternal malaria deaths were confirmed by autopsy in a substantial number of cases.[6] Postmortem evidence for malaria as a cause of death may be found more often with direct malaria deaths, but less frequently when malaria is an indirect cause.

There are good epidemiological data from Malawi and Kenya to suggest that pregnancy malaria and anaemia are more frequent in women with HIV infection.[1] These are important confounders related to indirect causes of malaria and maternal mortality and may relate to clinical observations in sub-Saharan Africa made over the past ten years, which indicate a worsening situation with dramatic increases in the MMR. In Malawi this has doubled from 620 to 1120 in 100 000 births. The absence of data on specific aetiology of maternal deaths for most of sub-Saharan Africa makes it difficult to identify the contribution of malaria-specific causes, although the present analysis would indicate that malaria has contributed to this increased maternal mortality during the 1990s. A study on female reproductive mortality in Dar es Salaam, Tanzania, between 1991 and 1993 showed that malaria was the third most common cause of female mortality in the Ilala district, where 18% of all female mortality was during the pregnancy period.[54] Similarly, in a community-based investigation in rural Zimbabwe during 1989 and 1990, malaria was the fourth major indirect cause (7.6%) of maternal deaths.[29]

For obstetric causes of maternal mortality, there is evidence that malaria has been associated with pre-eclampsia in Senegal[55] and with pre-eclampsia and eclampsia during the Ceylon epidemic.[33] A retrospective analysis from Papua New Guinea found a significant association with postpartum haemorrhage.[56] Case–control studies will be required to determine the contribution of malaria to these diseases.

Conclusions

Evidence from this review indicates that the percentage of maternal deaths in Africa attributable to malaria has ranged from 0.5–23.0% in hospital studies and 2.9–17.6%

in community studies. Outside Africa, the range for hospital studies in areas of low endemicity was 0.6–12.5%. Malaria-related MMRs in Africa during the last three decades have ranged from 1–215 in 100 000 births for hospital studies and 19–634 in 100 000 births for community studies. This variation partly relates to differences between study samples, but also to variation in malaria endemicity and use of and access to health services. This is nowhere better illustrated than in the sugar estates of Guyana between 1937 and 1960, when malaria control leading to eradication confirmed the wide-ranging influence of endemic malaria on maternal mortality.

There is a significant association between MMRs and all-cause mortality, suggesting that malaria-attributable mortality rises sharply above 50 in 100 000 births when all-cause mortality exceeds 400 in 100 000 births. Estimates of the contribution of direct and indirect malaria deaths to this mortality are difficult to segregate, especially as pregnancy-related nutritional anaemia and HIV comorbidity confound these classifications. The analysis by secular trend supports a tentative conclusion that maternal malaria deaths have increased since the emergence of the HIV epidemic and drug-resistant falciparum malaria in Africa.

Although malaria is an avoidable cause of maternal mortality, we are far from establishing a satisfactory model linking mortality to malaria transmission or to interventions. Early detection, accurate diagnosis and treatment are essential prerequisites for reducing the incidence of death. Practical aspects of interventions (choice of antimalarial drugs, distribution of impregnated bed-nets) need to be integrated into other disease-control programmes, as well as antenatal care. Provision of adequate antenatal and delivery care and strengthening of emergency obstetric services are essential. Training of staff in adolescent healthcare packages that include attention to the problem of malaria in pregnancy will be important, as well as community education programmes.

Acknowledgement

This work received financial support from the European Commission Research Directorate fifth framework programme on community activities in the field of research, technological development and demonstration for concerted actions and thematic networks (contract no: PREMA-EU – ICA4-CT-2001-10012).

References

1. Steketee RTW, Nahlen BL, Parise M, Menendez C. The burden of malaria in pregnancy in malaria-endemic areas. *Am J Trop Med Hyg* 2001;64 Suppl 1–2:28–35.
2. Brabin BJ, Rogerson S. The epidemiology and outcomes of maternal malaria. In: Duffy PE, Fried M, editors. *Malaria in Pregnancy, Deadly Parasite, Susceptible Host.* London: Taylor & Francis; 2001. p. 27–52.
3. Molineaux L. Malaria and mortality: some epidemiological considerations. *Ann Trop Med Parasitol* 1997;91:811–25.
4. Graham W. Maternal mortality: levels, trends and data deficiencies. In: Feachem RG, Jamieson DT, editors. *Disease and Mortality in Sub-Saharan Africa.* Oxford: Oxford University Press; 1991. p. 101–16.
5. Lawson JB. Maternal mortality in West Africa. *Ghana Med J* 1952;1:31–6.
6. Granje AC, Machungo F, Gomes A, Bergstrom S, Brabin BJ. Malaria-related mortality in urban

pregnant women in Mozambique. *Ann Trop Med Parasitol* 1998;92:257–63.
7. Macpherson TA. A retrospective study of maternal deaths in the Zimbabwean black. *Cent Afr J Med* 1981;27:57–60.
8. World Health Organization. *Maternal Mortality – A Global Factbook*. Geneva: WHO; 1991.
9. World Health Organization. *International Statistical Classification of Diseases and Relative Health Problems. 10th revision. Vols 1 and 2*. Geneva: WHO; 1992.
10. Guyatt HL, Snow RW. The epidemiology and burden of *Plasmodium falciparum*-related anemia among pregnant women in sub-Saharan Africa. *Am J Trop Med Hyg* 2001;64 Suppl 1–2:36–44.
11. Yoseph S, Kifle G. A six-year review of maternal mortality in a teaching hospital in Addis Ababa. *Ethiop Med J* 1988;26:115–20.
12. Costa CMM. La mortalité maternelle dans la région ded Befata (unpublished report). Ministry of Public Health. Guinea-Bissau; 1989.
13. Boerma JT, Mati JKG. Identifying maternal mortality through networking: results from coastal Kenya. *Stud Fam Plann* 1989;20:245–53.
14. Solange M. Mortalité maternelle dans le Firaisana de Belmoty-Toliara [dissertation]. Antananarivo: University of Antananarivo; 1989.
15. Drissen F. Maternal deaths in twelve Malawi hospitals in 1989 (unpublished report);1990.
16. Songane F. Analise des casos de mortes maternas ocorridas nos primeiros 7 meses de 1984. Maputo Hospital Central Boletin Informativo do Servico de Ginecologia Obstetricia, February 1985 and F160 Congress, Berlin, September 1985.
17. Granje CL, Machungo F, Gomes A, Bergstrom S. Adolescent maternal mortality in Mozambique. *J Adolesc Health* 2001;28:303–6.
18. Lawson JB, Lister UG. Clinical report of the Department of Obstetrics, University College, Ibadan. 1 April 1953 – 31 December 1954. London: Vail and Co. Ltd.
19. Courtney LD. Maternal parity, haemoglobin lead, mortality rate, labour and complications in a tropical centre. *Journal of the Irish Medical Association* 1974;67:159–61.
20. Gueye A. *Report de la deuxième mission d'identification pour la reduction de la mortalité maternelle au Sénégal*. Government of the Republic of Senegal/United Nations Development Programme/WHO. University of Colombia; 1989.
21. Williams B. *Maternal Mortality in Sierra Leone*. Freetown: Ministry of Health; 1979.
22. Baldo MH. Maternal mortality in the Sudan. Inter-regional meeting on the prevention of maternal mortality, 11–15 November 1985, Geneva. Report of the World Health Organization. Unpublished document FHE/PMM/85.95.
23. Mtimavalge LAR, Lisasi D, Ntagabaliwe WK. Maternal mortality in Dar-es-Salaam, Tanzania 1974-1977. *East Afr Med J* 1980;57:111–8.
24. Armon PJ. Maternal deaths in the Kilimanjaro region of Tanzania. *Trans R Soc Trop Med Hyg* 1979;73:284–8.
25. MacLeod J, Rhode R. Retrospective follow-up of maternal deaths and their associated risk factors in a rural district of Tanzania. *Trop Med Int Health* 1998;3:130–7.
26. Kampikaho A. Maternal mortality in the hospitals of Kampala (unpublished report); 1987.
27. Crowther CA. Maternal deaths at Harare Maternity Hospital during 1983. *S Afr Med J* 1986;69:180–2.
28. Crowther CA. Prevention of maternal deaths: a continuing challenge. *Centr Afr J Med* 1986;32:11–14.
29. Fawcus S, Mbizvo MT, Lindmark G, Nystrom L. A community based investigation of causes of maternal mortality in rural and urban Zimbabwe. *Centr Afr J Med* 1995;41:105–13.
30. Ministry of Health, Zambia. Family Health Programme. Maternal Mortality. Workshop on UNFPA-funded family health programme – reformulation exercise, 18–19 August 1988, Lusaka.
31. Mhango C, Rochat R, Arkutu A. Reproductive mortality in Lusaka, Zambia, 1982–83. *Stud Fam Plann* 1986;17:243–51.
32. Ahmed Y, Mweba P, Chintu C, Grange JM, Ustianowski A, Zumla A. A study of maternal mortality at the University Teaching Hospital, Zambia: the emergence of tuberculosis as a major non-obstetric cause of maternal death. *Int J Tuberc Lung Dis* 1999;3:675–80.
33. Wickramasuriya GAW. *Malaria and Ankylostomiasis in the Pregnant Woman. Their More Serious Complications and Sequelae*. Oxford: Oxford University Press; 1937.
34. Giglioli G. Changes in the pattern of mortality following the eradication of hyperendemic malaria from a highly susceptible community. *Bull World Health Organ* 1972;46:181–202.
35. Jarquin JD, Roults FK. Epidemiología y prevención de la muerte materna institutional en El Salvador 1983–1987 (unpublished report), San Salvador; 1989.
36. Yam A. Maternal mortality yet to be minimised. *Asia-Oceania J Obstet Gynaecol* 1986;12:79–87.

37. Kyi MK. Maternal mortality at the Workers Hospital, Rangoon 1983–1987. *Austr N Z J Obstet Gynaecol* 1988;159:80–3.
38. Rattanaporn P. The internal factors affecting maternal mortality [dissertation]. Bangkok: Mahidol University; 1980.
39. Nosten F, ter Kuile F, Maelankirri L, Dedudt B, White NJ. Malaria during pregnancy in an area of unstable endemicity. *Trans R Soc Trop Med Hyg* 1991;85:424–9.
40. Abdulghani NA. Risk factors for maternal mortality among women using hospitals in Yemen Arab Republic (unpublished report); 1990.
41. Mola G. Maternal deaths Papua New Guinea 1984–86. *Papua New Guinea Medical Journal* 1989;32:27–31.
42. Campbell GR. Maternal mortality at Goroka Base Hospital. *Papua New Guinea Medical Journal* 1974;17:335–41.
43. Sholapurkar SL, Gupta AN, Mahajan RC. Clinical course of malaria in pregnancy – a prospective controlled study from India. *Trans R Soc Trop Med Hyg* 1988;82:376–9.
44. Menon RT. Pregnancy and malaria. *Medical Journal of Malaysia* 1972;27:115–19.
45. Gray RH. The decline of mortality in Ceylon and the demographic effects of malaria control. *Popul Stud* 1974;28:205–29.
46. Harrison K, Rossiter LE. Maternal mortality. *Br J Obstet Gynaecol* 1985 Suppl 5:100–15.
47. Greenwood AM, Greenwood BM, Bradley AK, Williams K, Shenton FC, Tulloch S, *et al.* A prospective survey of the outcome of pregnancy in a rural area of the Gambia. *Bull World Health Organ* 1987;65:635–43.
48. Shulman C, Dorman E, Brabin BJ. Malaria in pregnancy. In: MacLean A, Regan L, Carrington D, editors. *Infection and Pregnancy*. London: RCOG Press. 2001. p. 124–36
49. Duffy P. Immunity to malaria during pregnancy: different host, different parasite. In: Duffy P, Fried M, editors. *Malaria in Pregnancy, Deadly Parasite, Susceptible Host*. London: Taylor & Francis; 2001. p. 71–126.
50. Greenwood BM, Greenwood AM. Snow RW, Byass P, Bennett S, Hatib-N'Jie AB. The effects of malaria chemoprophylaxis given by traditional birth attendants on the course and outcome of pregnancy. *Trans R Soc Trop Med Hyg* 1989;83:589–94.
51. National Committee on Confidential Enquiries into Maternal Deaths, Department of Health, Republic of South Africa. *Third Interim Report on Confidential Enquiries into Maternal Deaths in South Africa. Changing Patterns in Maternal Deaths 1998–2000.* Pretoria: NCCEMD, Department of Health, Republic of South Africa; 2000, p. 32.
52. Brabin BJ. An analysis of malaria in pregnancy in Africa. *Bull World Health Organ* 1983;61:1005–16.
53. Brabin BJ, Hakim M, Pelletier D. An analysis of anemia and pregnancy-related maternal mortality. *J Nutr* 2001;131:604S–615S.
54. Urassa E, Massawe S. Mgaya H, Lindmark G, Nystrom L. Female mortality in reproductive ages in Dar es Salaam, Tanzania. *East Afr Med J* 1994;71:226–31.
55. Sartelet H, Rogier C, Milko-Sartelet I, Angel G, Michel G. Malaria associated pre-eclampsia in Senegal. *Lancet* 1996;347:1121.
56. Piper C, Brabin BJ, Alpers MP. Higher risk of post-partum haemorrhage in malarious than non-malarious areas of Papua New Guinea. *Int J Gynaecol Obstet* 2001;72:77–8.
57. Nair LS, Nair AS. Effects of malaria infection in pregnancy. *Indian J Malariol* 1993;30: 207–14.
58. Singh N, Shukla MM, Sharma VP. Epidemiology of malaria in pregnancy in central India. *Bull World Health Organ* 1999;77:567–72.

Chapter 7

The contribution of anaemia

Nynke van den Broek

Introduction

Anaemia in pregnancy is a common and worldwide problem that deserves more attention. For many developing countries, prevalence rates of up to 75% are reported. Anaemia is frequently severe in these situations and can be expected to contribute significantly to maternal mortality and morbidity. This chapter focuses on anaemia in pregnancy in developing countries with particular reference to sub-Saharan Africa. After a discussion of definitions, screening for anaemia and prevalence, the relationship between anaemia and maternal mortality and morbidity will be reviewed.

Definitions

As a result of the normal physiological changes in pregnancy, plasma volume expands by 46–55%, whereas red-cell volume expands by 18–25%.[1,2] The resulting haemodilution has, perhaps wrongly, been termed 'physiological anaemia of pregnancy'. There are insufficient data to give physiological limits for the expected haemodilution. In most published studies, the mean minimum normal haemoglobin in healthy pregnant women living at sea level is 11.0–12.0 g/dl. The mean minimum by WHO criteria is 11.0 g/dl in the first half of pregnancy and 10.5 g/dl in the second half of pregnancy.[3,4] In the only well-conducted longitudinal study that could be found of the 'hydraemia' of pregnancy in iron-replete healthy pregnant women, 10.4 g/dl was the lowest recorded value.[5]

Anaemia in pregnancy is further divided into mild anaemia (haemoglobin [Hb] 10.0–10.9 g/dl), moderate anaemia (Hb 7.0–9.9 g/dl) and severe anaemia (Hb <7.0 g/dl).[4] The definition of severe anaemia in the published literature, however, varies and this may also be defined as Hb <8.0g/dl. There has been some debate about the relevance of the various cut-off points, whether different cut-off points should be used for different populations[5–8] and the need to adjust for populations living at high altitude.[9]

Screening

Screening for anaemia in pregnancy is useful for a variety of reasons. It may be helpful to collect baseline data on prevalence and severity in a given population, to assess the effects of supplementation with iron tablets, antimalarial prophylactics or anthelminthic treatment. At primary-care level, estimation of haemoglobin concentration can help to determine whether referral is necessary for more detailed investigation and treatment.

An accepted standard of practice is that all women have at least one measurement of their haemoglobin levels during the course of pregnancy. In industrialised countries or in the private sector in developing countries this is usually performed by electronic (automated) counter. In developing countries, these methods are often simply not available even at tertiary level. Either screening for anaemia may not be carried out at all or assessment of whether a pregnant woman is anaemic or not may be limited to inspection of the conjunctiva by the nurse or midwife for the presence of pallor during antenatal visits. By far the majority of pregnant women in sub-Saharan Africa will be screened for anaemia by this method.

There are few published papers reporting on the accuracy of screening for anaemia using clinical inspection of conjunctiva in pregnant women. In a large study conducted in women attending a rural antenatal clinic, sensitivity was 33.2% and 39.7% for haemoglobin values of ≤ 11.0 and ≤ 10.0 g/dl respectively. Values obtained were better for the lower range of haemoglobin values but did not exceed 62.1%.[10] A study from Mozambique reported a sensitivity of 31.5%, with anaemia defined as a packed cell volume ≤ 30.[11] In a smaller study from Kenya, examination of the conjunctiva was reported to have 62–69% sensitivity for detecting severe anaemia (Hb <7.0 g/dl) in a study population with a high incidence of severe anaemia (16%).[12]

Studies in children and in healthy ambulatory adults have also demonstrated poor accuracy. In children under five years of age a definite diagnosis of anaemia was correctly made in 5–42% of cases and a diagnosis of probable anaemia was correctly made in 24–64% of cases by conjunctival inspection.[13] When palm, tongue and nail-bed were examined in addition, accuracy improved. However, in this study a low cut-off point (8 g/dl) was used to define anaemia and it could be argued that this constitutes severe anaemia. Gjorup *et al.*[14] obtained a sensitivity of 27–44% at cut-off points of 10g/dl and 11 g/dl, respectively, in adults. The probability of detecting anaemia did not exceed 0.75 even when inspection was carried out by trained physicians. Substantial interobserver variability has also been reported.[14,15] Even when used in combination with a conjunctival – or anaemia – recognition card, sensitivity remains low except when anaemia is severe.[16,17]

Conjunctival inspection in pregnant women may be particularly inaccurate as a result of increased peripheral vasodilatation. It may be possible to improve the accuracy of screening for anaemia using conjunctival inspection in pregnant women by improved training and assessment of more than one physical sign of pallor. Further work would be needed to assess this.

In the absence of a functioning automated (Coulter) counter several alternative methods for measurement of haemoglobin concentration are available.[18] Both the portable haemoglobinometer (HemoCue, HemoCue Ltd, Dronfield, UK) and copper sulphate methods have been re-evaluated for use in pregnancy.

The HemoCue method was used by midwives as part of routine antenatal clinic care in a rural setting. Sensitivity was 80–97%, with specificity of 79–99% depending on the cut-off point used. The HemoCue method is well-liked by healthcare workers and it requires minimal training. It is a non-dilutional method, i.e. there is no mixing of blood with chemicals. It only requires a few drops of blood obtained through a finger-prick and measurement of haemoglobin concentration (Hb) can be done immediately at the patient's side. The small portable machine works either on batteries or from a mains electricity supply. In practice, however, it is still too expensive for use in the primary healthcare setting in most developing countries.[10,19–21]

The copper sulphate method has also been evaluated recently for use in antenatal clinic settings.[22–25] Use of the copper sulphate method relies on the preparation and availability of a solution of copper sulphate of known specific gravity. It is a non-dilutional method. The test is generally carried out by laboratory technicians rather than the nurse or midwife. There is a fixed range of haemoglobin values for which the blood sample can be tested, e.g Hb <8.0 g/dl or <10.0 g/dl or 8.0–10.0 g/dl.

In response to the need for a simple, cheap but accurate method for the estimation of haemoglobin concentration, a new colour scale was recently developed by the WHO.[26] This is an adaptation of the original Talquist scale,[27] which can to this day be found in remote clinics in many areas of sub-Saharan Africa.

Improvements to the new WHO scale include in particular a much improved set of ten colour standards corresponding to the colour of bloodstains of various haemoglobin concentrations (range 3.0–14.0 g/dl). Initial assessments suggest that the Haemoglobin Colour Scale is simple to use and acceptable to healthcare workers in rural areas.

Assessment in an antenatal population with high prevalence of anaemia by comparison with Coulter counter measurements gave sensitivities of 75.4% and 81.6% for cut-off points of Hb 11.0g/dl and 10.0g/dl respectively. Specificity was 47.2% and 45.3% respectively but improved to 76.4% for Hb <8.0g/dl and 98.5% for Hb <6.0g/dl. The sensitivity of the WHO colour scale as a screening tool to detect anaemia was consistently better than if conjunctival inspection was used for screening.[10]

The value of each screening test within a specific setting depends on the necessity of performing an assessment without the resources of a more accurate method and on cost–benefit considerations. Any method of screening for anaemia should be cheap, simple to operate, acceptable to both patients and staff, require a minimum of materials and give immediate accurate results. In situations with limited resources and poor technical support, a simple screening tool is likely to perform better than sophisticated methods that depend on correct dilution and preparation of standards or on power supply.

Prevalence

It has been estimated that over 50% of the pregnant women in the world have a haemoglobin level indicative of anaemia. In industrialised countries, anaemia in pregnancy occurs in less than 20% of women. This does, however, still reach the level of public health significance (≥ 10%). Published rates of prevalence for developing countries range from 35–72% for Africa, 37–75% for Asia and 37–52% for Latin America.[28–30] Not only is anaemia common; it is often severe. From the published reports available, it can be estimated that 2–7% of pregnant women have values of less than 7.0g/dl, and, probably 15–20% have values of less than 8.0g/dl.

Those authors who publish their range of Hb values not infrequently report on patients with values well below 5.0g/dl.[30–32]

At the African Regional Consultation on the Control of Anaemia in Pregnancy in 1989, it was recommended that simple studies of prevalence and aetiology should be undertaken for each region.[33] Up-to-date information from many countries is, however, still scanty; the few published studies often describe small sample sizes and are usually from hospital-based populations. There is a lack of data from rural areas. It has been suggested that the prevalence of anaemia may depend on the season, increasing in relation to malaria transmission in the wet season or in relation to increased food shortage at the end of the dry season but published prevalence rates rarely reflect measurements performed all year round.

With the realisation that prevalence rates remain high, it has been suggested that interventions should be focused on identified 'at-risk' groups. Suggested target groups have been women with severe anaemia,[34] adolescents,[35,36] primigravidae[35,37,38] or, conversely, multigravidae.[35,39]

One large study[30] from southern Malawi that was conducted over 12 months showed a higher prevalence of both anaemia (Hb <11.0 g/dl; 72%) and severe anaemia (Hb <7.0g/dl; 4.0%) in rural pregnant women (57%) compared with urban women (3.6%). Prevalence of anaemia in primiparae was slightly increased for both all anaemia (Hb <11.0 g/dl) and severe anaemia (Hb <7.0g/dl) but the effect of targeting primiparous women alone for interventions would mean that at least 65% of anaemic women and over 50% of all women with severe anaemia would be excluded.

In a review on maternal health during adolescent pregnancy, it was suggested that pregnant adolescents might be particularly at risk for anaemia.[40] Ogbeidi *et al.*[35] report a similar observation from Nigeria. However, the number of women studies was extremely low in these reports. Second, the influence of age has often not been separated from the effect of (primi-)parity. When the effect of age was examined separately from gravidity, adolescents were not found to be at increased risk of anaemia in southern Malawi.[30]

Most other studies from Africa also report that age alone is not an important determinant of haemoglobin values.[31,37,41,42]

Although there was no effect of parity on haemoglobin levels in studies from Tanzania,[31] an increased risk in primigravidae has been documented by a number of other workers.[37,43]

The explanation most frequently given is an increased susceptibility to malaria in primigravidae.[39,43] However, Matteelli *et al.*[39] reported that although malaria was associated with anaemia in primigravidae, the highest prevalence of anaemia was in multiparous patients. Seasonal variations in anaemia prevalence for both multiparous and primigravid women was suppressed in women who received malaria prophylaxis in a study from Mali.[44] If only primiparous women were targeted for malaria prophylaxis in Blantyre, 40% of women with peripheral parasitaemia at time of booking would be missed. Presentation in the malaria season and young age, rather than low gravidity, were found to be risk factors for malaria in this population.[30]

In 1993, the World Bank ranked anaemia as the eighth leading cause of disease in girls and women in developing countries.[45] Although anaemia is assumed to be less common in non-pregnant women, there is a lack of data on the prevalence of anaemia in this population group. Studies are also needed to assess the association between anaemia in pregnancy and pre-pregnancy haemoglobin levels.

Effects

Each year more than 500 000 women die from pregnancy-related causes, 99% of these in developing countries.[46] Estimates of maternal mortality resulting from anaemia range from 34/100 000 live births in Nigeria to as high as 194/100 000 in Pakistan.[4,28] In combination with obstetric haemorrhage, anaemia is estimated to be responsible for 17–46% of cases of maternal death.[47–49] A review of symptoms associated with maternal deaths in Bangladesh led researchers to conclude that anaemia had played a secondary role in nearly all cases.[50] Anaemia is probably a chronic rather than acute condition in many cases. There is a resulting compensatory shift of the oxygen dissociation curve to the right. Thus women with very low haemoglobin concentrations may be seen in the antenatal period without the expected overt symptoms of cardiac failure. They will, however, easily become tired by any form of physical activity and may decompensate, e.g. as a result of labour. Should any adverse event such as bleeding occur, their risk of death is high.

There is a need to clarify the relationship between haemoglobin levels (anaemia prevalence) in a population and maternal survival and pregnancy outcome. The available data on the association between anaemia and maternal survival are limited and there are serious methodological flaws in most of the studies, as pointed out by Rush.[51] In order to clarify the relationship between haemoglobin level, maternal survival and pregnancy outcome, measurement of haemoglobin levels needs to be carried out in a representative population of pregnant women at the beginning of pregnancy. Women need to be followed up prospectively until the end of pregnancy (and ideally until six weeks postpartum). It must be noted that pregnancy outcome will also be related to the underlying causes of anaemia (e.g. HIV, iron deficiency, recurrent antepartum haemorrhage) and to the effect of any supplementation or treatment received.

Most of the published studies report on outcome for hospital-based patients. In developing countries, this is rarely representative of the population as a whole. In particular, conclusions about association or causality drawn from a single measurement during delivery in hospital must be considered flawed. In many cases, haemoglobin concentration may have been measured only because of, for instance, a prior history of bleeding, fever or suspected malaria, which may be the reason for referral to the hospital in the first place.

It must also be noted that there are currently no agreed international standards or sets of criteria for attributing death to anaemia. It is in fact often difficult to establish accurately the cause of death in situations where clinical information is incomplete and data collection is not standardised. Thus, in many cases, the only two laboratory tests that may have been available to clinicians could be a haemoglobin concentration and a peripheral blood slide for malaria parasitaemia. Death from anaemia may sound better than death from haemorrhage, in that the latter could be perceived as the result of the health facility's inability to provide adequate care. Finally, level of access to emergency obstetric care and in particular to blood transfusion and the quality and speed of care received are of prime determining importance. Thus a study from Indonesia[52] illustrated the much higher risk of maternal death in anaemic women from rural areas than from urban areas, possibly as a result of problems with timely access to obstetric care. Morbidity resulting from anaemia is similarly difficult to establish. Diminished work capacity and physical performance have been reported as a result of anaemia.[53,54] Iron-deficiency anaemia leads to abnormalities in host defence and neurological dysfunction.[55,56] Increased risks of premature labour[57–59] and low birthweight[57,60,61] have also been reported in association with anaemia in pregnancy. Both are common problems in developing countries and contribute significantly to high perinatal mortality. However, most published work on this comes from industrialised countries where anaemia is much less of a problem and much less severe in nature. Confounding factors such as poverty, poor antenatal clinic attendance and recurrent infection, which can themselves result in low birthweight and prematurity, are seldom examined at the same time. Further research on the effect of anaemia *per se* on birthweight and prematurity is therefore necessary to establish a clear causal relationship.

It has been reported that higher haemoglobin concentrations are also likely to result in poor obstetric outcome.[57,62,63] This may, however, have been primarily the result of failure of adequate plasma expansion[64,65] and further work is needed in this area.

In developing countries, an association can be expected between anaemia or iron deficiency and increased risk of perinatal and infant mortality and morbidity. Several studies have reported a relationship between maternal and cord blood haemoglobin levels and iron status.[66–71] Delays in mental and psychomotor development have also been described in anaemic compared with non-anaemic infants.[72]

Aetiology

Relatively few studies have comprehensively assessed the aetiological factors responsible for anaemia in pregnancy in sub-Saharan Africa. This is probably for three main reasons: first, the lack of adequate diagnostic facilities in many institutions in developing countries; second, the frequent complexity of the aetiological pattern such that, for example, infection and nutritional deficiency coexist. Chemical measurements of iron and folate status are influenced by inflammation, and there is a lack of clearly defined and validated cut-off points for the diagnosis of deficiency in these circumstances.[73–75] Evaluation of suitably stained bone marrow aspirates may then be necessary to provide meaningful results.[76,77] Third, the relative contribution of each aetiological factor can be difficult to assess in pregnancy when maternal physiological changes alter the parameters used for the diagnosis of anaemia.[2,78,79]

Despite the lack of stringent criteria and definitional problems, pregnancy anaemia in sub-Saharan Africa is most often believed to be the result of nutritional deficiencies, especially iron deficiency.[80,81] Folate deficiency has been described in West Africa.[82] Recent studies have suggested that nutritional deficiency in other vitamins can also contribute to anaemia. Studies from Indonesia indicate that Vitamin A deficiency may contribute to anaemia in pregnancy.[83,84] Vitamin B12 deficiency was found to be an unrecognised but important cause of anaemia in Zimbabwe.[85]

Although the contribution of malaria is generally acknowledged, the role of other chronic infections has been discussed[86] but not extensively studied in pregnant women. In the last decade, HIV infection has become more prevalent and it must now be considered a possible aetiological factor.[87,88] A recent study from Malawi[89] illustrates the complex interaction between multimicronutrient deficiency and infection.

In many pregnant women, anaemia is probably caused by a combination of disease including micronutrient deficiency such as iron deficiency and infections such as HIV and malaria. In this respect, the laboratory parameter of haemoglobin concentration (Hb) can perhaps best be seen as a general marker of underlying morbidity.

Thus, possible aetiological factors responsible for anaemia are multiple and their relative contributions can be expected to vary by geographical area, as well as by season. Knowledge of the relative importance of different causes should form the basis for intervention strategies.

Conclusions

In many areas of the world, as many as 75% of women are anaemic during pregnancy by WHO standards (Hb <11.0g/dl). Many have severe anaemia (Hb <7.0 g/dl or <8.0 g/dl). It is not known whether most women enter pregnancy already anaemic or whether anaemia develops primarily during pregnancy.

Successful management of anaemia in pregnancy depends on accurate and acceptable methods of detecting anaemia, assessing its severity and monitoring response to treatment. From the available published data, it is not possible to identify a specific 'at-risk' group and therefore it should be policy that all women are offered screening.

Detection of anaemia often relies solely on conjunctival inspection, which is probably insufficient. The introduction of cheap but accurate screening tools should be encouraged.

There is a lack of studies measuring haemoglobin levels prospectively before and during pregnancy with assessment of maternal mortality and morbidity. Thus, it is not possible to indicate which level of haemoglobin is particularly associated with adverse outcome. However, on the basis of the available evidence it seems reasonable to assume that the risk of maternal mortality in developing countries is increased, especially with severe anaemia.

In women with mild to moderate anaemia, timely treatment is likely to prevent the development of more severe anaemia and therefore reduce the need for blood transfusion with its associated risks. It is possible that prevention and/or adequate treatment of anaemia in pregnancy may also improve pregnancy outcome with regard to reduced incidence of premature labour and low birthweight but studies are needed to assess this.

Factors that contribute to anaemia include both micronutrient deficiency and infection. The complex pattern of interaction between the two requires further study. Anaemia in pregnancy is probably very often the result of a combination of micronutrient deficiency and infection, and haemoglobin concentration can perhaps be regarded as a 'marker of morbidity' in these situations.

Acknowledgement

I would like to thank Dr EA Letsky for her helpful comments.

References

1. Letsky EA. The haematological system. In: Hytten F, Chamberlain G, Broughton Pipkin F, editors. *Clinical Physiology in Obstetrics*. Oxford: Blackwell Scientific Publications; 1998. p. 71–110.

2. Letsky EA. Blood volume, haematinics, anaemia. In: de Swiet M, editor. *Medical Disorders in Obstetric Practice*. 3rd ed. Oxford: Blackwell Science; 1995. p. 33–70.
3. World Health Organization. Nutritional Anaemias. Technical Report Series no. 503. Geneva: WHO; 1972.
4. World Health Organization. *Prevention and Management of Severe Anaemia in Pregnancy*. Geneva: WHO; 1993.
5. Leeuw NKM de, Lowenstein L, Hsieh YS. Iron deficiency anaemia and hydremia in normal pregnancy. *Medicine Baltimore* 1966;45:291–315.
6. Johnson-Spear MA, Yip R. Hemoglobin difference between black and white women with comparable iron status: justification for race-specific anaemia criteria. *Am J Clin Nutr* 1994;60:117–21.
7. Dallman PR, Barr GD, Allen AM. Hemoglobin concentration in white, black and oriental children: is there a need for separate criteria in screening for anemia. *Am J Clin Nutr* 1978;31:377–80.
8. Berti P, Leonard WR. The merits of race-specific standards. *Am J Clin Nutr* 1994;60:616.
9. Berger J, Aguayo VM, San Miguel JL, Lujan C, Tellez W, Traissac MS. Definition and prevalence of anemia in Bolivian women of childbearing age living at high altitudes: the effect of iron-folate supplementation. *Nutr Rev* 1997:55:247–56.
10. van den Broek NR, Ntonya C, Mhango E, White SA. Diagnosing anaemia in pregnancy in rural clinics: assessing the potential of the Haemoglobin Colour Scale. *Bull World Health Organ* 1999,77:15–21.
11. Liljestrand J, Bergstrom S. The value of conjunctival pallor in the diagnosis of pregnancy anaemia in Mozambique. *J Obstet Gynaecol East Centr Afr* 1992:10:45–6.
12. Shulman CE, Levene M, Morison L, Dorman E, Peshu N, Marsh K. Screening for severe anaemia in pregnancy in Kenya, using pallor examination and self-reported morbidity. *Trans R Soc Trop Med Hyg* 2001;95:250–5.
13. Luby SP, Kazembe PN, Redd SC, Ziba C, Nwanyanwu OC, Hightower AW, *et al.* Using clinical signs to diagnose anaemia in African children. *Bull World Health Organ* 1995;73:477–82.
14. Gjorup T, Bugge PM, Hendriksen C, Jensen AM. A critical evaluation of the clinical diagnosis of anemia. *Am J Epidemiol* 1986;124:657–65.
15. Sanchez-Carrillo CI. Bias due to conjunctiva hue and the clinical assessment of anemia. *J Clin Epidemiol*1989;42:751–4.
16. Sanchez-Carillo CI, Ramirez-Sanchez T de J, Zambrana-Castaneda M, Selwyn BJ. Test of a non-invasive instrument for measuring haemoglobin concentration. *International Journal of Technology Assessment in Health Care* 1989;5:659–67.
17. Ghosh S, Mohan M. Screening for anaemia. *Lancet* 1978;1:823.
18. United States Agency for International Development. PATH: Program for Appropriate Technology in Health. Anemia detection in Health Services. Guidelines for Program Managers. Washington DC: USAID; 1996.
19. van den Broek NR, Kayira E, White SA, Medina A, Neilson JP, Molyneux ME. The accuracy of measuring haemoglobin concentration using a HemoCue haemoglobinometer: comparison with an automated method; in press.
20. Neville RG. Evaluation of portable hemoglobinometer in general practice. *BMJ (Clin Res Ed)* 1987;294:1263–5.
21. Hudson-Thomas M, Bingham KC, Simmons WK. An evaluation of the HemoCue for measuring haemoglobin in field studies in Jamaica. *Bull World Health Organ* 1994;72:423–6.
22. Politzer WM, Myburgh WM, van der Merwe JF. Haemoglobin estimation – reliability of the copper sulphate specific gravity v. the cyanhaemoglobin colorimetric method. *S Afr Med J* 1988;73:111–12.
23. Pistorius LR, Funk M, Pattinson RC, Howarth GR. Screening for anaemia in pregnancy with copper sulfate densitometry. *Int J Gynaecol Obstet* 1996;52:3–36.
24. Kegels G, Cornelis G, Mangelschots E, Van Brabant R, van Lerberghe W. Haemoglobin and packed cell volume measurement: the reliability of some simple techniques for use in surveys or rural hospitals. *Ann Soc Belg Med Trop* 1984;64:413–19.
25. Wilkinson D, Sach ME. Cost-effective on-site screening for anaemia in pregnancy in primary clinics. *S Afr Med J* 1997;87:463–5.
26. Stott GJ, Lewis SM. A simple and reliable method for estimating haemoglobin. *Bull World Health Organ* 1995;73:369–73.
27. Tallqvist TW. Méthode protique d'évaluation directe de la quantité d'hémoglobine du sang. *Archives of General Medicine* 1900;3:421–5.
28. World Health Organization. The prevalence of anaemia in women: a tabulation of available information. Geneva: WHO; 1992.
29. Sloan NL, Jordan EA, Winhoff B. Does iron supplementation make a difference? Working Paper

MotherCare Project. Virginia USA 1992;15.

30. van den Broek NR, Rogerson SJ, Mhango CG, Kambala B, White SA, Molyneux ME. Anaemia in pregnancy in southern Malawi: prevalence and risk factors. *BJOG* 2000;107 445–51.

31. Bergsjo P, Seha Am, Ole-King'ori N. Haemoglobin concentration in pregnant women. Experience from Moashi Tanzania. *Acta Obstet Gynecol Scand* 1996;75:241–4.

32. Fleming AF. The aetiology of severe anaemia in pregnancy in Ndola, Zambia. *Ann Trop Med Parasitol* 1989;83:37–49.

33. World Health Organization. Report of the African Regional Consultation on Control of Anaemia in Pregnancy, Brazzaville, Congo, September. WHO; 1989.

34. Sarin AR. Severe anaemia of pregnancy, recent experience. *Int J Gynaecol Obstet* 1995;50:45–9.

35. Ogbeide O, Wagbatsoma V, Orhue A. Anaemia in pregnancy. *East Afr Med J* 1994;71:671–3.

36. Beard JL. Iron deficiency: assessment during pregnancy and its importance in pregnant adolescents. *Am J Clin Nutr* 1994;59 Suppl 2:502–10.

37. Jackson DJ, Klee EB, Green SD, Mokili JL, Elton RA, Cutting WA. Severe anaemia in pregnancy: a problem of primigravidae in rural Zaire. *Trans R Soc Trop Med Hyg* 1991;85:829–32.

38. Selo-Ojeme DO. Anemia in pregnancy: case control study of risk factors. *Int J Gynaecol Obstet* 1997;59:53–4.

39. Matteelli A, Donato F, Shein A, Muchi JA, Leopardi O, Astori L, *et al.* Malaria and anaemia in pregnant women in urban Zanzibar, Tanzania. *Ann Trop Med Parasitol* 1994;88:475–83.

40. Scholl TO, Hediger ML, Belsky DH. Prenatal care and maternal health during adolescent pregnancy; a review and metanalysis. *J Adolesc Health* 1994;15:444–56.

41. Liljestrand J, Bergstrom S, Birgegard G. Anaemia of pregnancy in Mozambique. *Trans R Soc Trop Med Hyg* 1986;80:249–55.

42. Royston E. The prevalence of nutritional anaemia in women in developing countries: a critical review of available information. *World Health Stat Q* 1982;35:52–91.

43. Shulman CE, Graham WJ, Jilo H, Lowe BS, New L,Obiero J, *et al.* Malaria is an important cause of anaemia in primigravidae: evidence from a district hospital in coastal Kenya. *Trans R Soc Trop Med Hyg* 1996;90:535–9.

44. Bouvier P, Doumbo O, Breslow N, Robert CF, Mauris A, Picquet M, *et al.* Seasonality, malaria and impact of prophylaxis in a West African village I: effect of anaemia in pregnancy. *Am J Trop Med Hyg* 1997;56:378–83.

45. World Bank. *World Development Report: Investing in Health.* New York: Oxford University Press; 1993. p. 1–329.

46. World Health Organization. *Maternal Mortality Ratios and Rates.* Geneva: WHO; 1996.

47. World Bank, WHO, UNFPA. Preventing the tragedy of maternal deaths. A report on the International Safe Motherhood Conference Nairobi, Kenya, 1987. World Bank, WHO, UNFPA.

48. Harrison KA. Maternal mortality. *Trans R Soc Trop Med Hyg* 1989;83:449–53.

49. Harrison KA. Severity of anaemia and operative mortality and morbidity. *Lancet* 1988 June 18:1392.

50. Alauddin M. Maternal mortality in rural Bangladesh. The Tangail District. *Stud Fam Plann* 1986;17:13–21.

51. Rush D. Nutrition and maternal mortality in the developing world. *Am J Clin Nutr* 2000;72 Suppl:212–40.

52. Chi I, Agoestina T, Harbin J. Maternal mortality at twelve teaching hospitals in Indonesia: an epidemiologic analysis. *Int J Gynaecol Obstet* 1992;39:87–92.

53. Viteri FE, Torun B. Anaemia and physical work capacity. In: Garby L, editor. *Clinics in Haematology.* London: WB Saunders; 1974. p. 609–26.

54. Hallberg L, Scrimshaw NS. *Iron Deficiency and Work Performance.* Washington DC: International Nutritional Anemia Consultative Group; 1981.

55. Cook JD, Lynch SR. The liabilities of iron deficiency. *Blood* 1986;68:803–9.

56. Dallman PR. Iron deficiency and the immune response. *Am J Clin Nutr* 1987;46:329–34.

57. Garn SM, Ridella SA, Petzold AS, Falkner F. Maternal hematologic levels and pregnancy outcomes. *Semin Perinatol* 1981;5:155–62.

58. Klebanoff MA, Shiono PH, Selby JV, Trachtenberg AI, Graubard BI. Anemia and spontaneous preterm birth. *Am J Obstet Gynecol* 1991;164:59–63

59. Allen LH. Iron-deficiency anemia increases risk of preterm delivery. *Nutr Rev* 51;2:49–52.

60. Mitchell MC. Lerner E. Maternal hematologic measures and pregnancy outcome. *J Am Diet Assoc* 1992;92:484–6.

61. Harrison KA, Ibeziako PA. Maternal anaemia and fetal birthweight. *J Obstet Gynaecol Br Cwlth* 1973;80:798–804.

62. Steer P, Alam MA, Wadsworth J, Welch A. Relation between maternal haemoglobin concentration

and birth weight in different ethnic groups. *BMJ* 1995;310:489–91.
63. Murphy JF, O'Riordan JO, Newcombe RG, Coles EC, Pearson JF. Relation of haemoglobin levels in first and second trimesters to outcome of pregnancy. *Lancet* 1986;1:992–5.
64. Vause S, Maresh M, Khaled K, Howe D, Fleming AK, Houghton A. Maternal haemoglobin and birth weight in different ethnic groups. *BMJ* 1995;310:1601–2.
65. Huisman A, Aarnoudse JG. Increased 2nd trimester hemoglobin concentration in pregnancies later complicated by hypertension and growth retardation. Early evidence of a reduced plasma volume. *Acta Obstet Gynecol Scand* 1986;65:605–8.
66. Colomer J, Colomer C, Gutierrez D, Jubert A, Nolasco A, Fernandez-Delgrado R, *et al.* Anaemia during pregnancy as a risk factor for infant iron deficiency: report from the Valencia Infant Anaemia Cohort (VIAC) study. *Paediatr Perinat Epidemiol* 1990;4:196–204.
67. Hokama T, Takenaka S, Hirayama K, Yara A, Yoshida K, Itokazu K, *et al.* Iron status in newborns born to iron deficient anaemic mothers. *J Trop Pediatr* 1996;42:75–7.
68. Prual A, Galan P, Bernis de L, Hercberg S. Evaluation of iron status in Chadian pregnant women: consequences of maternal iron deficiency on the haematopoietic status of newborns. *Trop Geogr Med* 1988;40:1–6.
69. Yepez R, Calle A, Galan P, Estevez E, Davila M, Estrella R, *et al.* Iron status in Ecuadorian pregnant women living at 2,800 m altitude: relationship with infant iron stores. *Int J Vitam Nutr Res* 1987;57:327–32.
70. Gaspar MJ, Ortega RM, Moreiras O. Relationship between iron status in pregnant women and their newborn babies. Investigation in a Spanish population. *Acta Obstet Gynecol Scand* 1993;72:534–7.
71. Letsky EA. Maternal anaemia in pregnancy. Iron and pregnancy – a haematologist's view. *Fetal and Maternal Medicine Review* 2001;12:3159–75.
72. Walter T, De Andraca I, Chadud P, Perales CG. Iron deficiency anaemia: adverse effects on infant psychomotor development. *Pediatrics* 1989;84:7–17.
73. Hansen NE. The anaemia of chronic disorders – a bag of unresolved questions. *Scand J Haematol* 1983:31:397–402.
74. Baumann Kurer S, Seifert B, Michel B, Ruegg R, Fehr J. Prediction of iron deficiency in chronic inflammatory rheumatic disease anaemia. *Br J Haematol* 1995:91;820–6.
75. Cook JD, Baynes RD, Skikne BS. Iron deficiency and the measurement of iron status. *Nutrition Research Reviews* 1992;5:189–202.
76. Fleming AF. Anaemia in pregnancy in tropical Africa. *Trans R Soc Trop Med Hyg* 1989;83:441–8.
77. van den Broek NR. The aetiology of anaemia in pregnancy in West Africa. *Trop Doct* 1996;26:5–7.
78. Hytten F. Blood volume changes in normal pregnancy. *Clin Haematol* 1985;14:601–12.
79. Bentley DP. Iron metabolism and anaemia in pregnancy. *Clin Haematol* 1985;14:613–28.
80. Baker SJ, DeMaeyer EM. Nutritional anemia: its understanding and control with special reference to the work of the World Health Organization. *Am J Clin Nutr* 1979;32:368–417.
81. DeMaeyer EM, Adiels-Tegman M. The prevalence of anaemia in the world. *World Health Stats Q* 1985;38:302–16.
82. Fleming AF. A study of anaemia in pregnancy in Ibadan, Western Nigeria, with special reference to folic acid deficiency [dissertation]. Cambridge: Cambridge University; 1968.
83. Suharno D, West CE, Muhilal, Karyadi D, Hautvast GAJ. Supplementation with vitamin A and iron for nutritional anaemia in pregnant women in West Java, Indonesia. *Lancet* 1993;342:1325–8.
84. Karyadi D, Bloem MW. The role of vitamin A in iron deficiency anemia and implications for interventions. *Biomed Environ Sci* 1996;9:316–24.
85. Savage D, Gangaidzo I, Lindenbaum J, Kiire C, Mukiibi JM, Moyo A, *et al.* Vitamin B12 deficiency is the primary cause of megaloblastic anaemia in Zimbabwe. *Br J Haematol* 1994;86:844–50.
86. Yip R, Dallman PR. The roles of inflammation and iron deficiency as causes of anemia. *Am J Clin Nutr* 1988;48:1295–1300.
87. Fleming AF. The aetiology of severe anaemia in pregnancy in Ndola, Zambia. *Ann Trop Med Parasitol* 1989;83:37–49.
88. van den Broek NR, White SA, Neilson JP. The association between asymptomatic human immunodeficiency virus infection and the prevalence and severity of anemia in pregnant Malawian women. *Am J Trop Med Hyg* 1998;59:1004–7.
89. van den Broek NR, Letsky EA. Etiology of anaemia in pregnancy in south Malawi. *Am J Clin Nutr* 2000:72 Suppl 1:247–56.

Chapter 8

Lessons from the Confidential Enquiries in the UK

James Drife

Introduction

The original Confidential Enquiry into Maternal Deaths (CEMD) in England and Wales began in 1928,[1] when the national maternal mortality rate (MMR) was around 400/100 000 births[2] – similar to the global MMR today.[3] From its outset, the Enquiry set out to count maternal deaths and identify avoidable factors in each case. In 1952, the CEMD took on its present form[1] and since then each maternal death in England and Wales has been analysed in detail by a panel of clinicians. Every three years a report has been published stating the numbers of deaths from each specific cause and drawing lessons to improve clinical care and service provision.

The early triennial reports dealt with patterns of disease similar to those in many developing countries today. Those reports were slim volumes compared with recent CEMD reports and, although they contained the necessary data, they did not give a national MMR. In 1952–54, the MMR for England and Wales – counting 'deaths directly due to pregnancy and childbirth' – was 53.3/100 000 maternities, and by 1955–57 it had already fallen to 40.7.[4] For 1997–99, the figure was 5.0 direct deaths per 100 000 maternities.[5] In the first two CEMD reports, 40% of the deaths had 'avoidable factors'. Standards have risen over the years and currently 'substandard care' is identified in just over 60% of direct deaths.

The early years of the CEMD were a time of dramatic progress. In the 50 years between 1935 and 1985, the overall MMR in the UK fell from 400 to 12 per 100 000.[2] This is such a substantial and rapid change that it seems almost beyond our comprehension today, whether we are looking at it from the perspective of a developed or a developing country. Nevertheless, it has taken place within living memory and has been well documented in medical journals and in the successive reports of the CEMD. Can lessons be drawn from this experience that may help other countries in their efforts to reduce maternal mortality?

Why have the lessons not been learned?

Few, if any, attempts have been made to formulate such lessons before and it is worth asking why. One reason is that the CEMD has always focused on local issues. To begin with, there were three separate enquiries, into deaths in England and Wales, in Scotland and in Northern Ireland. To some extent, these remain separate but since 1985 their findings have been amalgamated into a single triennial UK report. In the 1990s, several European countries collaborated on a shared method of data collection but that project was time-limited and has not continued.[6]

A second reason is that the CEMD reports have been published as monographs distributed mainly to relevant professionals in the UK. Only limited attempts have been made to summarise their findings in peer-reviewed journals for an international readership.[7,8] It is perhaps understandable, therefore, that a review published in 2001 quoted UK data from as long ago as 1988–90.[3] Until 1998, the triennial reports were published by Her Majesty's Stationery Office (latterly the Stationery Office), which is not an international publisher. The current report, however, is published by the RCOG Press at the Royal College of Obstetricians and Gynaecologists (RCOG) and for the first time is available on the internet (www.cemd.org.uk).

The main reason, however, is the widespread perception that the public health problems of developed and developing countries are completely different. To a large extent, this is true. Major health problems in the UK and the USA include obesity, cardiovascular disease and degenerative disease, while in developing countries they include infection, infant mortality, undernutrition and anaemia. But the causes of maternal mortality are the same in all countries. The pattern of causes across the globe today – sepsis, haemorrhage, eclampsia and illegal abortion – is strikingly similar to that in the UK 70 years ago.

The conditions in developing countries today, however, are different from those in the UK in the 1930s. At that time, in spite of an economic depression, the UK was comparatively wealthy and had a democratic government and a well-developed transport infrastructure. Literacy rates were high among both men and women and women's status was improving. In 1918, married women over the age of 30 years were allowed to vote and, in 1928, the franchise was extended to all women over 21 years of age. The nation was therefore well placed and well motivated to take advantage of the medical advances that occurred during and after the 1930s.

Although the UK's past experience cannot be directly extrapolated to all countries today, this should not lead to medical nihilism. Doctors in developed countries may be accused of ignorance or oversimplification when commenting on the problems of developing countries but some of their observations may be valid.[9,10] Doctors in developing countries may be starved of resources to treat the poor but they should not assume that nothing can be done about maternal mortality until their country achieves economic parity with the West.[11]

General lessons

Lessons about specific causes of maternal death have been published in successive CEMD reports and some will be mentioned later in this chapter. First, however, I will attempt to summarise lessons from the CEMD's general approach.

The importance of measuring maternal mortality

In 2001, an editorial in the *Bulletin of the World Health Organization* asked: 'Is estimating maternal mortality useful?' and concluded that it was, despite limitations in data collection in many countries.[12] In 2002, the case for measuring maternal mortality was argued in the *Lancet* by Professor Graham, a participant in this Study Group.[13] It is regrettable that the case still needs to be made 50 years after the CEMD started from what seemed an obvious premise – that information is a prerequisite for action. Even data of limited accuracy can show where the major problems are and, more importantly, can motivate a response. In England and Wales in 1928, action was prompted by public disquiet over the nation's high MMR, not by concern about statistical subtleties.[14]

Even today, despite well-developed systems of death registration in the UK, the Registrar General's estimates of the MMR are inaccurate. As the CEMD developed over the years, it began to identify maternal deaths that had been missed by the official system, and it is now clear that the Registrar General underestimates the true MMR (see below). It has recently been suggested that in the USA the true MMR may be twice as high as that estimated from registration data.[3]

The value of continuity

From the start, the CEMD assumed that data collection and analysis would continue indefinitely. This contrasts with surveys elsewhere that have produced a 'snapshot' and a well-intentioned but vague recommendation that the survey should be repeated in a few years' time.

The value of continuity is not only that it allows change (or lack of change) to be monitored. Over the years, the quality of data collection has steadily improved as the requirement to report maternal deaths to the CEMD has become ingrained into clinical practice among public health doctors, obstetricians and midwives. In the early reports, as mentioned above, the 'gold standard' was assumed to be the number of deaths reported to the Registrar General. In 1955–57, the Registrar General recorded 1112 direct maternal deaths, of which 861 were the subject of the CEMD. In 1997–99, by contrast, the number of maternal deaths known to the Registrar General was 142 and the number known to the CEMD was 242.

While retaining the ability to compare each triennium with previous ones, the Enquiry has broadened its scope. Classification has been refined in line with the International Statistical Classification of Diseases and Related Health Problems; for example, the distinctions between 'direct', 'indirect' and 'fortuitous' (now 'coincidental') deaths were introduced in 1976–78. Chapters are added as the need becomes apparent – for example, a chapter on psychiatric conditions was introduced in 1994–96.[15]

From time to time, people have questioned the need for continuing the CEMD. Early in the 1990s, when observational studies were out of fashion and the UK's MMR seemed to have stabilised, the assessors had to argue the case for continuing the Enquiry. Happily, within a few years its value was again being recognised. Indeed, the 'confidential enquiry' method has now been extended to stillbirths, perioperative deaths and suicides among people with mental illness.[16–18]

A professionally led enquiry

Since its relaunch in 1952,[19] the CEMD has been run by doctors and, since 1994, by midwives as well. (The idea of midwifery assessors had been considered in 1952 but was rejected at that time.) Other specialists, such as statisticians, make essential contributions but there has been no change to the principle that the enquiry is professionally led. The number of medical specialties involved has increased over the years and now includes intensivists and psychiatrists, as well as anaesthetists, physicians, pathologists and public health doctors. Input from specialists in accident and emergency medicine and general practice is likely to be needed soon.

Professional insight is essential if clinical lessons are to be drawn. Assessors therefore need to be in active clinical practice and well regarded by their professional colleagues. They are appointed, not elected or nominated, although the Enquiry seeks the views of professional bodies. Assessors' names are published. Appointments are for a fixed term but are renewable.

This firm professional base has meant that over the years the CEMD has earned the respect of clinicians. Until recently, however, it paid insufficient attention to engaging health service managers at national and trust levels. This is now being rectified, as the CEMD has become part of the National Institute for Clinical Excellence (NICE), which requires managers to implement its recommendations.

Confidentiality

As a professionally led enquiry, the CEMD is subject to professional confidentiality. This principle is often misunderstood. Obviously the triennial reports are not confidential. They are on sale to anyone, including journalists, patients and lawyers. The process of the enquiry, however, is confidential. The professionals involved with each case fill in detailed report forms that are then scrutinised by the assessors. All the forms are destroyed when the final report is published.

Nowadays many people are suspicious of enquiries 'behind closed doors'. In a public enquiry, however, evidence is given in the legalistic atmosphere of a court or tribunal with the press looking on. Professionals giving evidence have to consider their reputations and the possible legal repercussions, and their attitude may be defensive. They may be represented by lawyers or trade union officials, who are unlikely to acknowledge shortcomings.

The CEMD, by contrast, wants professionals to comment frankly on what they think went wrong and how any failings could be avoided in future. Doctors and midwives are reassured that their comments will be read only by fellow professionals and that no written material is retained. Nevertheless, in today's atmosphere of litigation some professionals, particularly midwives, are now defensive in their comments to the CEMD. They need constant reminding that the object of the exercise is to improve care in the future, not to apportion blame for the past.

Substandard care

The CEMD does, however, identify 'substandard care'. Originally it identified 'avoidable factors' but this phrase was changed in the 1979–81 report, as it gave the impression that the death itself might have been prevented, which was not always the case. The CEMD's standards are exacting and 'substandard care' is a higher test than negligence (as defined by lawyers), misconduct (as defined by employers) or poor performance (as defined by the General Medical Council). As noted above, standards have risen over the years and the proportion of cases identified as linked with substandard care has tended to increase.

Identification of substandard care in a particular case does not result in feedback to the individual or hospital concerned. Professionals are expected to read the report and apply its anonymised lessons to their future practice. Even when the management of a case is particularly poor, there is no formal mechanism for taking direct action. If the CEMD reported staff to their employer or regulatory body, it could hardly expect frank co-operation from others in the future. Cases are anonymised by the time they are seen by national assessors, but the regional assessor knows the individuals concerned and could give informal advice. If a regional assessor felt that the public was at risk from a dysfunctional hospital or a sick or seriously substandard practitioner, action would be necessary. In practice, in the UK nowadays, individual cases reported to the Enquiry have almost always been reported to other bodies through other channels.

Co-operation with the Government

Although the CEMD is professionally led, it has always liaised with the Government. It was set up in 1952 through co-operation between the RCOG and what was then the Ministry of Health, later the Department of Health. The Enquiry is now part of NICE, whose recommendations, as mentioned above, are binding on NHS managers. Liaison between the CEMD and the Department of Health also means that recommendations can be linked with other government initiatives, for example on social exclusion or domestic violence. In the eyes of clinicians and the public, the link between the Ministry and the professionally led enquiry has enhanced the status of the CEMD. Even in today's cynical age, the CEMD's recommendations are still recognised as independent. For its part, the CEMD has to strike a balance between applying pressure and co-operating with politicians.

Evidence-based medicine

As mentioned above, the CEMD's recommendations have always been firmly based on numerical data. This is now called 'observational' or 'descriptive' research, and its value is being recognised after a phase of being undervalued. In the early 1990s, descriptive studies were regarded as much less valuable than comparative studies and the CEMD was criticised for lacking a control group. Although randomised controlled trials (RCTs) are the gold standard for comparing different types of intervention (or non-intervention) in relatively common conditions, they are difficult to apply to the management of rare events.

As life-threatening complications became rare in developed countries, multicentre trials were organised to include developing countries with high MMRs. The results of these studies have been of value in developed countries but it could be argued that they are not the best use of scarce resources in developing countries. The early CEMD reports have been criticised retrospectively because none of their recommendations was supported by RCT evidence. If, however, changes in practice had had to await well-designed RCTs, there might have been a much slower decrease in the MMR over the last 50 years; in other words, many more women might have died. Change was introduced on the basis of observational research and clinical analysis, and it is important that this method is still used where appropriate.

Focusing on what is important

Current CEMD reports are extremely comprehensive. The 1997–99 report not only analyses direct deaths but also devotes much space to indirect and coincidental deaths. This has become appropriate in the UK as the number of direct deaths has fallen, but the early reports were highly selective. They focused not just on 'true' maternal deaths (the term 'direct deaths' had not yet been introduced) but on a few specific causes, such as haemorrhage and hypertension. This may well be a useful approach for countries faced with a similar task today.

Implementation and audit

The original philosophy of the CEMD was that well-founded advice from respected professionals is likely to be followed by their colleagues. In the early years, doctors were expected to ensure the implementation of recommendations relating to services, such as staffing levels and blood banks. As NHS management has become more autonomous, the culture has changed. Hospital managers are now explicitly required to implement CEMD recommendations. The CEMD has always striven to ensure that its recommendations are challenging but achievable.

In the early 1990s, the Enquiry attempted to audit the implementation of its recommendations.[20] It does not have the resources to carry out detailed audit but its recommendations are fed into the standards set by other bodies, including the RCOG, the Commission for Health Improvement (CHI) and the Clinical Negligence Scheme for Trusts (CNST), who undertake systematic inspection of services.

Risk factors

The CEMD report form collects background information about each woman, including her age, parity, social class and ethnicity, allowing the Enquiry to build up a profile of risk factors. These are discussed in Chapter 10, which provides a corrective to any complacency that modern UK health care is equally accessible and effective for all women.

In the early reports, high parity and the extremes of age were recognised as risk factors, as was marital status. Risk assessment was particularly important when access to hospital delivery was limited, and the early reports repeatedly stressed the importance of hospital booking for women with identified risk factors.

Direct deaths

During the 50 years of the CEMD, the number of direct deaths has fallen but this decrease has not been linear and the rate has not been the same for all causes. Between 1937 and 1985 the overall reduction was logarithmic, with a halving every decade, leading to optimism in the 1980s that there would be 'a further decline over the next decades'.[2] The fall stopped abruptly, however, in 1985, after which there was a slight increase, leading to concern about the more relaxed style of maternity care being introduced at that time. Recently, however, there has been a renewed fall in direct deaths (although not in indirect deaths), showing that safety need not be compromised by the continuing trend towards midwife-led and community-based care.

In Table 8.1, column 1 gives the leading direct causes of maternal death as listed in the 1952–54 report and column 2 shows the change in the next triennium. It also shows a dramatic difference between the 1950s and the 1990s. Some causes, such as abortion and anaesthesia, almost disappeared (but not quite) while others, such as thromoembolism, showed a less marked reduction. When consecutive reports are compared, both in the 1950s and the 1990s, some causes (such as haemorrhage) show a reduction in both decades, while others, such as sepsis, show no short-term fall. Most of the causes listed in Table 8.1 are discussed in detail in other chapters, but some points will be made here, comparing the recommendations in the early years of the CEMD with those in recent reports. The early recommendations may still be relevant to countries in which the MMR remains high.

Hypertensive disease

The early years

From 1952 until 1957, hypertensive disease was the leading cause of direct death in England and Wales. By 1958–60, the number of deaths from this cause had more than halved, to 118. In the first two reports, over 50% of the deaths had avoidable factors, of which 'faulty antenatal care is by far the most serious and most frequent'.[1] The 1955–57 report commented that 'the faults recorded in this series would be regarded by most doctors as inexcusable in these days', and spoke out strongly against confinement out of hospital for older and highly parous women, 'especially when

Table 8.1. Numbers of direct deaths reported to the Confidential Enquiries into Maternal Deaths; Crown copyright material reproduced with permission of the Controller of HMSO and the Queen's Printer for Scotland

Cause	1952–54[a]	1955–57[a]	1994–96[b]	1997–99[b]
Hypertensive disease	246	188	20	15
Haemorrhage	188	121	12	7
Abortion	153	141	1	3
Thrombosis and thromboembolism	138	147	48	35
Anaesthesia	49	31	1	3
Sepsis	42	46	14	15

[a] England and Wales; [b] UK

previous pregnancies had been complicated by pre-eclamptic toxaemia'. Other factors were refusal by some women to accept the advice of a doctor or midwife, follow-up of women who failed to keep appointments and a shortage of hospital beds. To some extent, these problems are familiar to today's obstetricians.

The recent reports

Between 1994–96 and 1997–99, there was a further reduction in deaths from hypertensive disease, due mainly to a fall in deaths from pulmonary and cerebral oedema, which accounted for nine of the 20 deaths in 1994–96. It is gratifying that in the 1997–99 report few women died from mismanaged fluid balance but substandard care was still present in 80% of cases and further improvement is possible.

Haemorrhage

The early years

The early reports emphasised the risks of pre-existing anaemia and the importance of checking haemoglobin levels during antenatal care. Avoidable factors included unwise booking for home confinement and delay in summoning the obstetric flying squad. By 1955–57, deaths from postpartum haemorrhage were already falling and the report commented that the standard of management of the third stage seemed to have improved, that greater use was being made of the flying squads and that 'the increasing use of ergometrine as a prophylactic against the occurrence of haemorrhage may also have played a part'.

Reading these chapters of the early reports, it is striking how much practice in the UK has changed. Obstetric flying squads are now a thing of the past in the UK but may still be relevant in countries with other styles of maternity care.

Table 8.2. Deaths from haemorrhage; Crown copyright material reproduced with permission of the Controller of HMSO and the Queen's Printer for Scotland

Triennium	Deaths (n)
1970–72	27
1973–75	21
1976–78	24
1979–81	14
1982–84	9
1985–87	10
1988–90	22
1991–93	15
1994–96	12
1997–99	7

The recent reports

The 1994–96 report included three women who had refused blood transfusion for religious reasons. It gave detailed guidelines for the management of such cases, which are extremely distressing for the staff involved.

The 1997–99 report contained only seven deaths from haemorrhage. This is the lowest ever total and represents a remarkable achievement when the total number of maternities was 2 123 614. Once before, in 1982–84, deaths from haemorrhage reached single figures but then they rose again (Table 8.2), possibly because of complacency and a feeling that old lessons were no longer relevant. For example, in 1988–90 four of the five deaths from placenta praevia occurred at caesarean section operations performed by a registrar without direct consultant supervision.[21] This illustrates the role of the CEMD in monitoring standards once the MMR is low.

Abortion

The early years

Therapeutic abortion was illegal in the UK until 1967 and in the early years of the CEMD no practical recommendations were made about deaths from this cause. An illegal abortion was classed as an 'avoidable factor'. After abortion was legalised, the number of deaths began to fall but it was 12 years before the last death from criminal interference occurred. In the first two full triennia after 1967 Abortion Act, there were as many deaths from legal as from illegal abortion, showing that the widespread introduction of a safe procedure takes time. It is currently estimated that 78 000 women die worldwide from illegal abortion each year. The British experience shows that the total can be reduced by political as well as medical action.

The recent reports

Despite the number of terminations in the UK now being over 100 000 per year, deaths from abortion averaged 0.5 per year between 1994 and 1999, making abortion statistically much safer than continuing pregnancy. Of the three deaths in these six years, two were associated with surgical termination beyond 12 weeks of gestation.

Thromboembolism

The early years

In the early years of the CEMD, most deaths from pulmonary embolism followed normal vaginal delivery, because woman were routinely confined to bed for a week after hospital delivery. Once early mobilisation became the norm, the number of deaths fell, although there was little change in antenatal deaths from thromboembolism or in deaths after caesarean section.[21]

Table 8.3. Deaths from postpartum thromboembolism; Crown copyright material reproduced with permission of the Controller of HMSO and the Queen's Printer for Scotland

Days postpartum	After vaginal delivery		After caesarean section	
	1994–96	1997–99	1994–96	1997–99
0–7	0	1	3	3
8–14	3	2	3	0
15–28	3	4	6	0
29–42	4	3	1	1
43–365	1	8	1	1

The recent reports

Since 1985, thromboembolism has been the leading direct cause of maternal death in the UK (Table 8.3), in contrast with other countries in the developed world. Most of the deaths from this cause occur outside hospital, often several weeks after delivery, making ascertainment difficult. It seems unlikely that British women are uniquely susceptible to thromboembolism and more likely that ascertainment is better here than in other countries.

This cause of maternal death seemed highly persistent but the 1997–99 report has given grounds for optimism, with a sharp reduction in deaths after caesarean section following the publication of RCOG guidelines on thromboprophylaxis.[22] The report also showed that almost all the women who died from thromboembolism had obvious risk factors, such as obesity, postpartum pill use or long-haul air travel. It is inappropriate to offer all pregnant women thromboprophylaxis but the 1997–99 report opens up the possibility of reducing the number of deaths by targeting those at highest risk. Development of appropriate guidelines is now in progress (see Chapter 14).

Anaesthesia

The early years

In the 1950s, general anaesthetics were still being given to pregnant women by part-time GP anaesthetists or by junior doctors at an early stage of their training. The Faculty of Anaesthetists (now the Royal College of Anaesthetists) recommended that the most junior training grades should not work unsupervised on the delivery suite and, from the 1970s onwards, there was a trend towards regional rather than general anaesthesia for caesarean section. These were probably the main factors in a remarkable reduction in the number of deaths from this cause (Table 8.4).

The recent reports

Despite the UK caesarean section rate reaching 20%, the number of deaths from anaesthesia remains low. Some of the fatalities have involved women with severe underlying disease, and the finding of 'substandard care' in such cases reflects the exacting standards that today's anaesthetists set themselves.

Table 8.4. Direct anaesthetic deaths; Crown copyright material reproduced with permission of the Controller of HMSO and the Queen's Printer for Scotland

Triennium	Deaths (n)
1970–72	37
1973–75	27
1976–78	27
1979–81	22
1982–84	18
1985–87	6
1988–90	4
1991–93	8
1994–96	1
1997–99	3

Sepsis

The early years

Until 1935, puerperal sepsis was the leading cause of maternal death in the UK. The numbers of deaths from this cause fell precipitately after the introduction of effective treatment, in the form first of sulphonamides and then of penicillin. What is remarkable about the first report of the CEMD was that in 1952–54 deaths from this cause were recorded only in an appendix, as part of a comprehensive table of all causes. Only 17 years after sepsis had been the most feared complication of childbirth, it was not important enough to warrant its own chapter.

This phlegmatic attitude to what was by any standards one of the major triumphs of 20th century medicine was further underlined in the 1982–84 report, which devoted only nine words to the remarkable fact that for the first (and only) time in the UK, 'No deaths could be directly attributed to puerperal sepsis'.

The recent reports

Puerperal sepsis, due to overwhelming infection by the haemolytic streptococcus, is now a rare occurrence. Cases highlight the difficulty of dealing with diseases that are potentially curable but have become rare. In the 1994–96 report, a woman who delivered at home developed a pyrexia on the fifth day. The midwife called the GP, who thought the woman's condition was satisfactory. In the past, a puerperal pyrexia would have struck fear into both the midwife and GP, who would have seen fatal cases of puerperal sepsis. In this case, the woman was merely observed and she died the next day. A major function of the CEMD is to describe anonymised individual case histories so that others can learn from rare tragedies (Table 8.5).

Indirect deaths

Among 'indirect' deaths in the CEMD are some causes that in other countries might be regarded as 'coincidental'. In recent years, indirect deaths have risen steadily and,

Table 8.5. Deaths from sepsis; Crown copyright material reproduced with permission of the Controller of HMSO and the Queen's Printer for Scotland

Triennium	All genital-tract sepsis (n)	Puerperal sepsis (n)
1970–72	34	13
1973–75	19	8
1976–78	15	6
1979–81	8	2
1982–84	2	0
1985–87	6	2
1988–90	9	4
1991–93	11	4
1994–96	15	11
1997–99	14	2 + 2 late

although the rise now seems to have levelled off, in the 1997–99 report indirect deaths outnumbered direct deaths for the first time, because direct deaths had fallen. The reason for the past rise in indirect deaths may have been improved ascertainment but it is worrying that they are not yet showing the same fall as direct deaths. The category includes many conditions that seem difficult or impossible to prevent, e.g. cerebral haemorrhage and malignancy. However, it also includes cardiac disease, psychiatric disease and epilepsy, which are discussed elsewhere in this volume. Women with pre-existing medical conditions require special attention during pregnancy to avoid their care falling into a gap between obstetrician and physician.

Coincidental deaths

Coincidental deaths (formerly 'fortuitous' deaths) include road-traffic accidents, and the CEMD repeatedly emphasises the importance of wearing a seat belt correctly positioned for pregnancy ('over and under the bump'). This category also includes murder, usually committed by the woman's partner or ex-partner. Such cases of homicide are the tip of the iceberg of domestic violence (see Chapter 28) and the CEMD has an important role in raising awareness about this among professionals.

Conclusion

Reducing maternal mortality worldwide needs data collection to define where the major problems are, analysis of what can be done in practical terms and action based on both vision and realism. Valuable lessons can be learned from the UK experience. The fact that they have not so far been learned is due partly to a failure by the CEMD to publicise itself globally, and partly to an unwarranted assumption that global problems are different from those solved in the past in the UK. The essential characteristic of the CEMD is that it has been run for many years by people involved in clinical practice. Today, developing countries may learn particularly from the early reports, when the challenges facing the UK were more like those now facing doctors, midwives and politicians in many other countries.

References

1. Ministry of Health. *Reports on Public Health and Medical Subjects No. 103. Report on Confidential Enquiries into Maternal Deaths in England and Wales 1955–1957*. London: HMSO; 1960.
2. Department of Health. *Report on Health and Social Subjects No. 34. Report on Confidential Enquiries into Maternal Deaths in England and Wales 1982–84*. London: HMSO; 1989.
3. Hill K, AbouZahr C, Wardlaw T. Estimates of maternal mortality for 1995. *Bull World Health Organ* 2001;79:182–93.
4. Department of Health and Social Security. *Report on Health and Social Subjects No 11. Report on Confidential Enquiries into Maternal Deaths in England and Wales 1970–1972*. London: HMSO; 1975.
5. Drife J, Lewis G, editors. *Why Mothers Die 1997–1999. The Confidential Enquiries into Maternal Deaths in the United Kingdom*. London: RCOG Press; 2001.
6. Salanave B, Bouvier-Colle MH, Varnoux N, Alexander S, Macfarlane A . Classification differences and maternal mortality: a European study. *Int J Epidemiol* 1999;28:64–9.
7. Drife J. Maternal mortality: lessons from the confidential enquiry. *Hosp Med* 1999;60:156–7.
8. de Swiet M. Maternal mortality: confidential enquiries into maternal deaths in the United Kingdom. *Am J Obstet Gynecol* 2000;182:760–6.
9. Drife JO. We know why they die. *BMJ* 1996;312:1044.
10. Kale R. Maternal mortality in India. Maternal mortality is falling in India but at slower rate than in Britain. *BMJ* 1996;313:304.
11. Goodburn E, Campbell O. Reducing maternal mortality in the developing world: sector-wide approaches may be the key. *BMJ* 2001;322:917–20.
12. Buekens P. Is estimating maternal mortality useful? *Bull World Health Organ* 2001;79:179.
13. Graham WJ. Now or never: the case for measuring maternal mortality. *Lancet* 2002;359:701–4.
14. Loudon I. *Death in Childbirth: An International Study of Maternal Care and Maternal Mortality 1800–1950*. Oxford: Clarendon Press; 1992.
15. Drife J, Lewis G, editors. *Why Mothers Die: Report on Confidential Enquiries into Maternal Deaths in the UK 1994–96*. London: The Stationery Office; 1998.
16. Confidential Enquiry into Stillbirths and Deaths in Infancy. *Sixth Annual Report*. London: Maternal and Child Health Research Consortium; 1999.
17. National Confidential Enquiry into Perioperative Deaths. *Changing the Way We Operate. The 2001 Report of the National Confidential Enquiry into Perioperative Deaths*. London: NCEPOD; 2001.
18. Appleby L. *Safer Services: National Confidential Inquiry into Suicide and Homicide by People with Mental Illness*. London: DoH; 1999.
19. Godber G. The origin and inception of the confidential enquiry into maternal deaths. *Br J Obstet Gynaecol* 1994;101:946–7.
20. Hibbard B, Milner D. Auditing the audit – the way forward for the confidential enquiries into maternal deaths in the United Kingdom. *Contemp Rev Obstet Gynaecol* 1995;7:97–100.
21. Department of Health. *Report on Confidential Enquiries into Maternal Deaths in the United Kingdom 1988–1990*. London: HMSO; 1994.
22. Greer I. Epidemiology, risk factors and prophylaxis of venous thrombo-embolism in obstetrics and gynaecology. *Baillieres Clin Obstet Gynaecol* 1997;11:403–30.
23. Royal College of Obstetricians and Gynaecologists. *Thromboprophylaxis in Obstetrics and Gynaecology. Report of a Working Party*. London: RCOG Press; 1995.

Chapter 9

Maternal mortality: global overview II

Discussion

Discussion following the papers by Dr Mubiru, Professor Brabin, Dr Nynke van den Broek and Professor Drife

Lewis: Dr Mubiru, we were all struck by your presentation and, as I used to run the UK AIDS programme, I know the figures only too well. What you did not bring out was the reasons why Uganda in particular of the sub-Saharan African countries is reducing HIV. What have you done in Uganda to improve this appalling situation, and what can others learn from your experience?

Mubiru: I am sorry I missed that one out. What has taken place here is a community approach. This has come right from the President. He mentions HIV in every speech he makes, so public awareness is high. HIV prevention is constantly on the radio, television and on billboards. What has helped Uganda is accepting the fact that HIV/AIDS is with us and trying to find ways of dealing with it. People have not tried to hide facts about HIV/AIDS in Uganda, and it has helped people to know about this. Uganda has made use of some of the programmes, such as for the prevention of mother-to-child transmission and, although we have had many deaths, the infection rate has still gone down because of this awareness.

The reduction in HIV/AIDS is believed to be for several reasons: the openness about the HIV/AIDS epidemic from its inception; the mobilisation and intensive sensitisation about HIV/AIDS; the multisectoral approach that has involved everybody in addressing the problem at different levels, starting with the presidency; and everybody's support in the fight, particularly our development partners who have extensively supported research, especially educational programmes.

Greer: Following on from that, like Dr Lewis, I was humbled by your presentation, which demonstrates the enormity of the task that confronts you in Uganda. One of the things that struck me, as well as the public-health message that you are obviously getting over very well to your population, was the fact that in the UK AIDS has been transformed by anti-retroviral therapy. You would be hard-pressed to identify someone with HIV infection in the UK nowadays because they do not progress to things like pneumocystis carinii pneumonia in the same way as they did, say, 15 or 20 years ago.

Coming from the developed world, I wonder how best to help you get anti-retroviral therapy into Uganda, because if you are going to break the cycle of infection, surely the time to target people for anti-retroviral therapy would be pregnancy, when you have the prospect of reducing maternal to fetal or neonatal transmission? How acute is the problem with getting anti-retroviral therapy, and what can be done to try and improve the situation for you?

Mubiru: At the moment, the point of entry as far as obstetrics and gynaecology is concerned has been prevention of mother–child transmission. Previously there have been a number of studies and in one of those it was found that nevirapine, which is a single-dose treatment, was very effective.[1] Right now there is a nevirapine implementation programme that is going on because of the results that we obtained from this study. As far as mother–child transmission is concerned, several hospitals, now seven, are offering this service as part of improving prevention programmes, but there are still more studies to come.

For example, right now there is a SIMBA study in Africa, stopping infection from mother to child via breastfeeding – it is being carried out in other African countries such as Rwanda, in order to see if transmission during breastfeeding can be reduced. Many of our mothers still breastfeed, and they need to do so because of the nutritional problems in children. So a lot is being done but still we need more, especially trials targeting men. Via their spouses, we are trying to encourage them to come for testing.

In Uganda, efforts are being undertaken to encourage women and couples to test for HIV. In addition, voluntary counselling and testing in antenatal mothers has been initiated and is being expanded with efforts to give access to the service to those health units that have libraries. Access to anti-retroviral drugs remains a problem for the majority of affected individuals because, costs notwithstanding, many people do not know their serological status and do not want to be tested. Health education programmes need to be increased, together with counselling, in the hope that more people will be tested and get to know their status. Anti-retroviral drugs should also be provided more cheaply so that more individuals can access them.

De Swiet: I get the impression that you really do believe that pregnancy increases the risk of dying from HIV. In the developed world, with the availability of anti-retroviral drugs, that is not the case. I wonder what your feeling is about the degree of risk, and that really comes back to my original question. Are you ten times or 100 times more likely to die of HIV in pregnancy, compared to the non-pregnant state?

Mubiru: It depends on the level of infection and the degree of immunodeficiency. The main problem that we find in these mothers who die from HIV-related problems are the infections such as meningitis and tuberculosis that develop. Many of our mothers are healthy, but those with clinical AIDS have problems. I would not say in pregnancy that one has a ten-fold or hundred-fold risk of death but they are more at risk of dying than in non-pregnant state. This is generally because, apart from the HIV base that may exist, pregnancy in itself predisposes women in the developing world to a much higher risk of dying than the non-pregnant state. Women book late, have poor-quality antenatal care and do not all deliver with skilled providers. They are therefore predisposed to haemorrhages, sepsis and so on, especially if all this is compounded by undernutrition, anaemia or intercurrent infection. Then it is clear how a woman who is HIV-positive can be at a higher risk than a non-pregnant one.

De Swiet: This is your impression, but do you have data? I am not accusing you; I just wonder if there are data.

Mubiru: Yes, we have some departmental records. These are not published but we record data, and this is where we get some of this information.

MacLean: To continue the question as to how Uganda has been able to reduce HIV, you talked about the publicity that had been given to the issue. Clearly there must be some sort of intervention, and perhaps you could comment on whether it relates to an increasing use of barrier contraception, safe sex, or whether there are messages going out about monogamy versus promiscuity. Is there any message that can be taken from Uganda and used elsewhere, even in London?

Mubiru: All these points have come up during this publicity campaign. People are being encouraged to have safe sex; they are using barrier methods. People are being encouraged to be faithful to their partners; adolescents are encouraged to postpone sex until marriage and to avoid sex outside of marriage. All these things are being incorporated at different levels through different people in schools, and there are different health systems that encourage people everywhere. There are posters and there are different avenues for approaching this.

MacLean: Clearly these are messages that apply internationally. Why has it been so successful in Uganda and not elsewhere? Is it because we do not have the data elsewhere, or are people not as good at following the advice?

Mubiru: Initially many African countries did not accept that there was a problem of HIV/AIDS in their countries. Uganda was one of the countries that accepted that HIV/AIDS was a problem. From this basis, work has been done and a lot of help has come in to carry out research in Uganda, and also to convey these messages through the various media. The message from Uganda is: an early acceptance of the national HIV/AIDS problem; advocacy for prevention from the highest political level, which was actually a national commitment towards eradication efforts; a multi-sectoral approach that treated HIV/AIDS as a national disaster and a development issue, ensuring that it was the responsibility of all sectors.

Pattinson: You have talked a little about stigma, so you might be preventing women from becoming infected with HIV, but when they are infected does the stigma contribute significantly to their mortality because they are outcast? Has an HIV-infected woman become accepted in society, or are they still outcast if it is known?

Mubiru: Different programmes have been set up. One of the earlier programmes was the AIDS Support Organisation, and this mostly supported widows. They came up with programmes to encourage these mothers to have positive living, to be able to support themselves. They would look after cows, try to get an income for themselves and to have a positive outlook on life. Also there were programmes, for example the Uganda Women's Support for Orphans. There were different programmes that have come up to try and remove the stigmatisation.

Initially, when the HIV/AIDS pandemic had just broken out, that stigmatisation was there, but right now all these organisations have helped reduce that stigmatisation so that people go out and continue living. People are encouraged to eat properly, and to seek medical care if they have any problems. Nowadays it is not common to find AIDS patients, as it was in the past. People are looking after themselves, they are seeking medical attention and they are taking better care of themselves.

Although it is impossible to say with 100% certainty that there is no stigmatisation, the level is very low now. This is because in Uganda almost everybody has been affected by HIV/AIDS in one or more ways. So people have come to realise that the problem is close and more often than not, they are helpful to the woman and her family in terms of moral and material support.

Brabin: Could you tell us what role voluntary testing and counselling for HIV has played in the Uganda programme?

Mubiru: I am not in a very good position to tell you about the role, but it has helped mothers and couples to come forward. When the mothers come for screening, we encourage the spouses to come as well because there are programmes for prevention of mother–child transmission. Without the support of the spouses, they sometimes encounter problems in carrying out these programmes, but when the spouse is supportive we find there is better follow-up of these mothers; they are able to come. Most of these mothers get transport money from their husbands; they get that support and they are able to look after themselves better as a couple to avoid reinfection and new infection.

The major role is played by an ever-increasing number of people who now know their serological status. In some circumstances, this has helped individuals and couples to make very important decisions regarding themselves and families, i.e preparing the families for coping after the woman's death, decisions on reproductive goals, decisions to access drugs, mode of delivery, breastfeeding, etc. Finally, voluntary counselling and testing seem to be helping in the whole process of HIV/AIDS prevention.

Graham: Can I add to what Dr Mubiru was saying? One of the things that you quite rightly pointed out first of all was the importance of the political support and the profile given to the issues of HIV/AIDS. We have to acknowledge that as one of the significant barriers in the reduction of maternal mortality, in that we do not always have the same political support. I have just been looking at the statistics, and from the modelling exercise it looks as if the maternal mortality ratio (MMR) in Uganda is still over 1000 maternal deaths per 100 000 live births. I know that some of those figures are disputed, but nevertheless it is still quite high. The issue for us, then, is why do we lack that political commitment towards maternal mortality when another very significant cause can receive that commitment very quickly?

That is a big challenge for us because most of us are not politicians, although we have political roles in our various jobs. That is something that the Study Group needs to think about. The political dimension is very important; we see signs of progress in countries such as Uganda, where they can tackle and dramatically change something that is a major challenge, HIV/AIDS, and yet maternal mortality remains stuck. What is it about that lack of political commitment? That touches on some of the things that Professor Drife brought up.

MacLean: Professor Brabin, one of the alarming things is the rapidity with which, if someone has cerebral malaria, they fall ill and then die. One of the things that concerns me in our antenatal clinic patients is a series of people who, having saved up for holidays, go off – usually to sub-Saharan Africa – to do some climbing or whatever. They become incredibly concerned about whether or not they should take their anti-malarials and often fly off without taking the medication. Do Europeans who visit these countries deteriorate with the rapidity that you describe?

Brabin: If a non-immune mother acquires *Plasmodium falciparum* infection and she is pregnant, she could be dead within 48–72 hours.

MacLean: That is an important message for all our pregnant tourists.

Brabin: Quite a number of them telephone me in Liverpool. If they have taken my usual advice not to travel to these malarious areas then I have probably ruined more holidays for pregnant women going to the tropics than I care to think about. They are highly susceptible.

Neilson: I was fascinated by the data showing the difference in prevalence in malaria between primigravid and parous women, and also the decreasing prevalence during the course of pregnancy. I could not understand the biology of what you described as parity-specific immunity. I wonder if you could elaborate on what is going on there.

Brabin: There is a great deal of data that confirms that multigravida have enhanced immunity to *P. falciparum* infection for women living under high exposure to malaria, and that this immunity is age-independent. As it relates to their exposure to malaria in their first pregnancy, it is considered parity-specific. There is recent evidence that there are substrains of *P. falciparum* parasites that express red-cell receptors and these are selected out during pregnancy because they preferentially adhere to the placental syncytiotrophoblast. The receptors attach to placental chondroitin sulphate A. Because these strains are selected out in this way, the mother has the opportunity to develop specific immunity to those particular strains, which is recalled during a subsequent pregnancy.

It is a very exciting finding and one that some of my colleagues have been involved with in studies in Malawi.[2] There are probably other receptors, as well as chondroitin sulphate A. This appears to be a 'unique form of immunity' in pregnant women and is part of the explanation for parity-specific effects. I am sure there are other reasons as well, but that is about as much as we know at present.

De Bernis: I was very interested in that because I am surprised by the stress you place on the number of malaria-related maternal deaths. We are working in the WHO with World Bank malaria teams because we try to work together to ensure that at a national level antenatal care services are good for addressing not only the obstetric complication but also HIV and malaria as a priority. When we discuss malaria with people they always insist on the risk of low birthweight for the newborn and of anaemia for the mother – but they do not attribute so much importance to death.

My second point is about the link between malaria and diseases such as eclampsia. There was a paper in 1996[3] about the link between malaria and eclampsia in Senegal, and I know that there is research relating to the placenta, malaria and other malaria-related disease. I would like to hear from you about this.

Brabin: Thank you for those questions. Probably the WHO has not focused on malaria-related maternal mortality because there has never been an analysis of it. As I mentioned, the invitation to this meeting stimulated us to do some homework, and we may or may not have made some headway. We were surprised at the consistency of our estimates using different methods. The cynical explanation is that the errors in the individual methods were equivalent and so we came up with the same result. Some of the data seem to be fairly reliable because they are supported by autopsy definitions of death, which is perhaps more reliable than other ways of defining malaria deaths, because there is plenty of pathology that you can link to a malaria death.

If these calculations of burden have any significance, they would indicate that under conditions of high transmission an extremely significant contribution to maternal death is made by malaria.

In terms of seasonality, the data from Senegal showed in a case-control study that women who had pre-eclamptic toxaemia were significantly more likely to have placental parasites. The data were reported as a letter in *The Lancet* so it is hard to get a closer look at the details.[3]

More convincing is some of the historical data from the Ceylon epidemic that I mentioned, which was a devastating affair in which one in six women died in pregnancy. In those cases, toxaemia was closely linked to the malarial deaths, and there are quite good case descriptions.

There is a hint that there are links between pre-eclamptic toxaemia and malaria, but almost no work has been done on it.

De Swiet: I was very impressed by the reports that came out some time ago about the risks of severe hypoglycaemia in pregnant women who were given chloroquine for falciparum malaria. Then when I started chatting to some friends who were in the malaria business they said, 'everybody knows that'; everybody with malaria is likely to get hypoglycaemic if you give them chloroquine, and I wondered whether that was the case.

Brabin: It is not the case, at least not with chloroquine, but it is with quinine. Quinine can induce insulin and this leads to hypoglycaemia. As you say, this is so well-known now that, if you are using quinine, necessary precautions are usually taken. Deaths from hypoglycaemia in cerebral malaria are probably not that common in places where there are adequate facilities to manage women. Outside of those, they could be occurring.

De Swiet: Do you think it is a pregnancy-specific phenomenon or is it, as my friends say, something that happens whenever you use quinine to treat malaria?

Brabin: That is an interesting question. The difficulty in answering it with regard to children is that malaria itself induces hypoglycaemia. So you have hypoglycaemic individuals who you are treating with quinine and you cannot easily conduct randomised trials to sort that out.

Nelson-Piercy: Dr van den Broek, I wanted to ask a rather provocative question. If 50% of your women have iron-deficiency anaemia, could I challenge your recommendation to screen everybody and suggest that you may wish to treat everybody with iron anyway? This might allow the money that you would otherwise have used for screening to be used to tackle what the other 50% has. What do you do with the people that you find to be anaemic who are not iron-deficient? Do you screen them for the entire list of infections that you put up?

Van den Broek: It is a challenging question and I do not have the answers. I was talking about screening for anaemia rather than for iron deficiency, which are two different things. I forgot to say that most sub-Saharan countries advise that all women are given iron and folic acid supplements throughout pregnancy and probably more recently also in the postpartum period. That is happening, and I would certainly not say that it should not happen.

The idea that the anaemia is more than just iron deficiency is quite difficult to tackle, and there are groups who say you should not only give iron and folic acid but you should perhaps provide a multivitamin, including iron and vitamin C, vitamin A and so on. There are some trials on the way to see if that is more effective than iron alone.

We were only able to do a lot of this screening – and if you look up the studies in the literature there are not many – to see what other contributors there are in a particular population to anaemia because of research money. It is not possible to screen women for all these infections. Even something as common perhaps as malaria is not on offer for many cases. I am also not suggesting that now everyone needs to have a full differential diagnosis screen if they are anaemic.

However, I wonder if it is sensible to continue measuring haemoglobin in pregnancy by some screening method that is available and accurate enough, but to look at it as a general morbidity measure. If the patient's haemoglobin is lower than whatever you think it should be, you know that this is a high-risk factor for a number of underlying things and she could therefore be put in a higher-risk group, but that is a new idea and it has not been tried in practice.

MacLean: Can I ask you to continue that? If you are talking about screening, you presumably mean at the time of first contact or at booking. Would you comment about reassessing the patient later in pregnancy, and at what gestation?

Van den Broek: Ideally, if you get really involved in this anaemia topic, I would like to see people screened at the beginning of pregnancy. In practice, in many developing countries they do not come until they are about 16 or 20 weeks pregnant, which is possibly not a bad time to screen because haemodilution is also well under way. It would be very good to screen them before delivery because, if they are still anaemic whatever supplements you have given, the risk of death is presumably high if they also have a haemorrhage, given that they are in a rural situation.

Perhaps for their future health it would be useful to screen them when they come for the postpartum visits. Many women are encouraged to come the first week after delivery and the sixth week after delivery in these countries, even if they do not deliver in a health facility, to come to a health facility to receive some form of care. If you were able to look at haemoglobin you might be able to correct any remaining anaemia before they embark on a new pregnancy, which is probably when you will see them again. That is with only anaemia in mind and with a hypothetical situation where you have the facilities and the cheap screening test.

MacLean: If you are going to assess them prior to delivery, at what gestation? Clearly it is too late by 39 weeks. Thirty-four weeks? Or is that too soon?

Van den Broek: I don't know what would be a good time if you are working in a population with a high prevalence of anaemia. We have just discovered as part of a trial where we managed to follow women longitudinally that 25% deliver prematurely, and that was defined as delivering before 37 weeks. So it would have to be before 37 weeks. If you go too far back you could argue that they can get anaemic again before they come into delivery, so I don't have an easy answer.

Drife: I think you mentioned at some point about people not taking their tablets or not wanting to take the tablets. Is that for the same reasons as people in this country? Is it because it makes them constipated or produces adverse effects, or is there a dislike of taking tablets in general?

Van den Broek: I meant to say that it is often said that women in these countries refuse to take their tablets, whereas tablets are often not available. Part of this idea that is circulating comes from work in India where efforts were made to get people to take the tablets that were also made available. But they were described by the healthcare workers, nurses or midwives as leading to bigger babies – you would have a better, healthier and bigger baby – so the women's conclusion was that we therefore have a higher risk of obstructed labour. So the tablet was not sold very well, and this has gone to lead its own life and now the saying is very often that women do not want the tablets. The practicality of it is that very often the iron tablets are not available in these clinics.

Robinson: On the question of methodology for the confidential enquiries, as Dr Lewis and the people who run confidential enquiries into stillbirth and deaths in infancy know, we are constantly writing every time a report comes out to comment that there is a huge flaw in the procedure because there is no voice for the patient. You went into the details of how everybody is very frank because there is no litigation and there are no consumers on the sidelines.

Nobody talks about the inadequacy of the data that you are working with because, as we deal with complaints about maternal care, including the occasional death but also many stillbirths, and near-misses are becoming even more common, the first thing we advise people to do is to get the case notes. In all cases, but certainly where there has been a poor outcome, there is an immediate challenge on the accuracy of those notes not only from the woman concerned, if still alive or if it is a baby case, but from the family, the birth companions and witnesses and the other people who at antenatal appointments with them. There are also things that are routinely not recorded in notes: 'I told the midwife that I was worried about the fact that I didn't seem to be growing as much with this baby', which was not written down. There is assessment on the basis of an incomplete story.

This worries me particularly where we have faults or procedural difficulties because of patients' actions or inactions which, in South Africa, we see comes up in 48% of cases. One of the most common allegations throughout my 30 years in consumer activity in any complaint about healthcare is a counter-allegation: 'this patient did not turn up for appointments'. This is frequently challenged and indeed disproved, refuted.

What we are missing is subtlety of communication. Considering that round this table we all want to get the best possible job and to move on, we have to look at ways in which we can feed in patient voices. Very often, for the bereaved – in cases of maternal deaths and infant deaths – we suggest that people might wish to send in their story to the Confidential Enquiries into Stillbirths and Infant Deaths (CESDI) or the Confidential Enquiries into Maternal Deaths (CEMD), and they are enormously comforted by that. We are trying to get emotional resolution for them, and the fact that there is somewhere for their story to go in the hope that it will be used is tremendously therapeutic, even if one does not get much of an answer.

We understand the reasons why things evolved in the way they did. We are enormously grateful for the confidential enquiries. We all want to see them improved and, please, is there a way that the views of the people who are most directly affected could be fed into it? Obviously, if professionals are too challenged, nobody is going to want it, and we can understand why. We honestly think that there should be a way through and people are being a bit more defensive than they need to be, and there is a lot of sociological data available.

In view of the latest enquiries, which show the problems with people at the lowest end of the social scale, they are very high-risk; with travellers, and they are high-risk, we know that there are particular communication difficulties on both sides with these groups. This may not be the occasion, but for the future we would really like to work with you on this in any way we can.

Drife: It is a huge issue, as Ms Robinson knows. Looking at complaints elsewhere, we all have the perspective of looking at complaints either locally or, in my case, nationally with the General Medical Council, and you get an insight from the hand-written, sad sometimes, piece of paper or sometimes the long word-processed piece of paper, but you get a flavour of what the interaction was like. We are desperate to avoid this kind of confrontation of: 'the patient did not turn up; therefore there was nothing I could do'. Dr Lewis knows that we are still getting cases like that, and my reaction is, we can flagellate ourselves so much but sometimes it is necessary; you did not make it easy for the patient to turn up or you used that as an excuse rather than going and getting them. These are very valid points.

In a way, because the system has evolved over many years, it is easiest to continue it as it has been. One of the things is raising expectations. The other is the fact that someone sending in information – as maybe you have experience of saying – will not get a reply, or resolution from someone else. They may get resolution or help a resolution by writing it down and putting it in, in the hope and expectation that it will be used constructively. In other areas, we see people's resolution being put on hold, sometimes for years, by the lawyers because they are waiting for somebody else to make a judgement and it never comes or it is unsatisfactory and that is unhelpful.

Your point is very reasonable. Some of the saddest cases are people who do not have an advocate, anybody left who knew what was going on at all, where you cannot identify someone to send in the material. I agree that we should be looking at the practicalities.

Lewis: We should perhaps have this discussion somewhere else, but to let you know that as we have moved to the National Institute of Clinical Excellence, part of our new remit will be, first, to have patient representation or lay representation on our board and, second, we are exploring the whole issue of how we can obtain vignettes from relatives. We are moving slowly in the right direction.

Brabin: I have two questions. Some data were presented earlier about an association of MMR with ethnic origin – I think it was Professor Graham in Asians. Have you looked at these data in relation to Townsend scores for social deprivation?[4] I am particularly asking because some recent analyses that we have been doing on childhood asthma, for example, show the most alarming associations with Townsend scores indicating a close link with social deprivation. Does this apply to maternal deaths?

My second question is about maternal deaths from legal abortion. Have there been any deaths from legal abortion since 1987?

Drife: The way I look at it now when I am talking about the report is that the level of the care that can be provided in a developed country now is a matter of teamwork between the woman and the carers. Both parties to that caring process need to be pretty switched on, so if you have a barrier, whether it is economic, communication, ethnicity or whatever to that communication, that is my global way of looking at why things can go wrong. The figures were quite upsetting, when we finally got them out, for our country these days.

Over the last six years there have been four deaths from legal abortion, three in this report and one in the last. Sometimes there is the problem of classification, whether it was into sepsis or abortion or whatever, but it is of that order. My little hobby-horse about that is that two of the four were on surgical late termination, which is the standard method of terminating a mid-trimester pregnancy in the USA, whereas here there tends to be a split between medical and surgical. From a maternal mortality point of view, the late surgical terminations, which account for a small number of terminations overall, account for 50% of our deaths.

Oates: I got myself tangled up in Ireland a couple of weeks ago, as you probably know, when the referendum was defeated. It is quite extraordinary how people do not understand modern data. One of the accusations that was hurled against us was that there is no postmortem evidence beyond a few months that a termination of pregnancy had taken place. Is that true? As a psychiatrist I really would not know. Presumably if a death occurs within a few weeks of a termination it will register, but there is very little way of knowing.

As you may know, one of the main issues that was used in the Irish abortion referendum was that termination of pregnancy increases women's risk of suicide. One of the things that came back was how to know, because there were no suicides associated with termination and there have not been for the last three or four triennia, whereas one of the most common causes of maternal suicide was unwanted pregnancy.

Drife: It is very interesting looking back. One of the things *a propos* a question Dr Hall asked earlier was that the people who died at the left-hand side of that graph were married, middle-class women. They did a social breakdown of the deaths from termination in the 1952–54 report and they had a rather quaint classification of well-to-do, comfortably off, poorly off and destitute, and single or married, instead of social classes 1, 2, 3, 4 and 5. The biggest cell by far was the married, comfortably off women.

For the record it should be noted that the referendum was on whether, as I understand it, the risk of suicide should be accepted as grounds for termination of pregnancy in the Republic of Ireland.

Oates: It was whether to criminalise abortion specifically on the grounds of suicide.

Drife: The interesting thing, again as I understand it, is that in spite of what amounted to a three-line whip by the organisations opposed to abortion, the result of the referendum was not to criminalise abortion. I suspect that you had a view on that which was perhaps vindicated by the Irish public. The specific piece of misinformation that is put out is: don't we have the data? We believe we do have extremely good ascertainment in this country. The area that has been missing – as you know better than I do – is deaths from suicide, which has not been reported well. Now that those case reports have come in, we feel that we have plugged that gap in terms of ascertainment, so I do not believe we are missing many suicide cases.

Again, you would have the theoretical possibility of people who go back across to Ireland and commit suicide there, which would have to be a very unusual group, but theoretically that is possible. Again, for the record, one of the reasons that Ireland is able to maintain such an unusual position on abortion is because the ferry to England takes only a few hours to cross the English Channel, and Irish obstetricians are the first to acknowledge that.

Bewley: We have not had any change in the abortion law in this country for 34 years, and my thought about the surgical deaths is not whether it should be surgical or medical, but why do we not have abortion on demand under 14 weeks? We have not moved on that or on whether that could be something that might be recommended as a reform for morbidity and mortality purposes. I do not see how we can drive abortion-seeking and service provision to lower gestations unless we make a distinction in the law.

I was going to ask about where you think the confidential enquiries can evolve from here. One of the main criticisms with CESDI was the lack of denominator data, and with our new health-service managers we have to answer very difficult questions such as: how can you prove that the confidential enquiries have had any effect at all? They did not change anything on those graphs that were going down, and didn't medical practice just get better anyway, aren't we all just better doctors? We are passionately wedded to it and I find it very painful to think about it possibly not serving the purposes it did originally, but in a positive way how can it be improved from here?

Drife: The answer to the first question is that the opinion-formers or the movers and shakers are not wildly enthusiastic about revising the abortion law again because it creates a huge debate and huge passion and brings out the people who would like to change the law in the opposite direction. The result in the past has been that things have stayed much as they are. One of the worrying trends in Britain and the USA just now is that those of us who are children of the 1960s are going to retire soon and a whole generation of people has grown up who take the abortion law for granted and do not feel particularly strongly about it. People are choosing not to get involved in the provision of abortion services in our specialty. In a few years' time that might cause something of a crisis, so we might have to start looking at the law more constructively.

This was discussed at a meeting of the European Society of Contraception last week in Genoa, Italy, which I attended. There was a session in which abortion law was being addressed, and I was reminded that there is still an Abortion Law Reform Association in this country, although, to many people, it is a matter of 'been there, done that, let's go off and do something else'.

As far as moving on goes, I am in two minds. In one way I would like to see the CEMD extended to near-misses and controls where appropriate. I still do not really know how, but I would love to see that happen. On the other hand, if you broaden it or change its remit, you lose that wonderful sense of confidence that you know all the figures. You then move into slightly arbitrary figures relating to issues such as how bad is bad haemorrhage, who decided that the patient should go to the intensive care unit (ICU) and a slightly arbitrary denominator, or at least numerator, which could make it harder to feel confident about it.

Part of me thinks that if something is a necessary thing and has been refined, is it necessary to want to change it radically? It is like companies always wanting profits to go up. Why can you not be happy with a straight line if you are making a living? That is the philosophy but there are strong perceptions.

MacLean: If I can make a point, and it relates to cancer deaths and pregnancy, we have no feeling for the incidence of this problem that allows us to make any sort of analysis of mortality. When you are talking about the denominator that we need to establish, I accept that the definitions of hypertension or haemorrhage may vary, but there are some basic things, such as cervical cancer, that you can diagnose and you can determine the incidence. Yet there is no mechanism in this country to do that. There is in some of the Scandinavian countries through cancer registration. Maybe we will be able to do it in the future.

De Swiet: Forgive me for going back to what I said before, but it is apposite to what you say. Surely there are data for the risk of dying from cervical cancer if you are not pregnant? The same thing could therefore be said for the risk of dying from dissecting aneurysm if you are not pregnant, and even for some direct deaths like thromboembolism if you are not pregnant. That would contribute to the impact of the report.

Drife: That is hugely important, and controls in that sense are indeed the next step. I was speaking to our local hospital, which is always a stimulating experience when physicians are in the audience, and asking me how many epileptic women would die anyway, and apparently quite a lot do. To make that comparison with all the medical conditions would be highly appropriate.

Lewis: Obviously we are taking the question of near-misses very seriously; we know we have to move on. We are being asked to consider it and we are going to fund, if not set up their database of admissions to ICU. This meeting needs to recognise that the confidential enquiries are funded on peanuts. They are run by me basically at nights and weekends and our money has been cut. We are being reviewed again by the National Institute of Clinical Excellence and I have no idea what will happen. They have told us we will stay, but I can guarantee you that we will have no more money, so that is less of me.

As part of the general recommendations, you may want to think about making a general recommendation about the future. I entirely agree that we need to look at near-misses and controls, but I am more worried about the future of what we have. Can I make a plea that you might want to think about that too?

Hall: I want to comment briefly on the issue of near-misses. There is a problem of ascertainment and definitions, but we are doing some research on that in Scotland at the moment. We have a pilot study under way and we have appointed a research fellow to look at the variations in the use of definitions and also to look at the evidence base for recommendations. The key thing is that we hope that it can all be done through the current risk-management structures eventually, once the research has been done. That is our hope. It would not be an enormously costly exercise.

In my view, with one exception, near-misses are the appropriate controls for maternal deaths. The one exception, of course, is thromboembolism because people do not necessarily present as desperately ill before they drop down dead with thromboembolism. With nearly every other condition, the antecedent period is the point at which they either become a near-miss or they become a death, and you can learn a lot from how the cases are managed. There has been useful experience from that in South Africa.

Tuffnell: Picking up on the risk-management side of things, one of the justifications for the confidential enquiries to continue is the development of the National Patient Safety Agency (NPSA), which encourages investigation into adverse events. Their present mechanism is to report what are called 'red events', which is where there are major adverse outcomes such as death or severe morbidity. The emphasis there is on taking a root-cause analysis of the single events that occur that large lessons can be learned from that. The confidential enquiries have been ahead of what the NPSA is now trying to establish for all clinicians, so it would be a nonsense to stop something that has been a forerunner of everything that is now being suggested for all conditions and all delivery of health care.

Lewis: Professor Drife, I do have a fundamental query on recommendation 3 (under 'Health policy and education', p. 413), 'Estimating the maternal mortality ratio is an essential component of health care for women'. I don't think it is the best use of scarce resources in very poor countries and the money used could be better diverted to local programmes that make a real impact on the ground. Of course it is a good idea where feasible, but I don't think it should be top priority absolutely everywhere. I would prefer to see this recommendation deleted if possible but would be grateful for others' views and comments.

De Bernis: Dr Gülmezoglu and I would like to strongly support the comment made by Dr Lewis regarding the MMR. We agree that this indicator, while extremely powerful and precious, is also very difficult to measure for both conceptual and practical reasons. So it could be detrimental to state that measuring maternal mortality is necessary to implement and monitor maternal health programmes. There is international agreement on the need to use intermediary or process indicators for monitoring progress towards maternal mortality.

Pattinson: I have a few comments regarding this recommendation. Establishing a CEMD set-up that calculates the MMR is in my opinion of minor importance, as the first priority is to collect the deaths and describe the pathology and substandard care associated with them. However, if the process is to continue and be of benefit, just describing the problems is not enough. The object of describing the problems is to make recommendations to improve the situation. The best way to measure whether the recommendation are having an effect is to examine the MMR. After all, that is the objective of the whole enquiry, to reduce MMR. Consequently, I believe that, once the CEMD system is established, work on establishing a denominator must come much higher up the priority list. A country can start by doing it only in specific areas where the collection of deaths is pretty complete and then expand to other areas as they improve their data collection system. Obviously the deliveries per institution should be collected before the home births are attempted. The institutional deliveries should be relatively easy to collect and we will start to have a usable denominator. In South Africa, we are to an extent hamstrung by our lack of a denominator (deliveries) because we are unable to show or even discuss the effects of the recommendations. The third full CEMD report from South Africa will have a reliable denominator and the MMR will be calculated.

One of the dangers of a CEMD system is that it will end up just describing the problem and not be an active agent for change (in Africa we have multitudes of studies describing the problems without any action being taken). Ideally, the CEMD once established is just a system to monitor effect. The causes and avoidable factors are known and do not change rapidly, the proportion of cases with avoidable factors might decrease, and that should then be reflected in the MMR. It is essential in countries with AIDS problems to divide the deaths into direct and indirect and any improvement of care will probably be seen in the direct causes. Finally, how can we monitor the effect without measuring it and, if the objective is to reduce the MMR, then surely it must be measured? Perhaps the recommendation could be changed to something like 'Estimating the MMR is an essential component of health care for women and attempts should be made to calculate the MMR once the CEMD system has been established. This will enable the effect of the process to be effectively monitored'.

Graham: I can see where Drs Lewis, de Bernis and Gülmezoglu are coming from, but also Professors Pattinson and Drife. So, how about rephrasing it as 'Monitoring trends in maternal health outcomes and relevant measures is crucial to identifying, enhancing and sustaining effective intervention strategies'? If we wish to relate this specifically to the CEMD, we could add 'where feasible, these outcomes should be tracked through routine mechanisms, such as a CEMD'.

References

1. Guay LA, Musoke P, Fleming T, Bagenda D, Allen M, Nakabiito C, *et al.* Intrapartum and neonatal single-dose nevirapine compared with zidovudine for prevention of mother-to-child transmission of HIV-1 in Kampala, Uganda: HIVNET 012 randomised trial. *Lancet* 1999;354:795–802
2. Fried M, Nosten F, Brockman A, Brabin BJ, Duffy PE. Maternal antibodies block malaria. *Nature* 1998;395:851–2
3. Sartelet H, Rogier C, Milko-Sartelet I, Angel G, Michel G. Malaria associated pre-eclampsia in Senegal. *Lancet* 1996 Apr 20;347:1121.
4. Townsend P, Philimore P, Beattie A, editors. *Health and Deprivation: Inequality and the North.* London: Croom Helm; 1988.

SECTION 3

INEQUALITIES AND MORBIDITIES

Chapter 10

Risk factors for maternal deaths in the UK

Gwyneth Lewis

The global picture

The UK and other developed countries, unlike many parts of the world, have low maternal mortality rates. Globally, however, over 600 000 women die each year of pregnancy-related conditions. While the overall global maternal mortality rate is 27 deaths per 100 000 live births, in developing countries it is nearly 20 times higher, at 480 deaths per 100 000 live births. In some regions, it may be as high as 1000/100 000 births.[1] The main causes of death in developing countries are shown in Figure 10.1.

The rates for the countries with the highest maternal mortality rates still far exceed those in the UK at the end of the 19th century.[2] Women in these countries die usually because they are not provided with the health care that they need, either through a lack of basic facilities or through an inability to access the local healthcare services. Only 53% of women in developing countries receive assistance from a doctor or midwife and many give birth alone. Some women are denied access to care because of cultural practices of seclusion or because responsibility for decision making falls to other family members. In some cases, the failure of support for pregnant women by families, partners or their government also reflects the societal value placed on women's lives. Thus, in developing countries, the overwhelming risk factor for maternal mortality is the lack of access, for whatever reason, to even basic clinical or public health care. Addressing these inequalities and reducing the maternal mortality in these countries is a leading priority for the World Health Organization (WHO).[3]

In developed countries, these causes of maternal death are now extremely rare. In the latest report of the UK Confidential Enquiries into Maternal Deaths (CEMD),[2] the leading cause of maternal death from a condition directly attributable to pregnancy was pulmonary embolism, which does not even appear in the list of causes for developing countries. The main causes of deaths in the UK are shown in Figure 10.2. Deaths from conditions indirectly associated with pregnancy, including pre-existing maternal disease, now outnumber deaths from direct causes. A record linkage study described in the report also suggests that deaths from suicide may well be the leading cause of maternal death overall. The overall maternal mortality rate in the UK (including deaths from indirect causes such as suicide and some malignancies, which are not included as

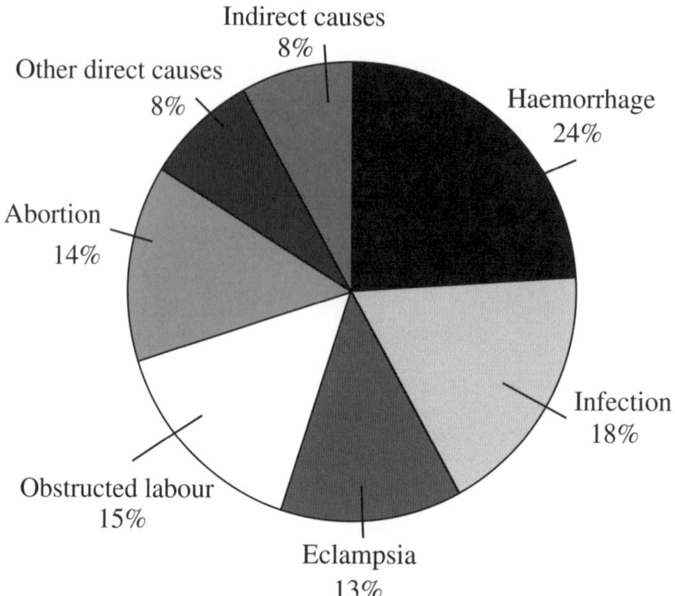

Figure 10.1. Major causes of maternal mortality in the developing world, 1999

maternal deaths in other countries' statistics) was 11.4/100 000 maternities. Chapter 8 provides a more detailed description of the main causes of maternal death in the UK.

A low maternal mortality rate should be no cause for complacency. There are still crucial lessons to be learned and implemented in developed countries to reduce maternal and neonatal morbidity and mortality rates still further. Some of these are clinical lessons that are described elsewhere in this book, but equally important are the findings relating to inequalities in health and social justice that are described in this chapter.

Maternal morbidity

Maternal deaths are the tip of the iceberg of maternal morbidity and, by extension, it appears logical that reducing amenable risk factors for maternal deaths should reduce the numbers of women who experience significant medical or psychological problems during or after birth, sometimes with long-lasting or permanent sequelae. A number of studies have been published on the incidence of severe maternal morbidity, or 'near-misses', but comparison between them is difficult because of the inclusion criteria used. The death to near-miss ratio in these studies ranges from 1:5[4] to 1:118.[5] These studies and the difficulties in their interpretation are discussed in Chapter 21 of the latest CEMD report.[2] More comprehensive studies on obstetric near-misses will be

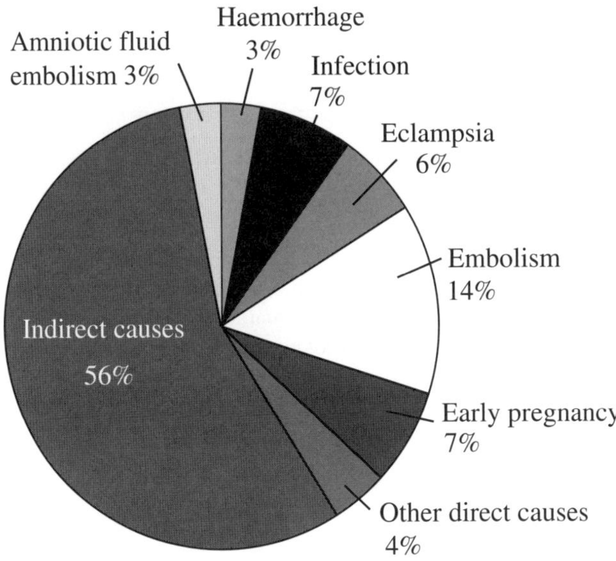

Figure 10.2. Major causes of maternal mortality in the UK, 1997

undertaken both in Scotland and, as part of the future CEMD work programme, in England, Wales and Northern Ireland.

The UK Confidential Enquiry into Maternal Deaths

The UK Confidential Enquiry into Maternal Deaths, now in its 50th year, has been increasingly widening its scope, with the aim of identifying further possible risk factors for maternal deaths in order to improve services for pregnant and recently delivered women. The latest report, because of the development of sophisticated coding programmes with the Office for National Statistics (ONS), has for the first time been able to evaluate more fully social and lifestyle factors that may have played a part in the death. These findings are of great concern, showing that the maternal mortality rates among the socially excluded, including women from lower socio-economic classes, very young girls and specific ethnic groups, are higher than those among the population as a whole. A summary of the findings shows that:

- women from the most disadvantaged groups of society are about 20 times more likely to die than women in the highest two social classes
- non-white women are, on average, twice as likely to die as white women; many of these women spoke little English

- in many cases, professionals used family members to interpret; there were several difficult cases where children were used inappropriately to interpret intimate personal or social details of the mother and vital information was withheld
- a disproportionate number of women from the traditional travelling community were likely to die
- 12% of all the women whose deaths are included in this report declared that they were subject to violence in the home; 20% of the women who died had booked for maternity care after 24 weeks of gestation or had missed over four routine antenatal visits.

Other factors are also associated with an increased risk of death, for example being under 18 years of age and increasing maternal age and parity. Many women in this Enquiry were also obese and/or smoked.

Risk factors for maternal deaths

Pre-existing maternal ill health

The fact that in the UK indirect deaths from complications that may arise from pre-existing medical or psychological disease now outnumber deaths from direct obstetric causes underlines the significant contribution that coexisting maternal physical or psychological comorbidity can have on the outcome of the pregnancy for both mother and child. Women with significant disease benefit from personalised multidisciplinary antenatal care, for example through combined diabetic, epileptic or cardiac clinics, or through a referral to an obstetric physician. The provision of services for women at risk from mental illness or substance misuse is discussed in Chapter 28.

Age

Maternal mortality is closely related to maternal age, as shown in Table 10.1. A recent survey of severe maternal morbidity[5] also found a correlation between age and risk of severe maternal morbidity, with women over 34 years of age being found to be at highest risk.

Maternal deaths are also more common in younger women. In the latest CEMD report, five school-age girls died aged 16 years or less and a total of 14 young women died aged 18 years or less. All but one were severely socially excluded. Four of the five girls aged less than 16 years had been in the care of social services, but three of these were homeless and 'living rough' at the time of their death. All but one of the deaths in women aged between 16 and 18 years were also characterised by social exclusion. Seven had suffered repeated episodes of domestic violence from within their own family and several of these also had suffered sexual abuse.

Parity

Maternal deaths are also more common in multiparous women, as shown in Table 10.2. For more robust analysis, the rates have been calculated for all maternal deaths by age

Table 10.1. Maternal deaths by age, UK 1985–99 and rate per 100 000 maternities[2]

Age (years)	1985–87	1988–90	1991–93	1994–96	1997–99	Overall 1985–99	
	(*n*)	(*n*)	(*n*)	(*n*)	(*n*)	Total (*n*)	Rate
< 20	15	17	7	15	19	71	8.2
20–24	47	38	30	40	35	190	7.2
25–29	53	74	87	71	61	346	9.0
30–34	60	57	61	70	66	314	11.5
35–39	35	31	36	53	50	205	20.7
40+	13	18	7	11	13	62	35.5
Not stated			1	8	4	9	
Total	223	238	229	268	242	1200	12.1

between the years 1991–99. Because of the large numbers of missing data for the triennium 1988–90, it has only been possible to calculate the overall rate from the data for the last three triennia.

Reproductive health

Although the findings should be interpreted with caution, because of the small numbers involved, the latest CEMD report found a maternal mortality rate of 20.1/100 000 twin maternities and 21.5/100 000 triplet maternities compared with a maternal mortality rate of 11.2 for singleton pregnancies.

Figures from the Human Fertilisation and Embryology Authority (HFEA), which are published on a financial-year basis, show that for the three financial years April 1997 to April 2000, there were 20 658 maternities from *in vitro* fertilisation (IVF). Using these data as a proxy for January 1997 to December 1999, the period of the latest report, a maternal mortality rate of 48.4/100 000 IVF maternities can be estimated. As with multiple births, because of small numbers these results need to be interpreted with caution. In future, the CEMD will continue to collect information on this group of women with the aim of providing a more robust data pool to facilitate more rigorous analysis.

Table 10.2. Number of maternal deaths and rates per 100 000 maternities by parity, UK 1991–1999[2]

	1991–93		1994–96		1997–99		Total 1991–99	
Parity	(*n*)	rate	(*n*)	rate	(*n*)	rate	(*n*)	rate
0	76	8.0	100	10.6	106	12.2	282	6.2
1	58	7.4	63	7.5	60	8.4	181	10.4
2	51	13.0	50	9.7	49	12.8	150	21.8
3	17	12.2	26	16.4	19	14.9	62	26.6
4+	18	25.6	13	10.8	16	37.7	47	35.0
Not stated	9		16				25	
Total and overall rate	229	9.8	268	12.0	242	11.4	747	11.3

Ethnicity

Many studies from other developed countries have shown higher mortality rates among women from ethnic minority groups. African American women have been shown to have a three times greater risk of maternal death than white women[6] and, in France, immigrant women are at twice the risk of death.[7]

In the UK, it has been difficult to identify mortality rates precisely among specific ethnic groups because ONS data for the mothers' ethnic groups have been confined to country of birth. It is not yet possible to calculate maternal death rates directly by ethnic group, as many mothers are second-, third- or more generation women born in the UK. However, ethnic group information is now being collected as part of the Hospital Episode Statistics (HES) system for England that was not complete for the years covered by the last CEMD report. There was 63% HES coverage of births by ethnic group for the period 1997–99.

Using the 1997–99 distribution by ethnic group as a best estimate for the period covered by the report led to the estimates of maternal death rates by ethnic group for England. Because specific coding was often incomplete, the ONS codes for 'Black African', 'Black Caribbean', 'Black Other' and 'Black Mixed' were grouped together, as were those from the Indian subcontinent.

As Table 10.3 shows, there was an increased risk of maternal mortality for all non-white groups. Women from India, Bangladesh and Pakistan appear to have a three times higher risk for the years 1997–99 and black women (a composite of Black African, Black Caribbean, Black Other and Black Mixed) have a one and a half times as great a risk. In the 1993–96 CEMD report,[8] the findings for these two groups were reversed, with black women, particularly recently arrived refugees, having a three times higher risk.

In some cases, the care received by women from ethnic minority groups was of an exceptionally high standard; in other cases it was poor. Some of these women were recently arrived immigrants who were pregnant on arrival in the UK and many did not speak English. Several were late in booking and others were poor attenders at antenatal clinics. Some constantly moved address during their pregnancy, making community follow-up difficult.

Table 10.3. Number and estimated rates of maternal deaths by ethnic group, England 1997–99[2]

Ethnic group	*Direct* and *indirect* maternal deaths (n)*	Estimated maternities (n)	Estimated rate per 100 000 maternities
White	159	1442286	11.0
Pakistani/Indian/Bangladeshi	31	95638	32.4
Black African/Caribbean/Mixed/Other	16	97502	16.4
Asian and others	7	50409	13.9
Total*	213	1771421	12.0

*English deaths only

Nearly half of the women who booked after 20 weeks in pregnancy or who were poor clinic attenders came from an ethnic minority group. Half of these women did not speak English. Some women who first arrived in the UK in advanced pregnancy accessed the services relatively promptly despite a lack of English. On the other hand, in a very few cases, some 'mail-order' brides appeared not to have received any help from their husbands in accessing the antenatal services.

Less obvious risk factors were also found among women in certain ethnic minority groups. There were a number of deaths in which the desire to fulfil motherhood and a specific role in society meant that some women who knew they were at serious risk of dying from pre-existing cardiac disease minimised or ignored the seriousness of their symptoms.

Also, perhaps from concerns of stigmatisation, some families refused help from the medical, midwifery and psychiatric services, preferring to care for women with severe postnatal depression themselves.

Translation

In a number of maternal deaths, family members had been used as interpreters for women who did not speak English. Several of these were the woman's own children, who may have been the only family members who could speak English, having learnt it at school. The use of family members as translators causes concern because:

- the woman may be too shy to seek help for intimate concerns
- it is not clear how much correct information is conveyed to the woman, as the person interpreting may not have a good grasp of the language or may have withheld information; in some cases, the translator was a perpetrator of domestic violence against his partner, thus not enabling her to ask for advice or help
- in those cases where the woman's pre-existing medical condition meant that she was at significant risk of dying, it is not clear how much information was conveyed concerning the risks to her own health
- it is not appropriate for a child to translate intimate details about his or her mother and it is unfair on both the woman and child.

Travelling women

A striking finding was that six women who died between 1997 and 1999 came from the travelling community. This community has not been included to date as a separate class by ONS when collecting ethnic group data. They are included in the 'White' category. It is therefore not possible to estimate the risk of maternal death in this group of women, despite attempts by ONS to identify suitable denominator data for this report. Nevertheless, it is clear that this group is grossly over-represented when compared with the white group of women as a whole and it may well have the highest maternal death rate of all ethnic groups. From the level of care taken over completing the report forms for the Enquiry and the tone of some of the comments contained within them, it appears that this community is at particular risk of substandard care from health service professionals.

Social class

Reducing inequalities in health, including maternal and infant mortality, is one of the most urgent challenges facing healthcare systems in both developed and developing countries around the world. A key indicator of social deprivation and vulnerability is social class.

For the first time, the latest CEMD report was able to calculate the social class of women who had a maternal death. The highest scoring occupational code of either the woman or her partner, or the woman herself if she had no partner, was classified into one of the nine ONS categories now used to describe social class. The UK maternities by social class used as the denominator data were derived by using the 1999 England and Wales live births by social class and applying the social class proportions to the 1997–99 UK maternities.

The results are shown in Table 10.4 and confirm, as has long been suspected, that women in the lower social classes have a higher risk of maternal death. Women from the most deprived circumstances appear to have a 20 times greater risk of dying of 'direct' or 'indirect' causes than women from social classes 1 and 2.

Similar, but less stark, findings have also been found in other developed countries such as the USA. In a WHO report,[9] comparisons of maternal mortality rates were made between those women who were economically and socially supported and those who were not. A stark contrast was demonstrated, with the most vulnerable women experiencing mortality rates ten times higher than the overall mortality. Vulnerability was classed as having insufficient financial and social support, poor diet and/or housing, substance misuse, poor access to health care and, in some instances, belonging to a minority ethnic group.

Domestic violence

Domestic violence is associated with maternal death, severe morbidity, fetal death, miscarriage, depression, suicide and alcohol and drug abuse.[2] Apart from the personal costs of domestic violence, family life and relationships suffer. Children are often involved as a result of experiencing violence between their parents. Up to 36% of children of violent relationships witness their mothers being assaulted.[10] This has profound short- and long-term effects on the child.

The 1994–96 report of the Confidential Enquiries into Maternal Deaths[8] estimated that one in three women experience domestic violence at some point in their lives, perhaps one in ten in the last year. Four in five women who are murdered are killed by a current or an ex-partner. About 30% of domestic violence starts during or just after pregnancy. The key indicators for violence, particularly in the obstetric setting, are:

- late booking
- poor/non-attendance at antenatal clinics
- repeat attendance at antenatal clinics, the general practitioner's surgery or accident and emergency for minor injuries or trivial or non-existent complaints
- repeat presentation with depression, anxiety, self-harm and psychosomatic symptoms
- minimisation of signs of violence on the body
- poor obstetric history

Table 10.4 Social class of women by type of death, estimated maternal mortality rate and relative risk, UK 1997–99[2]

Social class	Direct deaths (*n*)	Indirect deaths (*n*)	Direct/ indirect combined deaths (*n*)	Rate per 100 000 maternities	95% Confidence interval	Coincidental deaths (*n*)	Late deaths (*n*)	Total deaths (*n*)	Rate per 100 000 maternities	95% Confidence interval
1	3	2	5	2.94	0.96, 6.87	0	8	13	7.65	4.07, 13.08
2	9	16	25	4.19	2.71, 6.18	5	20	50	8.37	6.21, 11.04
3	13	18	31	15.21	10.33, 21.59	4	15	50	24.53	18.21, 32.34
4	9	24	33	5.32	3.66, 7.47	4	13	50	8.06	5.99, 10.63
5	14	12	26	8.31	5.43, 12.17	3	18	47	15.01	11.03, 19.96
6	8	4	12	11.35	5.87, 19.83	1	3	16	15.14	8.65, 24.58
7	0	7	7	23.81	9.57, 49.05	0	1	8	27.21	11.75, 53.61
8	1	4	5	38.96	12.65, 90.91	1	0	6	46.75	17.16, 101.75
9	48	49	97	135.46	109.85, 165.25	11	29	137	191.33	159.32, 223.33
Not stated	1	0	1			0	0	1		
Total	106	136	242	11.40	29	107	378	17.8		

- unexplained admissions
- non-compliance with treatment regimens or early self-discharge from hospital
- the constant presence of partner at examinations, who may answer all the questions for her and be unwilling to leave the room
- apparent evasiveness or reluctance by the woman to speak or disagree in front of her partner.

Studies have shown a variable incidence of abuse among pregnant women. A recent review article reports a range of 0.9%–20.2%[11] in studies mainly from the USA or Scandinavia. Until now, there have been no published studies in the UK, although there are preliminary reports of rates between 1.8–5.8%.[12] Higher rates are elicited in response to direct questioning by health professionals[13] and repeated questioning, compared with questions asked only in response to clinical suspicion.[14]

Forty-five of the 378 women whose deaths were investigated for the 1997–99 triennial CEMD report self-reported a history of domestic violence to a healthcare professional who was caring for them. This represents 12% of all cases. This percentage is undoubtedly an underestimate of the actual prevalence of violence among this group of women, as in none of the 378 cases was a history of violence actively sought through routine questioning as part of the social or family history at booking.

Domestic violence was fatal for eight of these women. It is also possible that two other women died as a direct result of physical violence. Half the girls or young women aged under 18 years who died were in violent, dependent relationships and four had been sexually abused in the past. All except one girl aged 16 years or under had also been abused, mainly by a family member. In all these cases, the healthcare staff knew the violence that the woman was suffering and some women were offered exceptional support. In other cases, little or no health or social service support was offered.

Many of the women reporting violence booked late or were poor attenders at the antenatal clinic. It was unusual for these women to be actively followed up. In many cases, it appears that little or no help was offered concerning the violence. In some cases, family interpreters were used inappropriately and there was some evidence of family 'secret-keeping'.

The use of simple screening questions, for example at antenatal clinics and where there may be an index of suspicion, is recommended. The last CEMD report, like this chapter, recommends that routine questions be asked about violence as part of the social history taken at booking, in line with the recommendations from the Royal College of Obstetricians and Gynaecologists.[15] Evidence from practice, where this has been followed, suggests that most women do not mind being asked when it is explained to them that the same enquiry is being made of all women because domestic violence is so widespread and often hidden. The Department of Health in England has published a resource manual for healthcare professionals, which gives guidance as to how this might best be achieved.[16] The Department of Health has also published an interagency guide on working together to promote the welfare of children.[17]

Access to healthcare services

In the latest CEMD report, over one-fifth of the women who had a death directly or indirectly attributable to an obstetric cause did not receive optimum antenatal care, in that they booked late or were described as poor attenders (missing four or more visits) at the antenatal clinic. These women had double the maternal mortality rate of women who died of unrelated causes. In the vast majority of cases, these women were not actively followed up when they failed to attend the clinic.

Women who book late

Twenty percent of the women who died from direct and indirect causes booked after 20 weeks of gestation. A disproportionate number of these women came from non-white ethnic groups. Virtually all had multiple indicators of social exclusion.

HES data show that women from non-white ethnic groups were twice as likely to book later than 20 weeks of gestation. Late bookers constituted about 8% of the white pregnant population and 17% of the non-white pregnant population. Among the women who died from direct or indirect causes of maternal death, 20% of those who booked late were from non-white ethnic groups compared with 12% of white women.

A recent survey of patterns of booking for antenatal care in nine maternity units in England and Wales found that primiparous women at high obstetric risk were 13.4% more likely to fail to book for antenatal care by ten weeks of gestation than the low-risk reference group.[18] Further, they were 34.3% more likely to not have booked for antenatal care by 18 weeks of gestation. High obstetric risk included coexisting medical illness, previous poor obstetric history, obesity, substance misuse and teenage motherhood. The association between high obstetric risk and late initiation of care was not as striking for multiparous women. The following characteristics were associated with failure to book by ten weeks: maternal age, smoking status, ethnicity, type of hospital at booking, the planned pattern of antenatal care and planned place of delivery. The association was exacerbated between clinical and sociodemographic characteristics for women who had failed to book at 18 weeks of gestation and was reduced concerning provider characteristics.

The study also found that women from ethnic minority groups were found to be up to five times as likely to fail to initiate care by 18 weeks, the odds ratio increasing if the woman was multiparous. Although the findings are not directly comparable to the CEMD report, this study adds value to those findings in that it shows that women who were already at higher risk of obstetric or medical complication were more likely to book late, and thus more likely to suffer adverse health outcomes.

Poor attendance at antenatal clinics

In addition to the 20% of women who booked late, a further 13% of women who died from a direct or indirect cause were poor attenders at antenatal clinics; poor attendance being defined as missing four or more visits. Most were socially vulnerable, with overrepresentation from women from ethnic minority groups. A recent study of the sociodemographic determinants of the number of antenatal visits[19] has shown that women from minority ethnic groups make 9.1% fewer antenatal visits than women of white British origin.

Factors are:

- pre-existing disease

- substance misuse
- social deprivation
- ethnicity
- late booking
- poor attendance at antenatal clinics
- domestic violence.

Conclusions and key recommendations

The importance of seeking antenatal care early in pregnancy should be indicated as part of health education and promotional materials for all groups in society. The planning and delivery of maternity services should focus on approaching each woman as an individual with different social, physical and emotional needs, as well as specific clinical factors that may affect her pregnancy. Her pregnancy must not be viewed in isolation from other important factors that may influence her health or that of her developing baby.

Antenatal services should be flexible enough to meet the needs of all women. The needs of those from the most vulnerable and less articulate groups in society are of equal, if not greater, importance. Many women in this report found it difficult to establish or maintain access to the services and follow-up for those who failed to attend was poor.

When planning new methods of service provision, it is helpful to involve women who might have difficulties in using the services. Where this has been done, antenatal clinic attendances have significantly improved.[20] Such flexibility may require imaginative solutions in terms of the timing and setting for antenatal clinics and the provision of outreach services.

At booking, a risk and needs assessment should take place to ensure that every woman has a flexible care plan adapted to her own particular requirements for antenatal care. This should be reviewed regularly.

Health professionals who work with disadvantaged clients need to be able to understand a woman's social and cultural background, act as an advocate for women and overcome their own personal and social prejudices and practise in a reflective manner. All healthcare professionals should consider whether there are unrecognised but inherent racial prejudices within their own organisations, in terms of providing an equal service to all users.

References

1. World Health Organization. *Reduction of Maternal Mortality*. A joint WHO/UNFPA/UNICEF/World Bank statement. Geneva: WHO; 1999.
2. Drife J, Lewis G, editors. *Why Mothers Die, 1997–99. The Confidential Enquiries into Maternal Deaths in the UK*. London: RCOG Press; 2001.
3. World Health Organization. Making pregnancy safer – a health sector strategy for reducing maternal and perinatal morbidity and mortality. (Discussion paper.) Geneva: WHO; 2001.

4. Mantel GD, Buchmann E, Rees H, Pattinson RC. Severe acute maternal morbidity: a pilot study of a definition of a near-miss. *Br J Obstet Gynaecol* 1998;105:985–90.
5. Waterstone M, Bewley S, Wolfe C. Incidence and predictors of severe obstetric morbidity: case control study. *BMJ* 2001;322:1089–94.
6. Hoyert D, Kochanek K, Murphy S. Deaths: final data for 1997. *Natl Vital Stat Rep* 1999;47:1–104.
7. Atrash HK, Lawson HW, Ellerbrock TV, Rowley DL, Koonin LM. Pregnancy related mortality. In: Wilcox, Marks JS, editors. *From Data to Action. CDC's Public Health Surveillance for Women, Infants and Children*. Washington DC: US Department of Health and Human Services, Public Health Services, Centres for Disease Control and Prevention; 1994. p. 141–54.
8. Drife J, Lewis G, editors. *Why Mothers Die. The 1993–96 Report of the United Kingdom Confidential Enquiries into Maternal Deaths*. London: HMSO; 1998.
9. World Health Organization. *World Health, 51st year*. No. 1, Feb–Jan 1998. IX. Geneva: WHO; 1998.
10. National Children's Home. *Action for Children. The Hidden Victims: Children and Domestic Violence*. London: NCH; 1996.
11. Bacchus L, Bewley S, Mezey G. Domestic violence and pregnancy. *The Obstetrician and Gynaecologist* 2001;3:56–9.
12. Bacchus L, Bewley S, Mezey G, Haworth A. Domestic violence in pregnancy: does use of a screening instrument increase detection? Unpublished data.
13. Gazamararian JA, Lazorick A, Spitz AM, Ballard TJ, Saltzman LE, Marks JS. Prevalence of violence against pregnant women. *JAMA* 1996;275:1915–20.
14. Gielen A, O'Campo PJ, Faden RR, Kass NE, Xue X. Interpersonal conflict and physical violence during the childbearing year. *Soc Sci Med* 1994;39:781–7.
15. Bewley S, Friend J, Mezey G, editors. *Violence against Women*. London: RCOG Press; 1997.
16. Department of Health. *Domestic Violence: Resource Manual for Healthcare Professionals*. London: DoH; 2000 [www. doh. gov. uk/domestic.htm].
17. Department of Health. *Working Together to Safeguard Children: A Guide to Inter-Agency Working to Safeguard and Promote the Welfare of Children*. DoH/Home Office/DfEE. London: DoH; 1999 [www.doh.gov.uk/domestic.htm].
18. Kupek E, Petrou S, Vause V, Maresh M. Clinical, provider and sociodemographic predictors of late initiation of antenatal care in England and Wales. *BJOG* 2002;109:265–73.
19. Petrou S, Kupek E, Vause S, Maresh M. Clinical, provider and sociodemographic determinants of the number of antenatal visits in England and Wales. *Soc Sci Med* 2001;52:1123–34.
20. Hepburn M, Elliott L. A community obstetric services for women with special needs. *Br J Midwifery* 1997;5:485–8.
21. Hepburn M. Horses for courses: developing services for women with special needs. *Br J Midwifery* 1997;5:482–4.

Chapter 11

Severe maternal morbidity in the UK

Susan Bewley, Charles Wolfe and Mark Waterstone

Introduction

Maternal mortality has been used as a measure of the success of obstetric intervention, but is now too rare for use in local practice in the developed world.[1,2] Severe maternal morbidity, or 'near-miss', has been suggested as an alternative measure.[3,4] For clinicians, avoidable maternal death should remain a central focus of attention. Maternal mortality rates are important as a measure of the impact of pregnancy on populations. They are purported to be sensitive measures of the quality of maternity services, although their utility is increasingly being questioned.

From mortality to morbidity

Mortality rates vary worldwide by orders of magnitude. They may be inadequate outcome measures of the quality of maternity services because:

- maternal mortality is rare in developed countries (i.e. low incidence and low impact)
- any lessons learned are anecdotal to any particular unit because the events are so occasional (although the collection may be valuable when collated and effectively disseminated)
- there is a natural bias towards less treatable and untreatable diseases with higher mortality-to-morbidity ratios (such as amniotic fluid embolism and cardiac disease rather than more common problems such as haemorrhage)
- concentrating on death may have diverted attention from the real impact of pregnancy on morbidity and other quality-of-life issues for mothers, babies and families.

Many more women are affected by severe and minor morbidity. Research attention is beginning to focus more on the impact of these events on women's longer-term health and on her baby and family. With greater understanding of the profound long-term biological and psychological effects of early life-events, we have the potential to impact positively or negatively on the health of future generations.

Conceptual difficulties with morbidity

Death is (relatively) easy to define and ascertain. Across clinical medicine, anything less than death is acknowledged to be difficult to define as an outcome and becomes blurred by subjectivity (of the patient, professional and health setting). Physiological characterisation of disease is generally easier where it is tightly defined and within agreed borders (for example APACHE scoring on intensive care units). There is currently no accepted definition of maternal or obstetric morbidity, and this is partly because of the spectrum of problems as shown below, with no easy distinction between categories of endpoints (apart from death). Considering that even after 50 years the Confidential Enquiries into Maternal Deaths (CEMD) is still modifying its definitions and ascertainment (see Chapter 8 and Chapter 10), it is hardly surprising that this is an evolving enterprise.

There is a huge range of pregnancy outcomes and outcome measures might be constructed in a hierarchy of severity:

1. death
2. 'near-miss'
3. severe morbidity
4. minor obstetric morbidity
5. sociocultural difficulties around major life event
6. normal physiological experiences and adaptation of pregnancy, lactation, puerperium.

A distinction between normal physiological symptoms of pregnancy and its pathology is difficult. To obtain good natural history data requires large, prospective and long-term cohort studies rather than looking back after birth or forward with very short time-scales. This is important for symptoms such as depression or urinary and faecal incontinence and has particularly bedevilled postpartum work, leading to the confounding of association and cause. Vaginal childbirth (rather than pregnancy, birth or life-event) is currently being blamed for many ills and conditions that occur (and recover) after childbirth, although only a fraction are caused by perineal trauma or the management of delivery.

Endeavouring to distinguish morbidity caused by, rather than associated with, pregnancy, another classification might be to mirror the direct/indirect/coincidental terminology of mortality reports. For example, the long hospital admission of a woman with pre-eclampsia or placenta praevia would be classified as direct, whereas the breathlessness due to pregnancy-exacerbated mitral stenosis might be indirect. Road accidents would be fortuitous.

A similar subdivision might be attempted by organ system or pathology. Researching a single morbidity (such as pregnancy in cystic fibrosis or HELLP syndrome [haemolysis, elevated liver enzymes and low platelets]) would be examples of this approach. For the full spectrum across the range of outcomes, another example would be postnatal bleeding. Bleeding is physiological in the third stage and puerperium but haemorrhage can be small, massive or fatal. Another psychological spectrum ranges from physiological wellbeing, serenity and joy during and after pregnancy through distress (e.g. caused by socially unacceptable pregnancy, single teenage motherhood or adoption), through mild and severe depression to suicide.

Lastly, in terms of the use of healthcare, we want to look at the drivers and predictors that make women move up or down the scale of outcomes. It is only by doing this that we can truly measure the effectiveness of interventions and quality of care.

Severe obstetric morbidity

With this understanding of the conceptual complexity of moving from mortality to morbidity indicators, we can tentatively start with the severest morbidity. The term 'near-miss' has the virtue of encompassing the emotional impact of the severest cases, and the concept of a life saved. However, it is probably inappropriate if we eventually wish to include all types of pathology, understand movement up and down throughout the range of morbidity or practise risk management. For example, what would constitute a 'near-miss' suicide? A prolonged severe depression or a failed small overdose?

Work so far has largely concentrated on the severest of pathology, involving direct obstetric causes and has been pregnancy- and hospital-based. Table 11.1 summarises studies on 'near-miss' and severe morbidity and their methodological strengths and weaknesses.

Problems with published work

Studies of severe maternal morbidity have generally

- been small-scale and undertaken in a small numbers of units
- been retrospective
- been hospital-based
- restricted analysis to intensive care admissions or the characteristics of obstetric intensive care patients
- used subjective and different clinical definitions (including management variables that are open to bias depending on available facilities available and local customs)
- provided widely different estimates of incidence
- not provided data on the predictors or outcome of severe maternal morbidity.

Collaborative Study of Severe Morbidity

The aim of the Collaborative Study of Severe Morbidity (COSMO) was to perform a

Table 11.1. Studies assessing maternal morbidity

Author	Date	Study type		Definition	Denominator	Cases	Rate/1000	Location	Additional issues
Graham[19]	1989	Retrospective single unit	Cohort	ICU admissions	21983	23	1.00	Nottingham	1st five years of a new tertiary unit
Mabie[37]	1990	Retrospective, single unit	Cohort	ICU admissions	22651	200	8.80	Memphis	Specific obstetric ICU over three years
Stones[3]	1991	Retrospective, single centre	Cohort	Clinical	2164	19	8.70	Norwich	
Fitzpatrick[4]	1992	Retrospective, single centre	Cohort	ICU/CCU admissions	13018	7	0.50	Ireland	ITU situated in separate hospital
Kilpatrick[20]	1992	Retrospective, single centre	Cohort	ICU admissions	8000	32	4.00	San Francisco	Tertiary referral centre
Johanson[21]	1995	Retrospective single unit	Cohort	ICU admissions	4116	258	62.00	Cape Town	
Bouvier-Colle[22]	1996	Retrospective, population-based	Cohort	ITU admission	NS	435[a]	3.10	3 regions in France	
Bewley[23]	1997	Retrospective, single centre	Cohort	ITU admissions	6.039	30	4.00	London	
Filippi[24]	1997	Retrospective, single centre	Cohort	Clinical	4291	353	82.00	Benin, Africa	Includes 193 cases of 'dystocia'
Lapinski[25]	1997	Retrospective single centre	Cohort chart review	ICU admission	25000	1690	67.00	Toronto, Canada	
Baskett[26]	1998	Retrospective, single centre	Cohort	Transfer for 'critical care'	76119	55	0.70	Nova Scotia, Canada	Transfers only over 14 years
Mantel[27]	1998	Prospective, 2-centre	Population-based cohort	Acute organ dysfunction	13429	147	11.00	Pretoria, South Africa	1 year. Organ dysfunction not simply extreme event
Nasrat[28]	1999	Retrospective, single centre	Cohort	Postpartum TAH	NS	NS	1.22	Saudi Arabia	85 months
Sivalingam[29]	1999	Retrospective, single centre	Cohort	Clinical	9932	122	12.00	Malaysia	
Prual[30]	2000	Prospective multi-centre	Population-based cohort	Clinical	20326	1215	59.00	West Africa	19 months
Waterstone[31]	2001	Prospective, multi-centre	Population-based cohort	Clinical	48865	588	12.00	South East England	One year, thrombo-embolism excluded
MOMS B	Not published	Multi-centre, multi-country,	Population-based cohort	Clinical	182589	1843	10.00	Europe	Nine countries; incidence varies between 6.0–15.5

[a] includes 22 deaths; ICU = intensive care unit; CCU coronary care unit, ITU = intensive therapy unit, TAH = total abdominal hysterectomy

multicentre population-based study, using reproducible evidence-based clinical definitions of severe obstetric morbidity, to estimate the incidence of severe obstetric morbidity and, by the use of a control population, to investigate its predictors.[31] The aims were subdivided as follows:

- to develop standardised definitions for severe maternal morbidity and to estimate the incidence of these conditions in a population of Southern England with 50 000 deliveries a year
- to assess risk factors for these severe maternal morbidities
- within these disease categories, to estimate the predictive value of demographic and obstetric factors that predict the condition and outcome afterwards
- to determine the appropriateness of medical care within this group and develop strategies to increase appropriateness of care
- to quantify the use of resources from these conditions
- to assess longer-term morbidity (resultant maternal impairment, disability and handicap, and use of health services) following a severe obstetric event.

Developing definitions of severe obstetric morbidity

The first challenge was to develop definitions. A Medline search was performed using key words (severe maternal morbidity, obstetric intensive care, obstetric haemorrhage, uterine rupture, obstetric sepsis, HELLP syndrome, eclampsia, maternal mortality). Definitions were selected that were clinically based and routinely measurable, and that did not include management processes. Where no definition relevant to the specific condition was available (e.g. sepsis), the non-pregnant definition was modified to take into account the physiological changes occurring in pregnancy. The focus of this study was morbidity associated specifically with pregnancy and for which the management usually involves maternity care professionals. Conditions were not included if they were difficult to diagnose accurately, or ascertain completely, the most important examples being pulmonary and amniotic fluid emboli. Table 11.2 details the conditions investigated and their definitions.

The exclusion of thromboembolism

Although the COSMO study has been criticised for not including thromboembolism, this was a carefully considered exclusion. Albeit a leading cause of maternal mortality in the UK,[1,2] thrombosis is difficult to diagnose accurately in the non-fatal event. The clinical diagnosis of thrombosis, with haematological, invasive and non-invasive radiological and nuclear medicine techniques, differs widely by hospital and facilities. The method of diagnosis differs from unit to unit, and some units in the study region relied entirely on clinical suspicion. Unlike other conditions arising anew in pregnancy, thromboprophylaxis may already be in use in women with a past history (making the establishment of natural history and severe morbidity incidence difficult). Especially with first-trimester diagnosis, the pregnancy itself may not be known to maternity-service providers. Furthermore, as most cases occur in the postnatal period, many

Table 11.2. Definition of severe maternal morbidity in the Collaborative Study of Severe Morbidity; reproduced with permission from the BMJ Publishing Group[31]

Disorder	Definition
Severe pre-eclampsia	BP 170 / 110 mmHg on two occasions four hours apart, or BP > 170/110 mmHg once, **plus** ≥ 0.3 g in 24 hours proteinuria or ≥ ++ on dipstick; or BP diastolic > 90 mmHg **plus** proteinuria (as above) on one occasion **plus** one of the following: oliguria (< 30 ml/hr for two hours), visual disturbances (flashing lights or blurred vision), epigastric / right upper quadrant pain or tenderness, thrombocytopenia (<100 x 109/l), pulmonary oedema
Eclampsia[32]	Convulsions during pregnancy or in the first ten days postpartum together with at least two of the following features within 24 hours after the convulsions: hypertension (≥ 170/110 mmHg), proteinuria (at least + on random dipstick analysis or ≥ 0.3 g in 24 hours), thrombocytopenia (< 100 x 10^9/l), increased aspartate transaminase (≥ 42 u/l)
HELLP syndrome[33]	Haemolysis (abnormal peripheral smear, or raised total bilirubin (≥ 12 mg/l), elevated liver enzymes (raised aspartate transaminase (≥ 70 u/l), or raised γGT (≥ 70 u/l), and low platelets (< 100 x 10^9 /l)
Severe haemorrhage[34]	Either estimated blood loss of over 1500 ml, a peripartum haemoglobin drop of ≥ 4g/dl or an acute transfusion of ≥ 4 units of blood
Sepsis	The systemic response to infection manifested by two or more of: temperature > 38°C or < 36°C (unless after prolonged caesarean); heart rate > 100 bpm; respiratory rate > 20/min or PaCO2 < 32 mmHg; white cell count > 17 x 10^9 /l or < 4 x 10^9 /l or > 10% immature forms **plus** i) bacteraemia (i.e. positive blood cultures) **or** ii) positive swab culture
Severe sepsis[35,36]	Sepsis associated with one of: organ dysfunction, e.g. acute renal failure, hypoperfusion: e.g. lactic acidosis, oliguria, or acute alteration in mental state, hypotension: i.e. a systolic BP < 90 mmHg, or a drop of ≥ 40 mmHg, in the absence of other causes of hypotension
Uterine rupture	Acute dehiscence of the uterus leading to the emergency delivery of the infant

women present to physicians and never see an obstetrician. With movement of mothers and the lack of communication between primary and different secondary-care services, it was considered that deep-vein thrombosis and pulmonary embolus would have been difficult to ascertain and capture confidently. Thus it would be impossible to ascertain if any cases gathered represented an accurate reflection of the incidence. Despite all the above, definitions were developed in this study for thromboembolism. Only six cases that fitted the rigorous definitions were identified. As the study was planned to exclude these from the analysis, they were not considered.

Sampling frame for cases and controls

Cases included women from the South East Thames Region (UK) who delivered over 24 weeks of gestation between 1 March 1997 and 28 February 1998 and met the definition criteria for severe morbidity. Controls were women from the same region who delivered without severe morbidity. Cases were identified from all 19 maternity units within the region, and from six neighbouring hospitals to ascertain residents who delivered out of region. Cases were identified from multiple sources (maternity computer databases, labour ward and postnatal ward diaries, staff reporting and medical records). A single investigator (MPW) who visited the hospitals twice- to four-weekly reviewed all the medical records. Social categories were grouped using the UK Registrar General's categories: non-manual = Class I, and IIa and manual = Class IIb, III, IV and V.[5] Ethnic origin was grouped into 'white', 'black' = black African and Caribbean, and 'other' = all other ethnic groups.

As measures of socio-economic status (e.g. marital status, male partner's employment) alone are inadequate for pregnant women, data were collected on indicators of social exclusion. This concept is currently in use by the UK Government.[6] Social exclusion was present in this study when any of the following were identified in the notes: concealed pregnancy, extremely young age (less than 16 years of age), poor housing, low income ('on income support' written in notes), minor/child in local authority or state care (currently or in the past), in trouble with the law (currently or previously), living alone (partner abroad or 'unsupported' written in notes), unbooked, unwanted pregnancy, currently or previously in foster care, care order being considered on potential child, social worker involvement and drug or alcohol dependency.

Power calculations were performed to estimate the number of cases and controls required. If the incidence of hypertension postdelivery is used, a rise from 5% to 20% incidence of postpartum hypertension[7] will only require 180 women in total (cases and controls) for a power of 90% at the 5% level. The estimated number of deliveries in the study region was 50 000 and using the previous estimates of incidence of severe obstetric morbidity this would have given between 25 and 545 cases. A year's data collection was also used as this avoids seasonal variations when calculating incidence.

Four controls per case were selected in order to increase the power to detect any differences in predictive factors between cases and controls. This was undertaken as follows: a random list of all the unit numbers (1–19) was generated with each unit's chance of being selected weighted to take into account the number of deliveries per year. This was done to remove selection bias towards the smaller units. The unit numbers were grouped consecutively into four for each case. In each unit, a further two-digit random number was generated to select the woman to act as a control. This number matched the delivery number, with unit number 1 being the first woman to deliver that week. A 'week' ran from 00.00 hrs on Saturday and finished at 23.59 hrs on Friday.

Statistical analysis

Four forms of severe maternal morbidity were considered: severe haemorrhage, severe pre-eclampsia (including HELLP syndrome and eclampsia), severe sepsis and uterine rupture. For each of these the incidence of severe maternal morbidity was calculated with 95% confidence intervals. Unconditional logistic regression models were constructed with STATA® (Stata Corp, Texas, release 5, 1997) with severe maternal morbidity as the dependent variable. When analysing individual conditions all the controls were used. Unadjusted odds ratios were estimated using logistic regression for each of the data variables collected. Those variables with a significance level of $P<0.05$ were then included in a multivariate analysis. Also included were variables that were thought to be clinically important but, owing to factors such as small numbers, were not significant in the univariate analysis.

Age was grouped into five-year bands. In univariate analysis the only significant age band was aged 35 years and over and this was therefore used in the multivariate analysis.

Cases that had multiple pathology (e.g. both severe pre-eclampsia and severe haemorrhage) were only considered once in the incidence figures, and the most severe morbidity was counted. These cases were, however, used in the univariate and multivariate analyses for each morbidity involved.

Table 11.3 shows the demographic details of cases and controls. Odds ratios for severe maternal morbidity were adjusted for all of the variables shown.

Results

There were 48 865 deliveries and 588 cases identified, giving an incidence of severe obstetric morbidity of 12.1/1000 deliveries (95% CI 11.2–13.2). During the same period there were five direct maternal deaths attributable to the study conditions (three sepsis, one haemorrhage, one HELLP), giving a severe morbidity-to-mortality ratio (SMMR) of 118:1 (95% CI 97–140).

Table 11.4 shows the incidence of severe morbidity by condition. Although the population of South East England is not the same as the UK, an extrapolation of these incidence figures to the whole of the UK would give the following figures. With 2 197 640 in the 1994–6 CEMD, there would have been 14790 cases of severe haemorrhage, 10 197 of the combined hypertensive conditions, 769 of severe sepsis and 5472 of uterine rupture.

Table 11.3. Demographic data of cases and controls in the Collaborative Study of Severe Morbidity; reproduced with permission from the BMJ Publishing Group[31]

Category	Cases (*n* = 588)[a] (%)	Controls (*n* = 2350)[b] (%)
Ethnic group:		
White	76.2	84.5
Black	16.6	11.2
Other	7.2	4.3
Class:		
Non-manual	58.2	57.3
Manual	18.8	22.3
Unemployed	14.5	11.4
Unknown	8.5	8.9
Marital status:		
Married	59.3	59.5
Single supported	33.8	34.1
Single unsupported	5.5	4.6
Divorced	1.4	1.5
Unknown	0.0	0.4
Parity:		
Para 0	42.0	32.0
Para 1	26.0	30.0
Para 2	14.0	18.0
Para 3	18.0	20.0

[a] Mean age (years) 29.6 (± 5.8); [b] mean age (years) 28.7 (± 5.6)

Table 11.4. Severe obstetric morbidity in Collaborative Study of Severe Morbidity; reproduced with permission from the BMJ Publishing Group [31]

Category of morbidity	Cases (*n*)	Deliveries (%)
All cases	588	1.21
All 'pre-eclampsia'	224	0.46
Severe pre-eclampsia	187	
Eclampsia	12	
HELLP syndrome	25	
All 'haemorrhage'	327	0.67
EBL > 1500 ml	180	
Hb drop ≥ 4 g/dl	96	
Transfused ≥ 4 units blood	51	
Severe sepsis	17	0.04
Uterine rupture	12	0.03
Others[a]	8	

[a] others = acute fatty liver of pregnancy x 3, anaphylaxis, severe hypertension, isolated pulmonary oedema, anaesthetic-related complications x 2 (cardiac arrest, total spinal); EBL = estimated blood loss; HELLP = haemolysis, elevated liver enzymes and low platelets

Risk factors associated with the individual conditions studied are shown in Table 11.5. Few factors were independently significantly associated with developing severe sepsis or uterine rupture. Results from the analysis without the multiple pathology cases ($n = 47$) was similar to that with all cases.

Incidence findings

In COSMO, a large multicentre study using standardised definitions, the incidence of severe obstetric morbidity was estimated at over 12/1000 deliveries. This incidence is higher than previously estimated in developed countries (see Table 11.1), although the conditions studied do vary between studies. The incidence of eclampsia is not dissimilar to that reported for the whole of the UK by the British Eclampsia Survey. There do not appear to be such large discrepancies between morbidity in different settings that have so far been studied as have been found for mortality. This may just be an early ascertainment and definitional issue. Alternatively, it is possible that different health systems impact significantly differently in terms of saving lives from 'near-miss' cases.

There is debate surrounding what constitutes the 'gold standard' for a definition of severe obstetric morbidity. The definitions developed and used in this study represent a spectrum of severity of the morbidity under study and are open to modification. An example of this involves severe haemorrhage. The definition has components that cover measurable blood loss, haemoglobin drop and transfusion. Further work can identify those elements of the definition that are associated with poorer outcomes.

The incidence estimates are likely to be an underestimate of the true incidence as case ascertainment is unlikely to be complete, especially if events occur outside the delivery suite and are not recognised; this may be particularly true of the milder cases. However, several measures were used to minimise this loss of ascertainment. Data were collected

Table 11.5. Adjusted odds ratios for all cases and for each specific condition

Risk factors	Odds ratios (95% confidence interval)				
	All cases	Severe PET	Severe haemorrhage	Severe sepsis	Uterine rupture
Age ≥ 35 years	1.46 (1.11–1.92)	1.83 (1.24–2.70)	1.41 (1.03–1.95)	–	–
Booking blood pressure	1.23 (1.12–1.34)	1.36 (1.21–1.52)	1.18 (1.06–1.31)	–	–
Black race	1.16 (0.85–1.58)	1.83 (1.22–2.74)	0.97 (0.66–1.42)	0.33 (0.03–3.38)	–
Other race	1.93 (1.24–2.99)	2.43 (1.36–4.34)	1.82 (1.09–3.03)	7.02 (1.49–33.15)	–
Social exclusion	2.64 (1.69–4.11)	1.99 (1.07–3.72)	2.91 (1.76–4.82)	2.96 (0.53–16.58)	2.89 (0.22–37.71)
Smoker	0.68 (0.49–0.93)	0.47 (0.26–0.84)	0.65 (0.44–0.96)	3.56 (1.16–10.87)	–
Previous PET	1.52 (1.02–2.27)	3.79 (2.13–6.74)	–	6.61 (1.81–24.18)	1.30 (0.28–6.10)
Previous PPH	2.41 (1.53–3.77)	–	2.74 (1.69–4.44)	–	–
Hypertension	1.10 (0.63–1.95)	1.92 (1.04–3.56)	0.82 (0.37–1.80)	–	–
Diabetic	1.76 (0.43–7.20)	6.10 (1.13–32.75)	1.85 (0.38–9.14)	–	–
Multiple pregnancy	2.21 (1.24–3.96)	3.27 (1.61–6.63)	2.29 (1.20–4.37)	3.05 (0.34–27.52)	–
Antenatal admission	1.75 (1.37–2.23)	1.82 (1.30–2.54)	1.85 (1.39–2.47)	–	–
On iron at booking	5.53 (2.28–13.41)	253 (0.67–9.59)	5.98 (2.28–15.65)	29.48 (2.50–347.83)	–
On anti-epileptics at booking	5.31 (1.40–20.13)	4.99 (0.85–29.15)	5.75 (1.28–25.72)	16.17 (0.40–661.17)	35.50 (0.12–10472)
On anti-depressants at booking	4.30 (0.91–1.88)	–	10.55 (2.19–50.71)	–	–
IOL for post dates	1.36 (0.99–1.88)	–	1.38 (0.95–1.99)	–	4.84 (1.11–21.22)
IOL on medical grounds	2.45(1.68–3.57)	–	1.33 (0.87–1.07)	–	8.61 (1.47–50.33)
Oxytocin augmentation	0.99 (0.76–1.28)	–	1.61 (1.20–2.15)	–	–
Manual removal of placenta	9.60 (5.67–16.28)	–	13.12 (7.72–22.30)	–	14.62 (1.35–158.80)
Emergency CS	4.31 (3.39–5.49)	–	3.09 (2.29–4.17)	11.85 (4.42–31.73)	–

CS = caesarean section, IOL = induction of labour, PET = pre-eclamptic conditions including HELLP syndrome and eclampsia, PPH = postpartum haemorrhage, – = not included in multiple regression analysis as not significant in univariate analysis, contemporaneously, reducing the number of cases lost because of an inability to find notes or information. There were multiple site visits at frequent intervals, to collect data, and information about cases was obtained from several sources.

Morbidity-to-mortality ratio

The SMMR was 118:1. The SMMR is a possible new indicator of maternal care, and could be used to compare improvements in treatments more accurately than mortality data alone. It is simple to explain to women that over one in 100 pregnant women suffer a life-threatening event and that there are 118 events for each direct maternal death (95% CI 97–140), the majority related to obstetric haemorrhage and pre-eclampsia. This major health risk to childbearing women has been relatively underinvestigated. Severe obstetric morbidity is measurable and may be a more meaningful way to measure the impact and improvements in health care. A ratio should be treated with caution, however. Although it might be expected that the figures rise and fall equally, it is possible that they are independent, or that improvements in one part (e.g. obstetric interventions to save life) might increase another (e.g. massive haemorrhage or anxiety/depression).

Risk factors

The main predictors of severe maternal morbidity were demographic (age over 34 years, non-white ethnicity and social exclusion), general medical (diabetes and hypertension) and obstetric factors (previous postpartum haemorrhage, multiple pregnancy, antenatal admission and emergency caesarean section). Anaemia may be a predictor, as a woman taking iron at the time of booking increases the risk of severe morbidity five-fold overall.

One could argue that few of these predictors are amenable to change, but they may be useful in highlighting women who require extra vigilance. Previous studies have observed an increased risk of morbidity in women delivering their first child when aged 35 years and over.[8–14] The trend to defer childbearing in the developed world may lead to increasing maternal morbidity and women should be advised that deferring childbearing has maternal as well as fetal risks. Social exclusion is a major public health issue that applies worldwide. This is another study highlighting the fact that those least advantaged are most likely to suffer harm.[15] Smoking has a protective effect on severe morbidity in general and haemorrhage and pre-eclampsia in particular, but is a predictor for severe sepsis. The protection against pre-eclampsia has been noted previously;[16,17] however, the deleterious effects of smoking on the fetus are well documented. The five- and ten-fold risk of severe haemorrhage with anti-epileptics and antidepressants respectively is unexplained.

The only significant predictors of uterine rupture were induction of labour and manual removal of placenta. This may however be a function of the small numbers of cases observed. Although a previous caesarean section was a significant predictor, on univariate analysis this association was no longer significant after adjusting for other risk factors.

Can risk factors be categorised in any way?

There is a remarkable similarity between the risk factors for maternal death (see Chapter 10) and those identified for severe obstetric morbidity. Risk factors can be divided loosely into:

- those that are not amenable to change (e.g. race, spontaneous twinning)
- those that require social change (e.g. maternal age, social equity)
- those that are within the control of the healthcare professions (e.g. the care of complicated women and intervention rates).

In reality, the risk factors interact and some influences, such as the availability of contraception and abortion affecting maternal age at conception, are a combination of medical, political and social conditions.

The predictors most immediately amenable to change are obstetric intervention; specifically the risk of being a case from induction of labour and emergency caesarean section. The adjusted odds ratio of developing severe sepsis after an emergency caesarean is particularly high. Efforts to reduce the rapidly rising caesarean section rate would be justified by the consequent reduction of severe maternal morbidity.

What interventions might be offered to reduce morbidity?

Table 11.6 suggests some interventions based on known risk factors for morbidity (and mortality). Any deliberate programme to improve maternal morbidity should be evaluated as there are potential dangers. For example, a formal induction or caesarean section reduction programme might have adverse (or beneficial) effects on neonatal outcome. Pre-pregnancy counselling might have a paradoxical effect of improving care during pregnancy but increasing maternal morbidity overall if some women with serious medical conditions chose to become pregnant rather than remain involuntarily infertile. Although we want evidence-based care and policy-making, some interventions are testable (e.g. local teenage pregnancy reduction programme) whereas others are not (wholesale change in women's status leading to reversal of the trend to defer childbearing) and policy may have to be informed by common sense.

Identification of some possible outcome indicators and audit tools

The resources required to estimate the incidence and predictors of severe obstetric morbidity were considerable and required a standardised approach by a dedicated research obstetrician. Significant morbidities were identified, together with their predictors that could be estimated in further population and hospital samples.

The emergence of clinical governance in the UK lends itself to grappling with the issues of severe obstetric morbidity. National audits of induction or severe obstetric morbidity (such as we have had with the National Sentinel Caesarean Section Audit) could enable variations in their impact by unit (depending on type and size) and types of specialist to be estimated. Such national audits could be the basis for development of service frameworks for the management of severe obstetric morbidity. The time is

Table 11.6. Known risk factors for severe obstetric morbidity and their amenability to change

Risk factor	Potential for change
Race	None
Age	Women encouraged to have babies in age range of 20–35 years
	Teenage pregnancy reduction programmes
	Middle-aged pregnancy reduction programmes
	Infertility reduction programme (age, STD)
Multiple pregnancy	Licensing/rules re IVF
	Financial disincentive (insurance for neonatal costs)
	Selective termination of multiple pregnancies
Social exclusion	Governmental social equity programmes
	Access to contraception, abortion and antenatal care
	Targeted maternity care on basis of need
	Special services travellers, teenagers, mentally ill
	24-hour professional interpreters as standard of care
Induction	Keep rates down
	Evidence-based guidelines
	Directed national audit
Caesarean section	One-to-one midwifery care as standard
	Labour ward practice
	Caesarean section reduction programmes
	Directed performance indicators (e.g. ECV/VBAC)
	Vaginal delivery rates (adjusted/standardised)
Medical complications	Pre-pregnancy counselling
Diabetes	Specialist services during pregnancy
Hypertension	
Antihypertensives	
Antidepressants	
Antenatal admissions	Social and psychiatric history taking
Suicide	Violence reduction
	Training and support for midwifery staff
	Research into effective interventions
Previous PET/PPH	History – none
	Advice might change voluntary fertility intentions

ECV = external cephalic version, IVF = *in vitro* fertilisation, PET = pre-eclamptic conditions including HELLP syndrome and eclampsia, PPH = postpartum haemorrhage, STD = sexually transmitted disease, VBAC = vaginal birth after caesarean section

ripe for defining performance indicators of quality to compare units, and even individual clinicians (midwife, generalist, maternal and fetal medicine obstetrician). Purchasers of care and women themselves want better information than is currently being provided by organisations such as Dr Foster. Uptake rates of external cephalic version, vaginal birth after caesarean section, vaginal delivery in standard 'normal primigravida' and other such rates (if suitably adjusted for case-mix of populations) might be some evidence-based indicators that also relate to morbidity and longer-term outcome. The structural and process aspects of care that lead to severe obstetric morbidity require further research and unravelling.

The uncosted and hidden resources expended nationally on CEMD could to some agencies appear outmoded.[18] Introduced when maternal mortality rates had already fallen sharply, and continued falling, it has become an unchallengeable (but unproven) assertion that the Enquiry exerts a positive effect. The Enquiry is based on 'expert opinion' rather than any defined, let alone evidence-based, standards. It is not an audit that closes the loop around any aspect of care, barring local professional developments. The link with the national governance agenda is opaque, although it need not be if appropriately adapted. However, the issue of severe (less alone moderate) morbidity is of great clinical and public-health importance and requires attention. On the basis that it is highly likely that standards will continue to be driven up if more attention is paid to the previously hidden parts of the 'iceberg' of obstetric outcome, maybe it is time to let go of the icon of mortality and move on to the more pressing problem of morbidity.

References

1. Drife J, Lewis G. *Why Mothers Die. Report on Confidential Enquiries into Maternal Deaths in the United Kingdom 1994–1996*. London: HMSO; 1998.
2. Drife J, Lewis G, editors. *Why Mothers Die 1997–1999*. The *Confidential Enquiries into Maternal Deaths in the United Kingdom*. London: RCOG Press; 2002.
3. Stones W, Lim W, Al-Azzawi F, Kelly M. An investigation of maternal morbidity with identification of life-threatening 'near miss' episodes. *Health Trends* 1991;23:13–15.
4. Fitzpatrick C, Halligan A, McKenna P, Coughlan BM, Darling MR, Phelan D. Near miss maternal mortality. *Ir Med J* 1992;85:37.
5. Office for National Statistics. *Classification of Occupation*. London: HMSO; 1990.
6. Cabinet Office. Social exclusion. London: HMSO; 1999. [http://www.cabinet–office.gov.uk/seu/index.htm].
7. Nisell H, Lintu H, Lunell NO, Mollerstrom G, Pettersson E. Blood pressure and renal function seven years after pregnancy complicated by hypertension. *Br J Obstet Gynaecol* 1995;102:876–81.
8. Tan KT, Tan KH. Pregnancy and delivery in primigravidae aged 35 and over. *Singapore Med J* 1994;35:495–501.
9. Roberts C, Algert C, March L. Delayed childbearing – are there any risks? *Med J Aust* 1994;160:539–44.
10. Peipert J, Bracken M. Maternal age: an independent risk factor for cesarean delivery. *Obstet Gynecol* 1993;81:200–5.
11. Jonas O, Roder D, Chan A. The association of maternal and socioeconomic characteristics in metropolitan Adelaide with medical, obstetric and labour complications and pregnancy outcomes. *Aust N Z J Obstet Gynaecol* 1992;32:1–5.
12. Jonas O, Chan A, Roder D, Macharper T. Pregnancy outcomes in primigravid women aged 35 years and over in South Australia, 1986-1988. *Med J Aust* 1991;154:246–9.
13. Tuck S, Yudkin P, Turnbull A. Pregnancy outcome in elderly primigravidae with and without a history of infertility. *Br J Obstet Gynaecol* 1988;95:230–7.
14. Lehmann D, Chism J. Pregnancy outcome in medically complicated and uncomplicated patients aged 40 years or older. *Am J Obstet Gynecol* 1987;157:738–42.
15. Peacock J, Bland J, Anderson H. Preterm delivery: effects of socioeconomic factors, psychological stress, smoking, alcohol, and caffeine. *BMJ* 1995;311:531–5.
16. Cnattingius S, Mills JL, Yuen J, Eriksson O, Salonen H. The paradoxical effect of smoking in preeclamptic pregnancies: smoking reduces the incidence but increases the rates of perinatal mortality, abruptio placentae, and intrauterine growth restriction. *Am J Obstet Gynecol* 1997;177:156–61.
17. Klonoff-Cohen H, Edelstein S, Savitz D. Cigarette smoking and preeclampsia. *Obstet Gynecol* 1993;81:541–4.
18. Wolfe C. Maternal mortality. In: McColl AJ, Gulliford MC. *Population Health Outcome Indicators for the NHS. A Feasibility Study*. London: Faculty of Public Health Medicine; 1993. p. 139–42.
19. Graham SG, Luxton MC. The requirement for intensive care support for the pregnant population. *Anaesthesia* 1989;44:581–4.
20. Kilpatrick SJ, Matthay MA. Obstetric patients requiring critical care. A five-year review. *Chest* 1992;101:1407–12.
21. Johanson R, Anthony J, Dommisse J. Obstetric intensive care at Groote Schuur Hospital, Cape Town.

J Obstet Gynecol 1995;15:174–7.

22. Bouvier-Colle MH, Salanave B, Ancel PY, Varnoux N, Fernandez H, Papiernik E, *et al.* Obstetric patients treated in intensive care units and maternal mortality. *Eur J Obstet Gynecol Reprod Biol* 1996;65:121–5.
23. Bewley S, Creighton S. 'Near miss' obstetric enquiry. *J Obstet Gynecol* 1997;17:26–9.
24. Filippi V, Gandaho T, Ronsmans C, Graham W, Alihonou E. New tools for prioritising and evaluating safe motherhood programmes: the near-misses and the sisterhood method. Report to the Overseas Development Agency, May 1997 (from a letter in Lancet: Filippi V, Alihonou E, Mukantaganda S, Graham WJ, Ronsmans C, *et al.* Near misses: maternal morbidity and mortality. *Lancet* 1998;351:145–6).
25. Lapinski SE, Kruczynski K, Seaward GR, Farine D, Grossman RF. Critical care management of the obstetric patient. *Can J Anaesth* 1997;44:325–9.
26. Baskett TF, Sternadel J. Maternal intensive care and near-miss mortality in obstetrics. *Br J Obstet Gynecol* 1998 105:981–4.
27. Mantel GD, Buchmann E, Rees H, Pattinson RC. Severe acute maternal morbidity: a pilot study of a definition for a near-miss. *Br J Obstet Gynaecol* 1998;105:985–90.
28. Nasrat HA, Youssef MH, Marzoogi A, Talab F. 'Near miss' obstetric morbidity in an inner city hospital in Saudi Arabia. *East Mediterr Health J* 1999;5:717–26.
29. Sivalingam N, Looi KW. Clinical experience with management of 'near miss' cases in obstetrics. *Med J Malaysia* 1999;54:496–503.
30. Prual A, Bouvier-Colle MH, de Bernis L, Breart G. Severe maternal morbidity from direct causes in West Africa: incidence and case fatality rates. *Bull World Health Organ* 2000;78:593–602.
31. Waterstone M, Bewley S, Wolfe C. Incidence and predictors of severe obstetric morbidity: case control study. *BMJ* 2001;322:1089–94.
32. Sibai BM. Eclampsia. VI. Maternal-perinatal outcome in 254 consecutive cases. *Am J Obstet Gynecol* 1990;163:1049–55.
33. Sibai BM, Ramadan MK, Usta I, Salama M, Mercer BM, Friedman SA. Maternal morbidity and mortality in 442 pregnancies with hemolysis, elevated liver enzymes, and low platelets (HELLP Syndrome). *Am J Obstet Gynecol* 1993;169:1000–6.
34. Benedetti J. Obstetric hemorrhage. In: Clark SL, Cotton DB, Hankins GDV, Phelan JP, editors. *Critical Care Obstetrics*. 2nd ed. Boston: Blackwell Scientific Publications; 1991. p. 573–606.
35. Bone RC, Balk RA, Cerra FB, Dellinger RP, Fein AM, Knaus WA, *et al.* Definitions for sepsis and organ failure and guidelines for the use of innovative therapies in sepsis. *Chest* 1992;101:1644–55.
36. Bone RC, Sibbald WJ, Sprung CL. The ACCP-SCCM Consensus conference on sepsis and organ failure. *Chest* 1992;101:1481–3.
37. Mabie WC, Sibai BM. Treatment in an obstetric intensive care unit. *Am J Obstet Gynecol* 1990;162:1–4.

Chapter 12

Major maternal morbidity in South Africa

Robert C Pattinson

Introduction

The concept of 'near-miss' is extensively used in the airline industry. Any collision, near-collision or incident potentially involving the safety of the passengers and crew is referred to the airline authorities for review and recommendations, so that the problem can be prevented in the future. The airline industry takes these reports seriously and failure to act on the recommendations may lead to litigation. Today it is safer to fly in an aircraft than to cross a street.

Acute major maternal morbidity can be likened to this 'near-miss' – a severe life-threatening incident occurs during pregnancy but fortunately the patient survives. Chronic major maternal morbidity most commonly occurs in women who retain significant problems (such as vesicovaginal fistula, chronic renal failure and residual brain damage) resulting from the severe insult that occurred during pregnancy. Furthermore, those women with acute major morbidity are those most likely to die. It is therefore extremely important to reduce the number of women who develop acute major morbidity. The airline industry's approach can be used to reduce the prevalence of major morbidity.

Definition of major maternal morbidity

Before any discussion can take place, major maternal morbidity needs to be defined. Certain criteria must apply for the definition to be usable: it must be reproducible, easy to understand and not require investigations that would not normally have been performed (i.e. not use extra resources). Finally, in developing countries such as South Africa, where resources are limited, it also must not be resource-dependent. For example, admission of a pregnant woman to intensive care would normally be a simple method of identifying major acute morbidity, as is often the case in developed countries but, if intensive-care beds are scarce, patients who would normally be admitted would not gain access. These cases would thus be missed, leaving an important weakness in the health system unidentified.

Mantel *et al.*[1] put forward a definition of severe acute maternal morbidity (SAMM) that was suitable for use in a developing country and possibly also in a developed country. The definition is based on the concept that the progression from a healthy pregnancy to a maternal death follows a sequence of events: a clinical insult, systemic inflammatory response syndrome, organ dysfunction, organ failure and finally death. A woman with severe organ dysfunction or failure would usually die without adequate treatment or support. Intuitively, a patient with SAMM is an extremely ill woman (with severe organ dysfunction or failure) who would have died had it not been for good luck or good care. The next step is to define dysfunction and failure for each organ system, using clinical or frequently used biochemical markers (Table 12.1) that all secondary and tertiary hospitals perform routinely. Not all intuitive 'near-misses' meet the definition because of the management of the clinician, so a management-based category has been introduced to accommodate those women who the clinician felt to be at significant risk of organ failure or death and intervened by performing an emergency hysterectomy, or admitted the woman to intensive care. In recognition of anaesthesia being possibly a major source of 'near misses' that would also not be recorded, a specific category for anaesthetic problems was created. Failed tracheal intubation requiring anaesthetic reversal and severe hypotension (systolic blood pressure of less than 90 mmHg for more than 60 minutes) for complications associated with epidural and spinal anaesthesia are the anaesthetic markers.

Identification of women with SAMM in itself is of limited value. Recording the clinical insult or primary obstetric factor leading to the SAMM adds greatly to the value of auditing SAMM. The primary obstetric factor is the disease that set in motion the train of events that led to the 'near-miss'. For example, a woman who had severe pre-eclampsia and developed renal failure would have recorded renal failure as SAMM (or the 'near-miss' marker) and the primary obstetric cause as pre-eclampsia. Identifying the primary obstetric factor is important, as it indicates where preventive

Table 12.1. Definitions of severe acute maternal morbidity

Definition	Criteria
Organ system dysfunction	
Cardiac	Pulmonary oedema, cardiac arrest
Circulatory	Hypovolaemia requiring ≥ 5 units red cell transfusion
Immunological	Sepsis resulting in a hysterectomy or intensive care unit admission
Respiratory	Intubation and ventilation for ≥ 60 minutes, oxygen saturation < 90% for ≥ 60 minutes
Renal	Oliguria (<400 ml/24 hour) that does not respond to fluids or diuretics, serum urea ≥15 mmol/l, creatinine ≥ 400 μmol/l, or need for dialysis
Hepatic	Jaundice in the presence of pre-eclampsia
Metabolic	Diabetic ketoacidosis, hypoglycaemic coma, thyroid crisis
Coagulation	Acute thrombocytopenia requiring a platelet transfusion
Cerebral	Coma lasting ≥ 12 hours, or intracerebral or subarachnoid haemorrhage
Management-based	
Intensive care admission	Any
Emergency hysterectomy	Any
Anaesthetic accidents	Severe hypotension associated with regional anaesthesia: a systolic blood pressure < 90 mmHg for ≥ 60 minutes, a high spinal anaesthetic requiring intubation, or failed intubation requiring anaesthetic reversal

measures should be aimed. The 'near-miss' marker and the organ system dysfunction indicate the resources required to treat these women. The definitions of the primary obstetric cause are the same as those used in the Confidential Enquiry into Maternal Deaths in South Africa.[2]

Identifying and recording any substandard care that may have taken place gives valuable information on the functioning of the health system. The definitions of substandard care were also the same as those used by the Confidential Enquiry into Maternal Deaths in South Africa.[2] The definition takes into account not only failure in clinical care but also some of the underlying factors that may have produced a low standard of care for the patient. This includes actions by the woman herself, her family and community, which are outside healthworkers' control, and administrative problems such as inadequate transport and lack of facilities, for example, intensive care beds.

The process of collecting information is dependent upon the definitions used. If simple clinical markers are used as described above, the case can easily be flagged and discussed during the routine maternal morbidity and mortality meeting. A simple computer programme has been written to facilitate this and it allows for rapid analysis of the data. This reduces the labour involved in the audit process.

Other definitions of severe maternal morbidity have been put forward in the developing and the developed world. Prual *et al.*[3] defined severe morbidity according to the obstetric complication and the health services' response to the disease, such as days spent in hospital, blood transfusions, etc. In order to reflect the situation in West Africa, severe dystocia was included and defined as obstructed labour or prolonged labour requiring either instrumental fetal extraction or caesarean section and uterine rupture and other complications of prolonged labour, such as laceration of the perineum, pelvic fistulae or death. This definition reflects the resources available within the health services in West Africa and their definitions have to be determined within these confines. In the developed world, admission to an intensive care unit seems to be the most common way of measuring severe obstetric morbidity.[4] This definition would not be suitable for a developing country where intensive care units are extremely scarce. Furthermore, criteria for admission to intensive care units vary from hospital to hospital and even from consultant to consultant. Trying to establish a universal definition of severe maternal morbidity will be difficult but will have the advantage of allowing comparisons. For uniformity across countries, a system based on organ system failure has the best prognosis. If treatment responses to complications are used (such as admission to intensive care units), comparisons will not be feasible because the resources available in each country vary so widely.

Maternal morbidity and mortality audits in developing countries

Auditing maternal morbidity has two major advantages over auditing maternal deaths. First, maternal morbidity occurs over three times more frequently than maternal death; information on maternal care can therefore be gathered and analysed more rapidly, allowing for more rapid feedback and intervention. The second is that the woman can be interviewed to establish whether the health system failed or not. This is particularly valuable for women who have been referred from one institution to another, and especially for assessing care at the primary level. Often this part of the audit is not available in maternal deaths.

There is one major disadvantage to maternal morbidity auditing, which is that almost by definition women with SAMM are treated in secondary- and tertiary-level institutions. Women with SAMM who do not reach these institutions presumably die (if the definition is correct). If the point of analysing SAMM is to evaluate maternal care, maternal deaths from the whole area must also be collected and analysed. Exclusion of maternal deaths might give a false impression of how effectively the primary level of care is functioning because in SAMM all women reach secondary or tertiary care. Thus, important health system issues would not be identified.

The primary aim of confidential enquiries into maternal deaths is to identify inadequacies in all aspects of the health service and thus it is an audit of the quality of maternal care. The philosophy of these audits is that by analysing a few clearly defined cases, solutions to identified inadequacies will improve the quality of care of similar cases but also the care of other patients within the service. Confidential enquiries into maternal deaths have been associated with dramatic reductions of maternal deaths over time,[5] presumably because, having identified the problems, the health profession is in a position to act to improve the situation. To be effective, the information obtained has to be fresh and relevant to the current situation. Data that take too long to collect, that include insufficient numbers to analyse within an appropriate period of time or do not reflect major problems limit the usefulness of any audit. This numbers game can be remedied either by expanding the area of collection, for example to a whole province or country, which requires a large infrastructure and commitment by many people, or by expanding the definition of the clearly defined cases. Maternal mortality is easily defined, maternal morbidity less so, but with the definitions of Mantel *et al.*,[1] this can be reliably and repeatedly performed. Thus, by combining maternal morbidity and mortality audits, a more rapid analysis of maternal care can be obtained in a smaller geographical area, which requires fewer resources. In developing countries, it is more appropriate to use a combination of SAMM and maternal deaths as a system of auditing maternal care.

The continuing SAMM and maternal mortality audits in the Pretoria region are an example of this.[6] After two years, two major problems were identified. The first was that of transporting severely ill women over long distances from one province to another, resulting in delays to treatment and, thus, to more severe illness. Upgrading a secondary hospital within the referring province solved this problem. This allowed for better resuscitation before further referral, if needed, or, as was increasingly the case, full treatment of a less severely ill patient. The second major problem was the large number of women with SAMM due to complications of abortion. This was due to a lack of pregnancy termination services within the region. Within the following two years, the problem was partly solved by private institutions providing pregnancy termination services, resulting in a dramatic reduction in SAMM due to abortions. The Confidential Enquiries into Maternal Deaths would have detected neither of these two problems within the time period because the number of women dying from complications of abortion or transport delays was low.

Disease pattern of severe acute maternal morbidity

Major maternal morbidity has been surveyed in three areas of South Africa. These included rural and urban areas. Information on maternal deaths was collected and analysed at the same time.[7] The definitions of SAMM, the primary obstetric causes and

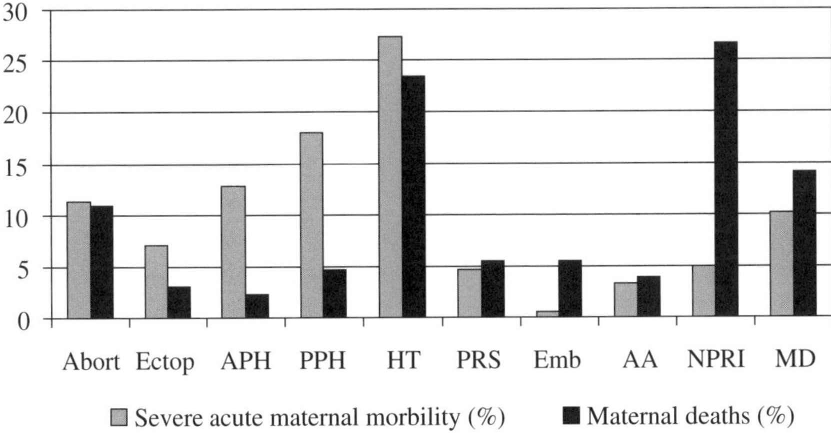

Figure 12.1. The primary obstetric cause of 'near-miss' and maternal deaths; AA = anaesthetic-related; Abort = abortion; APH = antepartum haemorrhage; Ectop = Ectopic pregnancy; Emb = embolism; HT = hypertension; MD = pre-existing medical disease; NPRI = non-pregnancy-related infection; PPH = postpartum haemorrhage; PRS = pregnancy-related sepsis

substandard care used to describe major maternal morbidity in South Africa are those given above.

Data relating to a total of 423 women with SAMM and 128 maternal deaths were collected over two years in the three sites. Interestingly, the primary obstetric causes of SAMM and maternal death did not correlate (Figure 12.1). The four most common causes of SAMM were complications of hypertension (27.2%), postpartum haemorrhage (18.0%), antepartum haemorrhage (12.8%) and abortion (11.3%), whereas the four most common causes of maternal death were non-pregnancy-related infections (26.6%), complications of hypertension (23.4%), pre-existing medical disease (14.1%) and abortion (10.9%). Significantly fewer women died after developing severe morbidity due to haemorrhage, but significantly more died after developing an embolism or non-pregnancy-related infections.

In order to compare the number of women dying from SAMM in different areas, with different diseases and organ system failures, a new 'mortality index' was created. It was defined as the number of maternal deaths divided by the sum of the women with SAMM and maternal deaths and expressed as a percentage (this is similar to the lethality rate of Bouvier-Colle *et al.*[4] and maternal morbidity:mortality ratio of Waterstone *et al.*,[8] although they differ in the definition of what constitutes a 'near-miss'). The mortality index gives an idea of what proportion of women with severe acute morbidity, as defined, will die. For example, the mortality index for hypertension in pregnancy is the number of women with SAMM due to hypertension in pregnancy divided by the sum of the women with SAMMs and maternal deaths due to hypertension in pregnancy. The mortality index for the various primary obstetric causes is shown in Table 12.2.

Table 12.2. A comparison of the primary obstetric cause between women with severe acute maternal morbidity and maternal deaths

Primary cause	Mortality index (%)
All cases	23.2
Direct:	
Abortion	22.6
Ectopic pregnancy	11.8
Antepartum haemorrhage	5.3
Postpartum haemorrhage	7.3
Hypertension	20.6
Pregnancy-related sepsis	25.9
Embolism	77.8
Anaesthetic-related	26.3
Indirect:	
Non-pregnancy-related infections	61.8
Pre-existing medical disease	29.5

The mortality index for non-pregnancy-related infections was high (61.8%). The category 'non-pregnancy-related infection' includes AIDS, tuberculosis, meningitis, malaria and pneumonia. The diagnosis of AIDS was made only if there was a positive HIV test and either an AIDS-defining condition or a CD4 count of less than 200/μl. The high mortality index in women with non-pregnancy-related infections indicates that women with an organ system dysfunction or failure have a poor prognosis. Women with AIDS are major contributors to non-pregnancy-related infections. This raises the question of what role intensive care plays in a resource-poor environment for women with SAMM and AIDS. This is an ethical and moral question that the community must take part in deciding. The debate is informed by the data provided by the mortality index. Researchers will need, as a priority, to investigate ways in which these women can be adequately treated, for example with short-course anti-retroviral drugs. The mortality index for women with SAMM following a pulmonary embolism (77.8%) is also high. This stresses the importance of identifying women at risk for deep vein thrombosis and providing preventive measures, even in a developing country. The mortality index for ante- or postpartum haemorrhage was low (5.3% and 7.3%, respectively, and 6.5% combined). However, the mortality index varied from 21.4% to 2.3% between the three sites (Figure 12.2). This large deviation warranted investigation and the information was provided by analysis of substandard care in each case. The great increase in the mortality index was found to be due to lack of blood transfusion facilities in the smaller hospitals in the Bloemfontein area and the delays in transporting the patients to the larger hospitals. Here, valuable information was identified that may lead to interventions in the health system in the Free State. The mortality index gives a measure of the health service's effectiveness at managing the disease process.

Organ failure and maternal death

Analysing the frequency of the different organ systems that were dysfunctional or failed in women who died or who had severe morbidity also gives us new insights

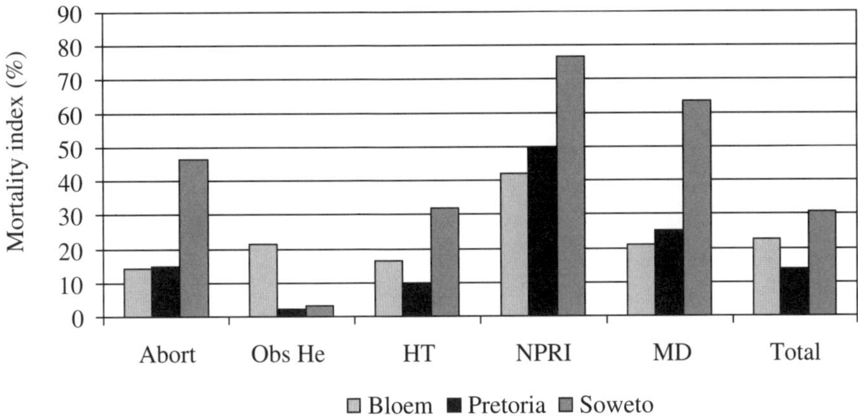

Figure 12.2. Comparison between the study sites and the mortality index per disease category; Abort = abortion; HT = hypertension; MD = pre-existing medical disease; NPRI = non-pregnancy-related infection; Obs He = obstetric haemorrhage

(Table 12.3 and Figure 12.3). The mortality where the central nervous or respiratory system was involved was high, with mortality indices of 60.3% and 42.0%, respectively. The majority of the central nervous system problems were related to intracerebral haemorrhage. Rapid control of hypertension is the only way to prevent this and severe hypertension must be seen as an obstetric emergency.

In developing countries, there is often considerable resistance to ventilating a patient. This is mainly due to the lack of ventilation facilities or the lack of intensive-care beds. This lack of facilities for ventilating patients contributed to the high mortality index. Recognition of the high mortality index led to the search for

Table 12.3. A comparison of the organ system dysfunction between women with severe acute maternal morbidity and maternal deaths; SAMM = severe acute maternal morbidity

Organ system dysfunction[a]	SAMM		Maternal death	
	(*n*)	(%)	(*n*)	(%)
Total	423		128	
Cardiac	98	23.2	34	26.5
Cerebral	23	5.4	35	27.3
Coagulation	61	14.4	5	3.9
Metabolic	1	0.2	2	1.6
Vascular (hypovolaemia)	177	41.8	21	16.4
Hepatic	7	1.7	1	0.8
Renal	62	14.7	7	5.5
Respiratory	47	11.1	34	26.5
Immune	48	11.3	23	18.0
Multiple organ failure	0	0	10	7.8

[a] More than one organ system dysfunction may apply in each case

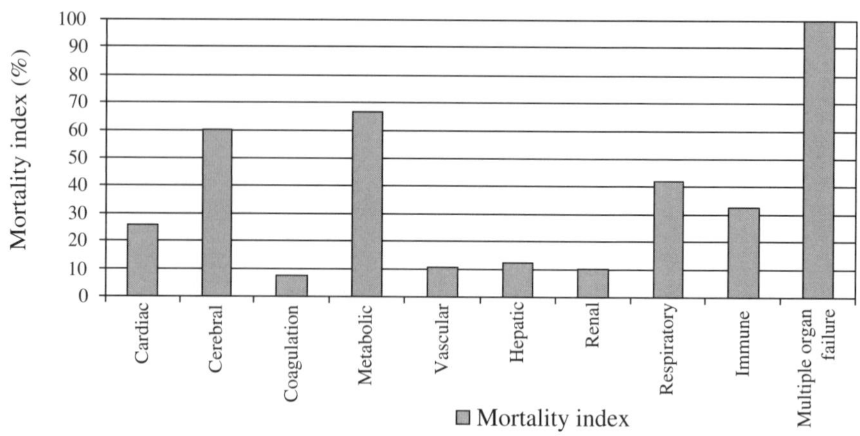

Figure 12.3. A comparison of the mortality indices of organ system dysfunction between women with severe acute maternal morbidity and maternal deaths

alternatives to ventilation and currently continuous positive airway pressure (CPAP) masks are being used to assist ventilation. CPAP masks do not need to be used in an intensive-care setting and may bring down the mortality index due to respiratory dysfunction.

Substandard care

Patient-orientated problems occurred in similar frequencies in both groups (Table 12.4). However, there were significantly more administrative problems in the women who died. This was mainly due to lack of facilities, such as intensive care beds, and to transport delays. There were similar proportions of substandard care by the health workers but in the maternal death group there was less accurate diagnosis and poorer monitoring of patients.

Maternal morbidity and mortality audits in developed countries

In developed countries, maternal deaths are now rare events and analysis of sufficient numbers of maternal deaths to obtain a meaningful picture of the health service takes a long time, limiting its value as a tool for improving maternal care. Rather than representing problems in the health service, maternal deaths in developed countries are unusual cases where the circumstances are so specific to the particular event that the information cannot be generalised. The basic premise that confidential enquiries into maternal deaths would give relevant information about maternal care in general seems to be no longer valid. There were only 106 direct and 136 indirect maternal deaths in

Table 12.4. A comparison of the avoidable factors, missed opportunities and substandard care between women with severe acute maternal morbidity and maternal mortality (SAMM)

Factor	SAMM		Maternal death		*P*
	n	%	*n*	%	
Total	423		128		
Patient-orientated	150	35.5	45	35.2	NS
Administrative	103	24.3	50	39.1	0.002
Medical personnel	219	51.8	70	54.7	NS
Initial assessment	30	7.1	16	12.5	NS
Problem recognition	40	9.5	22	17.2	0.0200
Management plan	109	25.8	29	22.7	NS
Monitoring	24	5.7	21	16.4	0.0002
Non-professional conduct	10	2.4	6	4.7	NS

NS = non-significant

the UK in 1997–99.[5] Are the lessons learned applicable to the majority of women? The biggest problem identified in the report[5] for the obstetrician was in the prevention or treatment of thromboembolism. Deaths from obstetric haemorrhage were rare, being five times less frequent than thromboembolism, and were the sixth most common cause of direct maternal deaths. In an audit of severe obstetric morbidity in the South East Thames Region,[8] obstetric haemorrhage was the most common cause. A similar picture emerges in France.[4] It seems that obstetricians in developed countries might consider SAMM as more applicable than maternal deaths to audits of maternal care.

Differing patterns of the causes of maternal death and morbidity

In the South African acute maternal morbidity study,[7] no correlation was found between the primary obstetric cause of maternal deaths and SAMM. Investigating women with SAMM cannot thus be used as a proxy for describing the disease pattern of pregnant women who die. Audits of women with SAMM and maternal deaths give different but complementary information. Analysing the differences between morbidity and mortality gives us a clearer picture of how the health system is functioning and where to concentrate efforts.

A population has a basic disease profile that is modified by the response of the health system to the disease profile (Figure 12.4). A few hundred years ago, the healthcare system for the whole population essentially consisted of the family and the first aid that they could provide. The most common cause of maternal death was probably haemorrhage and there would have been little difference between the primary obstetric causes of maternal death and SAMM (Figure 12.4A). To some extent, this is seen in the maternal death and morbidity profile in West Africa,[3] where haemorrhage is the most common cause of maternal death and morbidity. Subsequently, health systems developed and health 'safety nets' appeared where the patient with a problem would be seen and the problem solved or referred on to the next level. The primary, secondary and tertiary care levels act as the various safety nets. Where the system was incomplete (as in developing countries), patients would still fall through the safety net and die; however, the pattern of primary obstetric causes leading to maternal death would change (Figure 12.4B). The health system is now superimposed on the basic disease

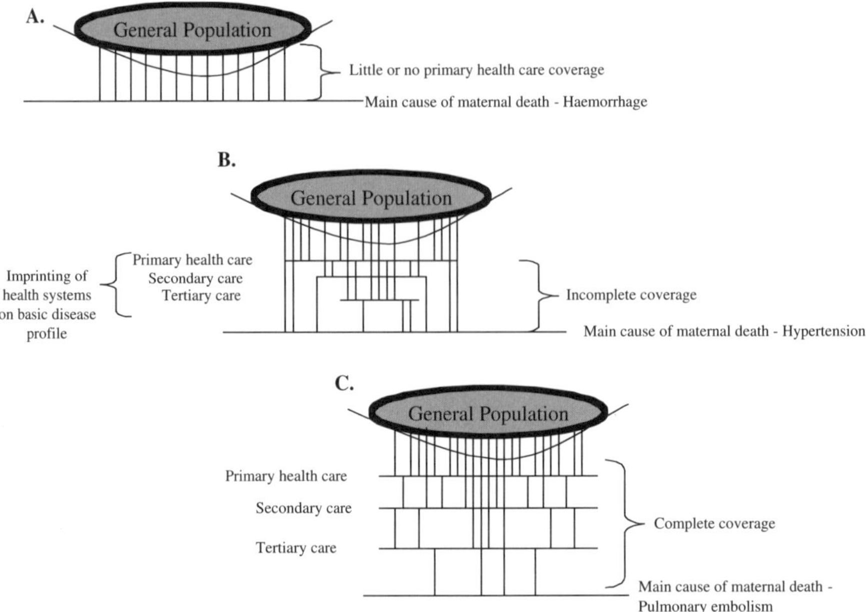

Figure 12.4. A diagrammatic representation of the effect of superimposing a primary healthcare system on the basic disease profile of a population with respect to maternal deaths

profile of the population and the most common causes of maternal mortality change. The most common direct cause of maternal death in the South African Confidential Enquiries into Maternal Deaths[2] was hypertension, but haemorrhage was still the most common cause of SAMM. Provision of oxytocics and blood transfusions by the South African health system prevents a large number of deaths from haemorrhage, so the importance of haemorrhage is reduced as a cause of maternal death while remaining high as a cause of SAMM. In a developed health system, fewer patients fall through the health system (safety nets) and there would be few deaths other than from rare diseases that the medical profession is not yet able to treat adequately (Figure 12.4C). In the UK, pulmonary embolism is the most common cause of maternal death,[5] but haemorrhage and complications of hypertension are still major causes of severe maternal morbidity.[8] Hence the pattern of maternal mortality reflects the level of development of the tiered healthcare system and severe maternal morbidity reflects the actual disease profile in the population.

Educational use of severe acute maternal morbidity definitions

An unexpected 'adverse effect' of developing the SAMM definitions and using them in the daily audit meeting was the evolution of the systemic approach to obstetric patients.[9] One of the most common areas of healthworker substandard care was non-recognition of a problem. In this approach, the clinicians managing a case were forced routinely to examine each organ system and any abnormality detected would trigger further specific investigations. Hence, a woman with a tachypnoea or abnormal breath sounds had to have her oxygen saturation measured using pulse oximetry and a chest X-ray immediately to investigate the respiratory system further. Any abnormalities would be investigated until a diagnosis was made and treatment instituted. This approach has since been adopted by the National Committee on Confidential Enquiries into Maternal Deaths for its protocols to prevent maternal deaths from common causes.[9]

Conclusion

Recording and analysing SAMM is a process that follows the same system of confidential enquiries into maternal deaths. When used in combination with an analysis of maternal deaths, it allows for a more rapid diagnosis of problems inside maternal care system within a smaller geographical area. This in turn allows for a swifter response to the problems and ultimately to an improvement in maternal care. The system is not resource-dependent, as the definitions used are based on clinical findings or laboratory investigations and require little manpower.

References

1. Mantel GD, Buchmann E, Rees H, Pattinson RC. Severe acute maternal morbidity: a pilot study of a definition for a near-miss. *Br J Obstet Gynaecol* 1998;105:985–90.
2. Department of Health. *Saving Mothers: Confidential Enquiries into Maternal Deaths in South Africa. 1998*. Pretoria: Government Printer; 1999.
3. Prual A, Bouvier-Colle MH, de Bernis L, Breart G. Severe maternal morbidity from direct obstetric causes in West Africa: incidence and case fatality rates. *Bull World Health Organ* 2000;78:593–600.
4. Bouvier-Colle MH, Salanave B, Ancel PY, Varnoux N, Fernandez H, Papiernik E, *et al.* Obstetric patients treated in intensive care units and maternal mortality. Regional Teams for the Survey. *Eur J Obstet Gynecol Reprod Biol* 1996;65:121–5.
5. Drife J, Lewis G, editors. *Why Mothers Die 1997–1999: The Confidential Enquiries into Maternal Deaths in the United Kingdom*. London: RCOG Press; 2001.
6. Vandecruis H, Pattinson RC, Macdonald AP. Changing patterns of severe acute maternal morbidity and mortality in the Pretoria region. *Eur J Obstet Gynaecol Reprod Biol* 2002;102:6–10.
7. Pattinson RC, Buchmann E, Mantel G, Schoon M, Rees H. Making sense and getting direction from 'near miss' and maternal mortality audits. Proceedings, 18th Priorities in Perinatal Care Conference, Buffelspoort Dam, North West Province, South Africa 1999.
8. Waterstone M, Bewley S, Wolfe C. Incidence and predictors of severe obstetric morbidity: case control study. *BMJ* 2001;322:1089–94.
9. Pattinson RC, Mantel G. A systematic approach to examining an ill pregnant patient. In: Moodley J, editor. *Saving Mothers. Policy and Management Guidelines for Common Causes of Maternal Deaths*. Pretoria: Government Printers; 2000. p. 6–23.

Chapter 13

Inequalities and morbidities

Discussion

Discussion following the papers by Dr Lewis, Dr Bewley and Professor Pattinson

Millward-Sadler: I wanted to ask Dr Lewis about the ascertainment of suicide, because that was a very stark change in the pregnancy-related deaths. I was slightly concerned because most of these suicides occur in the community rather than in hospital and so there will be great difficulty in ascertainment. Will we have that system of ascertainment from the Office for National Statistics (ONS) available to us for the Enquiry?

Second, how confident are you that these represent all the suicides? In my experience, coroners are becoming increasingly reluctant to pass a verdict of suicide when they hold an inquest.

Lewis: The ONS has agreed to continue this. It took us some time to set it up because it is a complicated database. As long as the funding comes through, we will be continuing. It is not just suicides – there are late cardiac deaths too. These data came in very late in the process of publishing the book and I am trying to produce a further paper on the other deaths that we missed. We had all the direct ones, but it was the suicides that we missed.

In the ascertainment for suicides we actually went for open verdicts too. We know that coroners find it difficult to write 'suicide', so we are going for all women who die within a year of birth, including open verdicts, violence, murder and other causes of death. This is really a foretaste of how we will improve the Enquiry in the future. It means a great deal more work for all of us, because we will pick up 200 extra cases that will need assessment.

The suicides are complicated because they take place in the community and it is difficult for us to identify them under our traditional pattern of notification. We have fabulous reporting by obstetricians and midwives – they have grown up with this Enquiry and so they know how to do it. Psychiatrists, community healthcare workers and general practitioners do not and, in any event, they may not be in touch with any of them. That is a good way of picking them up.

We are looking at ways – not this year, but perhaps next – of linking in with the Confidential Enquiry into Suicides and Homicides. They look at deaths but they, too, can only look at deaths from suicide in institutions where they can obtain death certificates. They, too, cannot identify deaths in the community, but we are working actively to try to improve that.

Millward-Sadler: I have a follow-up question related to that. Often, much of the information is only available through the police service and we obviously need to link in with that. They obtain what little clinical history there is in these situations. Do we have good links with the Home Office?

Lewis: Well, we have links with the Home Office. You have to sell extra work to government departments, because we are all overwhelmed with work. However, we have developed links with the Home Office and we are talking to them about engaging the police. This is extending the role of our Enquiry way beyond how it was ever envisaged. We know that we need to engage coroners. We know that we need – and I want – to engage social services as well in the reports. We are hoping to do this next time. We are working on the Home Office and the police, but you are quite right.

MacLean: Dr Lewis, could I ask you about ethnic backgrounds and whether there is any information about duration of stay in the UK? In other words, people who have been here for a generation and those who have recently arrived – whether they have come as legitimate refugees or are here illegally. I could imagine that they would be less likely to avail themselves of services, in case they were disclosed and deported. Do we have that information?

Lewis: We have limited information. As I said, until six years ago, we were not even allowed to discuss ethnic background because it was considered politically incorrect. The data collection systems in ONS do not include country of birth, just nationality. We rely on more information being given in our report. I have that information for most of our cases and I have to say that most of them are second or third generation. The African women come under the heading of refugee – we only have a very small number of asylum seekers who died, but I can identify the number. We need to improve our data collection but that is an NHS data collection problem and not just our data collection problem. We are pretty confident at the moment that most of these women were second- or third-generation women and they do not speak English.

Bewley: Two points. First, it strikes me that, if late booking is an issue, there is a very clear idea – like the French – of tying early booking into benefits.

The second point is about the definition of social exclusion. I am amazed that the new social class definition has the Armed Services as social class three, because it always used to be six and unclassified because it is very low. That looks wrong and I wonder whether there is an opportunity of changing that? There is also a need to hone down on the factors that really constitute 'social exclusion'. We were vague – we looked at the NHS website and some other ideas. If we can get that definition very tight, that will be very helpful clinically. There is no such thing as a 'difficult patient' – there are patients with difficult problems and, because of the inverse care law, here is a template for you and your services to worry about. That will give a focus around that definition of vulnerability or social exclusion, to the clinical coalface, and then be measurable.

Lewis: Yes, you are absolutely right. Social exclusion is the buzzword, and the

Government uses it in different ways. Social justice is actually our new term. In terms of being able to set something measurable, we are working with ONS certainly for this enquiry, and I hope to extend it through the National Service Framework on deprivation indices in relation to postcodes. We have been unable to obtain postcodes from records until very recently, for reasons of confidentiality. However, we are now allowed these and so we will have a proper deprivation index for maternal deaths. I hope that we will be able to roll that out, once we have worked out how to do it easily with what information the NHS collects, into a new NHS patient record.

Oates: Suicide research since the 1950s, when it started, has always been bedevilled by underascertainment. The 50% underascertainment in this study is entirely consistent with suicide literature. All respectable suicide researchers have to go into multiple sources of data collection and they have to consider open verdicts – that is entirely respectable.

Something that concerns me a little about the findings of the study is that it is highly likely that the earlier a death occurs by suicide in relation to childbirth, the more likely it is to be reported. We may find that the majority of these ONS-linkage deaths are in fact very late postpartum deaths. This is also true of drug abuse. When you start looking at deaths at 11 months postpartum, you begin to wonder what kind of messages they have for this kind of group, as opposed to where deaths are occurring at three or four months postpartum.

This clear distinction between early and late does not make sense to me and perhaps we should extend 'early' to 90 days or three months. If you look at the distribution of psychiatric deaths, mostly from suicide, by two-week blocks from delivery, you find that all the illnesses cluster within 90 days, so that this cut-off at 42 days misses them. From the psychiatric point of view, you could then probably afford to forget about the rest, because there is then this long space where nobody dies, and then they start coming in again at 11 months – and presumably for the rest of their lives. From the psychiatric point of view, the puerperium almost stops at about 90 days – and that would capture most of these.

My other question is, what can we do about having no psychiatric assessors? We have no access to psychiatric notes. Every one of these deaths will have had a suicide audit, and there will have been reports to coroners, but we have none of it.

Lewis: On the first point, about definitions of deaths, Dr Oates and I know only too well that we have to put our suicide deaths arbitrarily into the indirect chapter, or the late indirect chapter, depending on which day they happen to do it. That goes back to the question that I am concerned about, as to what is the definition of a maternal death. It is absolutely clear that maternal deaths extend beyond 42 days. We have been doing late deaths for many years and it is absolutely clear that a number of these should not actually be classified as late and ought to be included in our statistics. That is particularly the case for the deaths that you are concerned with.

When we look at the extra deaths that we picked up recently on the study, they were up to five months mainly and then they dropped off, and we had missed all those cases. So (1) is the World Health Organization definition and (2) is that, in terms of international statistics, do we have to carry on using this 42-day criterion for us to be marked against other countries? However, as I said earlier, we already include a large number of deaths that other countries do not – including suicides. We could run the psychiatric section from now on with a later timeframe, but we still have to pull out these deaths. So yes, you are absolutely right – we have to think about this.

Second, how do we carry out the case assessments? Two reports ago, I took over maternal death reports. Just as a matter of note, we no longer call them fortuitous deaths, but coincidental, because fortuitous implies something happy. There was a chapter on coincidental deaths. It was two pages long and there was one table which, at the bottom, said 'Suicides – 17' – and that was it. It is only for the last six years that we have been trying to get a handle on this and, as you know, I have no funding or resources. That is why I am trying to link in with some of the psychiatric assessors from the other enquiries. It is vitally important that we expand this role and this is a recommendation that we should make.

I am trying my best to find ways around it and, from now on, I am insisting that the incident report form and the suicide report form be sent to us – otherwise we will not accept them and the cases will go back. We are trying to improve this. We then have to find some of your colleagues who will be prepared to help us at no cost.

Robson: Could I ask you to explore a little the degree of causation, or association, between suicide and pregnancy? It may relate to some of the issues that Dr Bewley was talking about, and how morbidity impacts on suicide. If you take early suicide and late suicide, how does the relative risk of dying in the puerperium compare with the relative risk of dying outside of the one-year interval?

Oates: The suicide rate for women is 3.4/100 000, or about one-third of the rate for men. It has long been assumed that pregnancy and having a child under the age of two years is protective but, if you do standardised mortality rates, there are two groups of women who are at increased risk – increased above the rate of non-pregnant women. One group is the very young women in early pregnancy, which comes through quite clearly in the findings, and the other is women in the first 28 days following delivery. We have worked out – and this is not in the Confidential Enquiry – that the suicide rate of women with puerperal psychosis is 2.0/1000, compared to 3.4/100 000 of maternities.

Robson: What about the totality of the early puerperal population? What is the risk factor?

Oates: Two per thousand women delivered will suffer from a puerperal psychosis – an enormously elevated risk but of course it is still extremely small numbers and therefore escapes notice.

Van den Broek: My question is related to something mentioned by both Dr Lewis and Dr Bewley – age and risk and, in particular, the group of women below the age of 20 years.

It is quite interesting to see what problems there are with care in this country and developing countries, and that they overlap – such as in unwanted pregnancy, late or no antenatal care, illiteracy and lack of respect for the patient. Second, I note that there is a large volume of literature, also from developing countries, stating or contradicting that teenagers are at particular risk. If you separate out all these issues of not coming to antenatal care and not having an unwanted pregnancy and so on, is age still a risk factor? Can we give a clear recommendation on this yet?

Lewis: We could not separate out very young girls, because the numbers were too small to give an evidence-based recommendation. We were describing the circumstances in which these poor girls died, which were truly awful. One of my major recommendations is that they have simply lost touch with social care – it is not a healthcare issue, so much as that the social services were failing them. We should be alert to them, and perhaps we should alert social services to be particularly aware of the healthcare needs of very young girls – including contraception, abortion and follow up if they are admitted to hospital.

Dr Bewley mentioned *in vitro* fertilisation (IVF) and I would like to bring that in, because I am also responsible for the IVF policy. We have been trying very hard recently to get journalists to run stories in papers saying, 'If you are over 40, please try to forget IVF'. The first one that was sympathetic to our cause came out in the *Sunday Times* about three weeks ago. It is clear that IVF is causing problems for us and older women. We have this rule now about two embryos but, as you know, private clinics are still trying to get round that under certain circumstances. We are trying to address this, but we need to recognise that we cannot just tell women to hold off. I was 40 years old when I had my child, and many of us in this room are in the group that we are talking about stopping. We have to be more upfront with the public about the risks and we can be absolutely certain in telling women over the age of 35 years that they run higher risks of a range of problems, including maternal morbidity and mortality.

Robinson: I particularly wanted to come in on this question of social work. I was late yesterday because we had an extremely long meeting at the Department of Health, expressing our concerns, with some of our clients, about the devastation caused in families by intervention of social workers. We have not seen a beneficial intervention yet. There is no adequate evidence base – indeed, there is virtually no evidence base – of benefits of intervention. We have a number of families who, after contact with social workers and fear of future referrals, now do not go near any healthcare facility at all. The last three or four years have opened up a whole new world to us.

Following recent cases, where I have sat in with clients on meetings with social workers on conferences and so on, I will never call an NHS consultant arrogant again! I apologise for every time I have said it in the past, to each and every one.

Drife: That is most uplifting! Much appreciated!

Robinson: Looking through, when we have access to case notes – the quality, the bias and the sheer dishonesty! I say that, having sat in and made my own notes on meetings, and then accessed case notes. It is simply unbelievable.

As with healthcare, I know that we are not seeing a representative sample, but we are seeing samples where people have problems. However, when we have someone running a maternal death enquiry saying that we need to involve social workers, I would say they should think cautiously about this.

Lewis: I did not actually say social workers – my comment about the young girls was that they were already in care. We can dispute whether they should have been in care, but they were, and they were let down. In some ways, I am underlining what you are saying. We face a major learning curve. If we have women who are in touch with social services, then we are beholden to contact social services in the best way possible.

Marteau: I wanted to thank Dr Lewis for giving us such a strong example of the inverse care law. I have a comment and a question about staff attitudes. The message I took from Dr Lewis's presentation was that staff attitudes will be important in influencing the communication between staff and the women who have accessed care and the kind of care that they then have the influence to shape.

Thinking about what we know about people's attitudes towards helping, we have very little research about the attitudes of obstetric staff. I am thinking about the social psychology work on general attitudes towards helping behaviour, and there seem to be two core beliefs that drive people's attitudes towards whether or not we help somebody else. One of these is the extent to which we blame others for the situation in which they find themselves, and you seemed to be hinting that this could be a belief that might be influencing staff not to do all they could to help some of these women.

The other core belief that seems to influence people's attitudes towards helping, and whether we go out of our way to help others, is the extent to which we think doing something will make a difference. It may well be that one of the key attitudes here is born of a sense of helplessness. Those are some observations to flag up that it is terribly important for us to understand more about what is driving staff. Some of them are burnt out, and some have their own problems that prevent them from driving forward. However, for any initiative to be successful from the top down, right to service delivery, we have to become more sophisticated in understanding what is driving staff behaviour in this context. Are you aware of any initiatives that are looking at these kinds of issues?

Lewis: Yes. Staff attitude is a huge issue, and you know more about communications than I do. Some of the assessors around the table who have read the case notes will tell you about the dismissive tone and some of the attitudes.

Ms Robinson is able to say things that I cannot. I remember that when I first took the Enquiry over, it was an old-fashioned enquiry. Under 'substandard care', if you remember, it had 'women's actions'. The first thing that Ms Robinson did when I took it over was to telephone me and tell me that these women are not responsible, necessarily, for their actions. They are not the cause of their own substandard care and we have to understand what it is that stops them from seeking care or what has gone wrong. That was a very powerful message that she gave me and I have always worked with that. However, we have a long way to go to explain to most healthcare workers that people who default, discharge themselves early or do not take whatever medicine is prescribed actually have their own reasons for doing that, and that it is not necessarily a fault that can be blamed on them. We have to understand what makes people do that.

Drife: We have taken the first step of recognising that it is a problem. I have phrased it in some of my talks as 'How do you give care to people that you do not like?', which is what a professional does, of course.

De Swiet: My question directly follows on from Professor Marteau's and it is perhaps more sensitive, so Dr Lewis may choose not to answer it. Does the ethnicity of the healthcare provider seem to matter? I am thinking particularly of people who may have come from a different culture, who have quite different attitudes from those prevalent in this country.

Lewis: It is fairly obvious that, in some of our reports, you can tell the ethnicity of the healthcare provider from some of their comments. There were not many, but one or two examples.

Under the Data Protection Act and the new laws that are coming in, which will make this Enquiry even more difficult, we are not allowed to collect any information about the names or institutions of the healthcare provider, although we can state positions. Therefore, in order to be able to continue this Enquiry, I cannot collect this information. That is not a cop-out – that is the requirement I have to comply with.

Drife: It is very disconcerting sometimes.

Graham: I have two questions relating to possible follow-on work from the latest Confidential Enquiry into Maternal Deaths. Dr Lewis made the very important point about substandard care, which is a key element to which we need to refer in our recommendations. You commented that the level of substandard care had remained at the same level for an extremely long time. Internationally, one sees very similar levels of substandard care and in fact I showed some of those data yesterday. Will you be looking at how the pattern of that substandard care has changed over that time?

Second, there is an opportunity to look at some of the issues in the CEMD using more sophisticated techniques, such as multivariate analysis, in order to work out the relative importance of different explanatory factors. I mentioned Ibison's work yesterday,[1] which was based on the fairly old UK data and I am wondering whether you are considering repeating such multivariate analysis for the most recent CEMD, particularly as this can be an efficient way to deal with the problem of small numbers of cases. I realise that the CEMD does not itself necessarily have the resources to complete the analysis alone but perhaps collaboration with a research group might be one way forward.

Lewis: The sensitive point is that I have no money and I run this Enquiry by myself, as you might have gathered. It is up to the grace and favour of people I can persuade and whose arms I can twist, even to do the ONS study. I hope we will be able to change that.

In terms of substandard care, this is the 50th year of this enquiry, so we are about to write a major paper for the next book on substandard care. I am beginning to start unpacking that. This is important. We set our criteria for substandard care low, in a sense: we are being much more critical than we might be in some cases. However, the substandard care is the same thing – and I have been reading all the reports recently because I have to talk next week on 50 years of it. It is the same things all the way through.

Professor Drife showed the impact that the report has had on improving substandard care in some areas. For example, there are our thromboprophylaxis and haemorrhage rates, and we have not celebrated in this meeting the successes that we have demonstrated so well in the last report. This report has actually shown that guidelines work in a way that we have never seen in any other publication in this country for a long time.

Why it is still continuing – it is still the juniors, it is still misdiagnosis out of hours, the same old story. However, we must also look at the impact of the guidelines and remember that the recommendations that have come out of this report will have prompted the College to produce guidelines and had a significant effect on some women's health in this country.

Greer: I come back to the issue of age, which is tending to alter in terms of when women have their children. When you talk to women, the relative risk and the absolute risk that you present to them is still relatively modest. We may see that the relative and absolute risk is significant, but these women tend not to see these figures as very important – particularly when you balance that against the biological drive to have a child.

Obstetricians do not pay enough attention to age either. Similarly, I do not think they pay enough attention to body mass index (BMI). We see many women with very high BMIs encountering problems, but no one along the way treats them specially or differently, even though they have substantially higher levels of mortality and of morbidity, both for the mother and the fetus.

That brings me to the IVF scenario, where many older women are being allowed to conceive and yet they run substantial risks, as we would all agree. As far as I am aware, very few have pre-pregnancy counselling, at least by anyone with an interest in maternal medicine. They may have that counselling by someone with an interest in providing IVF, but I suspect that that is not the best practitioner to deliver that information.

I am concerned that, if we are to make a recommendation, we cannot say that women aged over 35 years should not have children, because these women will continue to have children and ignore us. However, we should perhaps recommend that women over 35 years going for things like assisted conception actually seek prepregnancy counselling and advice from people who understand the maternal problems of pregnancy. Many of these women have additional medical problems, which is very common, and often these are entirely ignored by the IVF people. A common scenario is women at a high thromboembolic risk being exposed to superphysiological levels of oestrogen, carrying a very high level of thromboembolism but with no prophylaxis in place.

I would like to see us push forward for better care for women over 35 years, seeing people who can deal with their problems, as opposed to trying to stop these women becoming pregnant. It is not a problem that will go away – I am aware that women over 40 years old are pushing hard to have more than three embryos put back under the human rights legislation, where they say that their clock is ticking away in terms of success with IVF. They therefore want three embryos put back and it is against the human rights legislation for them to be restricted in that choice. We will be faced with more and more difficult problems: we cannot stop it, but we can offer these women better counselling before pregnancy and better care during their pregnancy by making sure that they see people with particular expertise.

Drife: Thank you very much, Professor Greer. I will not ask Dr Lewis to comment on that, because it leads rather nicely on to Dr Bewley's presentation. I had made a note – if I could just ask Dr Bewley – about the relationship of age as a risk factor for morbidity. Could you remind me how age figured in your survey?

Bewley: Over 34 years, morbidity increased by 1.5 times and by nearly 1.8 for severe haemorrhage. That is for everybody over 35 years, and in my unit that accounts for 20% of women. It is extremely common, I agree. We can see from all these charts that, if it is 1.5 over 34 years, then it will be 1.6, 1.7, to whatever, and on and on upwards.

I agree with your comments about prepregnancy counselling. My feeling about the mechanism for that would be to make it a function of the HFEA to say that clinics will not be granted a licence until they can see their protocols for medical conditions A, B, C and D. We heard a recent story about a patient with cystic fibrosis having triplets and not even being referred for booking until 24 weeks, which is just a disaster. Licences should be withdrawn because those are bad doctors, offering no prepregnancy counselling and giving no consideration to the numbers of embryos put back in those situations. The mechanism for that must be the licensing of the clinics, and then age is one of many factors.

The biological drive to have children is very strong. What women do not realise in the demographic shift is that they are experiencing a clash between 'having it all' and deferring child-rearing. They are trying to have financial security and careers on the one hand and have children late, on the other, which results in more miscarriage, more infertility and more complications. We should not deal with individuals because that is far too painful. We need to think about how social policy affects the demographic shift.

I suspect that the demographic shift is related to the position of women in society, and there must be mechanisms to counteract it. Just as sex education in schools is thought to reduce teenage pregnancy, I suspect that general education about the dangers of having children late may focus women's minds that this is not something that can and should be deferred. We should call it a 'middle-age pregnancy reduction programme' – not to the individuals, because that will not stop them, but to get the demographic shift moved back.

Drife: It is quite spectacular, looking through the three reports and documenting the demographic shift – which one can do from the relevant chapters in consecutive reports. Over the 1990s, in a nine-year period, there was a dramatic shift. As you say, it is not a matter of grabbing a woman and sitting her down, but it is a matter of giving information beforehand.

Oates: I just have a comment. I find myself becoming quite annoyed when I hear the word 'choice' in this matter. As far as I know, the factor that is related to increasing maternal age is increasing female education. It is rather like, 'Don't put your daughter on the stage, Mrs Worthington'. As soon as you put your female child – and that applies to everyone in this room – through her 'A' levels, her age of first childbirth moves up. As soon as she goes to university, it goes up further. As soon as she has a higher professional qualification, it goes up again.

If the Royal College of Obstetricians and Gynaecologists is to make a public policy drive to reduce middle-age pregnancies, it will have to run a dating agency. Otherwise, what will happen to all these delightful, gorgeous junior doctors that I see floating around the place, who cannot get a bloke for love nor money? The more educated you are, the more conservative you become and most people these days do not have babies out of the blue – they wait for a bloke – but young blokes do not marry girls with degrees. The reason why these women are getting married later and later is because we have educated them.

Bewley: And men do not like it?

Oates: You said that, not me! But you cannot have your cake and eat it. The reason why we all have to have our menopauses treated is because we are now the mothers of very young children while we are having hot flushes, and so we have to put that off too.

Drife: I feel that we are in very deep water! It is such a huge issue that I am somewhat overwhelmed.

Robinson: On severe morbidity, I would particularly like to ask Dr Bewley a question about emergency hysterectomies. We are having more cases reported to us and supporting these women is tough. When one talks about maternal death, it is very hard to listen to women who say, 'They did that to save my life, but I would much rather be dead!' They say this over and over again. 'They did not give me a choice: I would rather be dead'.

The woman who came out of it well did have a choice, because she was under epidural and it was explained to her. She knew the situation and was party to the decision. She might have been the sort of woman who would have reacted well anyway, but we are finding it really tough out there – our work is becoming harder too. There does not seem to be automatic referral to appropriate services. I would like us to look more at long-term morbidity. Since, according to your earlier report and to what we are coming across, this has been increasing – for understandable reasons – does anyone have any ideas on this?

Bewley: We want to do a paper on hysterectomies – we had 34 out of the 50000, which gives a rate of about 7:10 000. I do not think there are so many reports in the literature to be able to say what is the rate and whether it is going up or not.

Regarding the fertility wishes of the women who had hysterectomies, but who had been planning further children, they had extremely high scores on the Edinburgh Postnatal Depression Scale later. This all makes sense. If more women had regional anaesthesia when you were discussing these things – marvellous – but hysterectomy is not usually a cool and calm situation. It worries me that it looks as though it is also associated with placenta praevia, which is associated with previous caesarean sections, and therefore there is a cycle of problems going on there. We have had an outbreak of placenta praevia locally with that.

Hall: This is a very simple point. The absolute risk for older women is very small, and women quite correctly perceive that, as Professor Greer said. I would certainly not want to be involved in any way with a programme for telling women off for being older. The relative risk may be increased but the absolute risk is very small. In exactly the same way, we counsel women about risks from the contraceptive pill, for example. We point out to them that the absolute risk is tiny – even if it might be increased, and there might be an increased risk for thromboembolism; in practical terms it is not actually very significant.

Neilson: Dr Bewley, you presented some fascinating data and some very interesting ideas. In your opinion, should there be a routine national system of collecting data about severe morbidity? If so, what sort of routine data collection systems would be required to capture that information?

Bewley: I do not know. I suspect that we are at too early a stage without good enough definitions to know what we should be doing. Talking about the work involved, this was a £75,000 grant with one researcher and two years of work. It is an enormous amount of work to do on a population basis. I do not think this can be done.

In the same way as we started with deaths and complications meetings, perinatal mortality and morbidity meetings, and these evolved into confidential enquiries on death – obstetric, surgical, stillbirths and infant deaths – a vast range. The scope of this is far wider. Looking at the value of local audit on near-miss is relatively easy. The national sentinel audits that we have seen on caesarean section – and we could apply that to some factors – might also be possible.

We need a great deal more research to give us a handle on the definitions and the incidence before we get into this. There are many initiatives around national maternity notes coming up again from the National Patient Safety Agency, and this is the opportunity to get that minimum dataset collected nationally. That would give us something to start just the number-crunching before we become too sophisticated.

Let me make one last comment about attitude. I was very interested that Dr Hall talked about 'telling off'. We have no hesitation about having teenage pregnancy reduction programmes, and you used the words 'telling off'. There is something going on here in attitudes to what is acceptable pregnancy and what is not acceptable pregnancy. The relative and the absolute risks of being pregnant at 18 or 16 years of age are exactly the same. All I suggest is that the Royal College of Obstetricians and Gynaecologists should say that the best time, biologically, for a pregnancy is between the ages of 20 years and 35 years, which is true. I do not want to tell these older women off – I just think that the demographic shift is bad for them.

Cooper: It would not surprise me if Dr Yentis might have been going to say the same thing. With regard to Ms Robinson's comment about caesarean hysterectomies – do not make the mistake of believing that it is just the patients who find it worrying – I can tell you that the healthcare professionals do. However, if you advocate that you want them done under regional anaesthesia, you will see more deaths – just so that the patient can be informed beforehand. Obviously, it is much better if you can predict those patients who will run into this problem and obtain consent beforehand, but it is never real until it happens. To have someone bleeding to death under regional anaesthesia just so that they can give consent? No, thank you.

Robinson: No, I was not advocating it. I was simply saying, coincidentally, that one woman who had not come out of it so badly happened to have been told beforehand that it was really necessary and had agreed. She therefore had the opportunity to refuse and had the right – as any woman has – to say 'I don't want that done. I would rather die!' She had the opportunity but she did not take it.

There are other women who say, retrospectively, 'I would rather have died'. Whether, at the time, they would have done, one does not know. We are not advocating it, but it was simply that on that occasion there was an element at least of prior knowledge, if not of real choice.

Tuffnell: I do not particularly want to get into swapping anecdotes, but I would just counter that consideration. I ended up doing a caesarean hysterectomy and tying off internal iliacs on a woman who my anaesthetist kept awake all the way through, even when she bled down to a haemoglobin level of 2 g/dl. That woman has been having enormous trouble with flashbacks about everything that happened ever since, as have I.

Drife: It is reality, when it intrudes into our discussions. It is uncomfortable.

De Swiet: I have a question on which I am sure Dr Nelson-Piercy should also comment. This relates to the throwaway comment that it was perfectly obvious – or something like that – that women on anticonvulsant drugs should have greater morbidity. In fact, the risk ratio, or however you expressed it, was a figure of five, which was the highest of the risk ratios, but I did not understand that. We know that people with epilepsy die, but I do not see why they should have more morbidity, unless 'epileptic drugs' is only a surrogate for social class.

Bewley: If I said that, I did not mean it. I may have been referring to all medical conditions – if you are hypertensive, if you are epileptic or whatever – and, in a way, it is not surprising that there would be more morbidity in a group that started off unwell. I have puzzled over why anticonvulsants should be related to haemorrhage – I do not understand the physiology of that. I am sorry if I said the wrong thing.

Nelson-Piercy: One possible explanation is that there are quite good prospective data suggesting that the caesarean section rate is higher in women with epilepsy, for several very complicated reasons.

Bewley: But that should have come out in the multivariate analysis. This is independent of caesarean section.

Drife: Professor Pattinson – a propos of the question asked of Dr Bewley – £75,000, one person to look after 19 units – we could do it nationally if we had 20 people doing the same thing, and costing 20 times as much, I guess, if there is a full-time person.

Pattinson: The way the system works is that every morning an audit is done within the institution. We have a single-page datasheet and then we put that on computer. That is how it is done – it is a routine part of our practice and part of our daily function, so it is not particularly difficult to maintain. We spent a fair amount of time trying to get the datasheet right but, once that was achieved, it ran on autopilot.

Drife: Is the information collected by you, or by somebody who goes round picking it up?

Pattinson: Each morning, if there was a near-miss, in that case it was flagged up and a report was written on it.

Hall: Professor Marteau mentioned briefly yesterday that the current risk management structures will certainly pick up all the cases that you would want for a near-miss enquiry. We find that the South African system, which is system-based plus intensive care, works very well – we are using that at the moment in Scotland on our maternity units and we do not find it is a problem.

Just trying to marry together the data from the South African and the London study, there is no scientific basis for having any particular threshold. With some things, such as cardiac arrest, it is all or nothing anyway, and so there is no difficulty there. However, if it is haemorrhage, you could make it any cut-off point that you want. One issue that you would have to consider is the number of cases that you could handle in terms of trying to look for substandard care. So there is no real scientific basis for that – it is a practical decision. Using the system-based structure, in most of the decisions there is no difficulty in identifying that there is a major organ problem.

De Swiet: My feelings are exactly the same as yours, Dr Hall. I was saying to myself that this is rather like gestational diabetes – there is no proper scientific definition of gestational diabetes, so let us make the cut-off at the level of abnormality that we can cope with. However, you could also turn it round and say that perhaps the ratio of morbidity to mortality ought to be 1:100, and then we could define major obstetric haemorrhage in terms of the figure that gives a 1:100 ratio.

Hall: You could certainly do that. I know that it is theoretically attractive to look at it, comparing one area with another, and that has been useful in South Africa. The ratio will be entirely dependent on what your cut-off point was for the incidence of severe morbidity.

Drife: One of the most interesting points was the way in which the severe acute maternal morbidities varied – the actual intrinsic variations.

Bewley: It would be very interesting to study one of the conditions, to answer the other question that was raised about standards of care. One reason why the standard of care has not changed is that the standard has gone up and 50% is the right motivating factor for health professionals. It is not that I would criticise the Confidential Enquiry, but the standard is that 'it might have been better if', by a group of experts in a room, and it has absolutely nothing to do with standards that are defined beforehand and then examined.

What was very nice about the model of either haemorrhage or depression or interventions such as caesarean sections is that you can actually set standards. It would be relatively simple to look at whether standards of care changed along that variable of size of postpartum haemorrhage (PPH), i.e. 1 litre, 2 litres, 3 litres etc., and how women reach the point of massive haemorrhage. There is some evidence out there and you could collect a group of experts and ask them to define the standards – how long to diagnose it, how long to get to the operating theatre, ergometrine as a drug of choice and so on. You could then put those standards in with large numbers and test them. That would be very helpful.

My worry about starting now on data collection based entirely on organ dysfunction is that it is hospital-based – although, in intensive care units and with Apache scores, that is manageable. However, it distorts the whole debate towards that – which may be fair enough. The nice point about Professor Pattinson's safety nets is that they show that you have the maximum effect if you get that primary care right. That primary care, and the primary caregiver, and the first intervention on PPH, I suspect, will be the most important. Therefore, we should look at the whole range of a common condition such as haemorrhage or depression, just we start to try to collect the near-miss data, but I am not sure that basing it on organ systems is right. I would hate to become entrenched in something when it is so early in terms of the definitions. Perhaps the system of the Confidential Enquiry into Stillbirths and Deaths in Infancy midwife also being the near-miss midwife in every single unit is a good one to adopt.

Drife: We are approaching something, but we will not achieve it before the coffee-break. I was going to adopt the non-evidence-based system that when the chairman's blood sugar drops below a certain level, that is when we stop. Let us give the last word to Dr de Bernis.

De Bernis: I have a question for Professor Pattinson: based on your experience, could you say a few words about how to implement this practice at a national level? We think that it is very important to improve the quality of care through these audits and near-miss enquiries. It is also a matter of making clear to practitioners that the quality of data is related to the quality of care, and vice versa, and we cannot imagine improving the quality of care without improving the reporting of cases and so on.

I do not know whether your experience is based on your decision to lead your service in this direction, or whether it is linked with national policies on recommendations. The World Health Organization is trying to support this activity at a national level. We are publishing a guideline to explain all these methodologies and to give practitioners the opportunity to choose the best strategy for them. However, the question is how to convince the leaders of maternity services to start in this direction, and to make this feasible on a daily basis of work.

Do you have any experience of that? Is there any recommendation that you can provide to us, to help countries to start on that?

Pattinson: In terms just of policy, our Government wants all institutions to run maternal and perinatal mortality meetings, so that is part of policy. As to how one institutes this in other places, I think you need an enthusiast. You need sentinel sites at the start; these then bring other people on board. If you wanted it in one country, you would start with a hospital where someone was keen: he would start it and talk to his colleagues and others then come on board. I do not see that you can ever say from the top down that you are going to institute this policy, because it has to be grown organically by enthusiasts.

Reference

1. Ibison JM, Swerdlow AJ, Head JA, Marmot M. Maternal mortality in England and Wales 1970–1985: an analysis by country of birth. *Br J Obstet Gynaecol* 1996;103:973–80.

SECTION 4

SPECIFIC PROBLEMS OF MORTALITY AND MORBIDITY I

Chapter 14

Venous thromboembolism and thrombophilia

Ian Greer

Introduction

Pulmonary thromboembolism (PTE) remains the leading cause of maternal mortality in the UK.[1] PTE arises from deep venous thrombosis (DVT), which is frequently not recognised clinically before PTE occurs. DVT is associated with a significant risk of recurrent thrombosis and deep venous insufficiency, as well as the acute morbidity and mortality of venous thromboembolism (VTE), while PTE carries a risk of subsequent pulmonary hypertension.

Epidemiology and pathophysiology

The incidence of DVT has been estimated at 0.615/1000 maternities in women under 35 years of age and at 1.216/1000 maternities in women over 35 years of age in the antenatal period and at 0.304/1000 maternities in women under 35 years of age and 0.72/1000 maternities in women over 35 years of age in the puerperium.[2] While antenatal DVT is more common than postpartum DVT, the event rate is higher in the puerperium.[2,3] Accurate data are available for fatal PTE because of the UK Confidential Enquiries into Maternal Deaths. The overall incidence of fatal PTE has fallen substantially from the early 1950s; however, the greatest reduction in the number of deaths has been in those following vaginal delivery. Nonetheless, in the last 10–20 years there has been no further reduction in fatalities after vaginal delivery[1] and the number of deaths during the antenatal and intrapartum period has changed little since the early 1950s despite major advances in identification of risk and thromboprophylaxis and diagnostic and therapeutic intervention over this same period. The total number of deaths following caesarean section had changed little since the 1950s until the RCOG guideline on thromboprophylaxis was published in 1995[4] and after its introduction the number of deaths fell dramatically. This highlights the usefulness of appropriate thromboprophylaxis following caesarean section and, perhaps more importantly, emphasises the need for better prophylaxis in the antenatal period and after vaginal delivery.

The major risk factors for VTE in pregnancy are:

- age of over 35 years
- caesarean section, particularly as an emergency in labour
- operative vaginal delivery
- body mass index (BMI) greater than 29 kg/m^2
- heritable or acquired thrombophilia[5]
- history of DVT or PTE
- gross varicose veins
- current infection or inflammatory process (e.g. active inflammatory bowel disease, urinary tract infection)
- pre-eclampsia
- immobility
- significant current medical problem (e.g. nephrotic syndrome, cardiac failure)
- paraplegia.

Following DVT, there is a risk of deep venous insufficiency. Over 60% of women will have objectively confirmed deep venous insufficiency following a treated DVT, and almost 80% will develop post-thrombotic syndrome. The odds ratio for developing venous insufficiency after a DVT has been estimated at 10.9 (95% CI 4.2–28.0) compared with 3.8 (95% CI 1.2–12.3) after a PTE.[6] The difference may be due to the thrombus clearing from the legs in those women with PTE, resulting in less extensive damage to the deep venous system.

Virchow's classic triad of factors underlying venous thrombosis – hypercoagulability, venous stasis and vascular damage – all occur in the course of normal pregnancy and delivery. Hypercoagulability is brought about by:

1. the substantial increase in levels of coagulation factors including von Willebrand factor, factor VIII and fibrinogen
2. an acquired resistance to the endogenous anticoagulant, activated protein C that occurs in almost 40% of normal pregnancies
3. a reduction in protein S, the co-factor for protein C[7]
4. impaired fibrinolysis through increases in plasminogen activator inhibitors 1 and 2, the latter being produced by the placenta.[8]

It is noteworthy that in the non-pregnant situation high factor VIII levels and resistance to activated protein C are associated with an increased risk of VTE. A substantial reduction in venous flow, as measured by ultrasound, occurs by the end of the first trimester, progressing to around a 50% reduction by the end of the second trimester, reaching a nadir at 36 weeks of gestation[9] and taking around six weeks to return to normal non-pregnant flowrates. Endothelial damage to pelvic vessels can occur during the course of vaginal delivery or caesarean section.

More than 70% of DVT in pregnancy are located in the iliofemoral region. This contrasts with the non-pregnant situation, where only around 9% of DVT are located in the ilio-femoral area, the majority being calf-vein thrombosis. This is important, as iliofemoral DVT are more likely to generate PTE than isolated calf-vein thrombosis. Almost 90% of DVT affect the left side in pregnancy. This contrasts with the non-pregnant situation, where only 55% occur on the left.[5,10] This may be due to compression of the left iliac vein by the right iliac artery and the ovarian artery, which cross the vein on the left side only.

Thrombophilia and venous thromboembolism

Thrombophilia is found in many women with a VTE in pregnancy. The major heritable forms of thrombophilia recognised currently include deficiencies of the endogenous anticoagulant proteins, antithrombin, protein C and protein S, abnormalities of procoagulant factors, particularly factor V Leiden and the prothrombin gene variant, prothrombin 20210A.

Hyperhomocysteinaemia has been linked to VTE in the non-pregnant situation[11] and is associated with homozygosity for a variation in the methylene-tetrahydrofolate reductase gene (MTHFR C677T), which occurs in around 10% of the UK population. This genotype is not directly linked to venous thrombosis, as it requires to interact with dietary deficiency of B vitamins and, in contrast to the non-pregnant situation, this genotype has not been associated with an increased risk of maternal VTE.[12–14] The lack of association might reflect the physiological fall in homocysteine levels seen in normal pregnancy or the effects of folic acid supplements.

Deficiencies of antithrombin, protein C and protein S, where the major components of the body's endogenous anticoagulant system are defective due to quantitative or qualitative defects, can underlie thrombotic problems in pregnancy.[15] These abnormalities have a combined prevalence of less than 1% in Europe (the prevalence of protein S deficiency has not yet been clearly established) and collectively they will be found in less than 10% of cases of VTE. Factor V Leiden produces resistance to activated protein C, the endogenous anticoagulant directed against factor Va and factor VIIIa. Activated protein C inhibits coagulation by proteolytic cleavage of these factors. With factor V Leiden, this resistance is due to a single point mutation in the factor V gene at the cleavage site where activated protein C acts. This results in a potentially hypercoagulable effect. Factor V Leiden has a prevalence of around 2–7% in Western Europe,[15] but can be identified in 20–40% of patients with VTE.[16] Activated protein C resistance, however, can be caused by problems other than factor V Leiden, including antiphospholipid antibody syndrome and other genetic defects in the factor V molecule, and it can also be acquired in pregnancy,[7] possibly due to increases in factor V and factor VIII. The so-called prothrombin gene variant (prothrombin 20210G) is present in around 2% of the population and associated with elevated plasma prothrombin levels, and it increases risk of venous thrombosis three-fold.[17] This variant is found in around 6% of patients with VTE and in 18% of those with a family history of VTE,[17] and it has been linked to gestational VTE.[14,18]

While heritable thrombophilias are present in at least 15% of Western populations[19,20] and underlie around 50% of episodes of VTE in pregnancy, the incidence of VTE is only around 0.1% in pregnancy. Therefore, the presence of a thrombophilia alone, even when combined with the physiological prothrombotic changes in coagulation and venous flow found in pregnancy, does not usually result in VTE. It is now clear that clinical VTE in women with thrombophilia reflects a multicausal event resulting from the interaction between congenital and acquired risk factors.[20] The level of risk will depend on the underlying thrombophilic defect(s), history of thrombotic events and additional risk factors such as obesity. It is important to establish the risk of thrombosis in pregnancy in women with thrombophilia to guide thromboprophylaxis.

Initial estimates for the risk of VTE in pregnancy in women with thrombophilia, in the absence of anticoagulant therapy, were high, for example up to 60% in antithrombin-deficient women.[15,21–23] Estimates for the risk of VTE in pregnancy are 3–10% for protein C deficiency and 0–6% for protein S deficiency, rising to 7–19% for protein C deficiency and 7–22% for protein S deficiency postpartum[15,21,22] However, these data came from observational studies of symptomatic thrombophilic kindreds that will overestimate the risk in asymptomatic kindred. Factor V Leiden has been found in up to 46% of women investigated for venous thrombosis in pregnancy[23] but, again, this reflects the investigation of women with VTE. Recent studies provide estimates for the risk of VTE in pregnancy in the more common thrombophilias; Gerhardt *et al.*[13] studied 119 women with VTE in pregnancy and 233 controls for the presence of congenital thrombophilia. The relative risk for thrombosis in pregnancy after adjusting for other key variables was 6.9 (95% CI 3.3–15.2) with factor V Leiden, 9.5 (95% CI 2.1–66.7) with prothrombin 20210G and 10.4 (95% CI 2.2–62.5) for antithrombin deficiency. Combined defects substantially increase risk, with an odds ratio estimated at 107 for the combination of factor V Leiden and prothrombin G20210A in pregnancy, which is higher than the risk of VTE when these defects are combined outwith pregnancy. Additional risk factors such as obesity were present in 25% of the cases, compared with 11% of controls. Women with recurrent VTE were more likely to have underlying combined thrombophilic defects, protein C or antithrombin deficiency, or prothrombin 20210A. This study also provided a positive predictive value for each thrombophilia, assuming an underlying rate of venous thromboembolism of 0.66/1000 pregnancies, consistent with estimates from Western populations.[19] These values were 1:500 for factor V Leiden, 1:200 for prothrombin 20210A and 4.6:100 for these defects combined. This work is complemented by a retrospective study of 72 000 pregnancies where women with VTE were assessed for thrombophilia[5] and where the underlying prevalence of these defects in the population was known. The risk of thrombosis was 1:437 for factor V Leiden, 1:113 for protein C deficiency, 1:2.8 for type 1 (quantitative) antithrombin deficiency and 1:42 for type 2 (qualitative) antithrombin deficiency. This study was recently extended[14] and reported an odds ratio of 4.4 (95% CI 1.2–16) for prothrombin G20210A, 4.5 (95% CI 2.1–14.5) for factor V Leiden, 282 (95% CI 31–2532) for antithrombin deficiency type 1 (quantitative deficiency) and 28 (95% CI 5.5–142) for antithrombin deficiency type 2 (qualitative deficiency) (Table 14.1).

There is no evidence at present to support routine universal screening of all pregnant women for thrombophilia. The natural history of many of these conditions, particularly in asymptomatic women, has not been established and we have not identified appropriate intervention. Furthermore, the cost of screening is significant and such screening would have to be shown to be cost-effective. In a recent assessment of the cost-effectiveness of screening for factor V Leiden in pregnancy universal screening was not found to be cost-effective.[24] There is a case for selective screening of women with VTE in pregnancy or who have a personal or family history of VTE, as around 50% of such women will have a thrombophilia.[19] There is a consensus view that women with a personal history of VTE and an underlying thrombophilia should receive

Table 14.1. Risk of venous thromboembolism (VTE) in pregnancy with thrombophilia

Thrombophilic defect	Odds ratio (95% CI) for VTE in pregnancy[a]	Relative risk (95% CI) for VTE in pregnancy[b]
AT deficiency Type 1 (quantitative deficiency)	282 (31–2532)	N/A
AT deficiency Type 2 (qualitative deficiency)	28 (5.5–142)	N/A
AT deficiency (activity < 80%)	N/A	10.4 (2.2–62.5)
Factor V Leiden	4.5 (2.1–14.5)	6.9 (3.3–15.2)
Prothrombin 20210A	4.4(1.2–16)	9.5 (2.1–66.7)
MTHFR C677TT	0.45 (0.13–1.58)	No increase in risk (RR not reported)

[a] based on a retrospective study of 93 000 pregnancies where odds ratios were calculated by screening women with VTE in pregnancy for thrombophilia and relating this to the known prevalence of these defects in the population[12]; [b] based on a study of 119 women with thromboembolism in pregnancy and 233 controls for the presence of congenital thrombophilia[12]; relative risk calculated after logistic regression to adjust for age, body mass index, oral contraceptive use, protein C and S activity, factor V Leiden, prothrombin G20210A, MTHFR 677TT and antithrombin activity

thromboprophylaxis during pregnancy and, in particular, the puerperium.[29] Screening for thrombophilia in patients with problems such as recurrent miscarriage, intrauterine death, intrauterine growth restriction and pre-eclampsia should also be considered in view of the growing evidence linking thrombophilia with these pregnancy complications.[19] If screening is to be used in these situations, it is important that we identify appropriate and effective interventions.

Recurrent venous thromboembolism in pregnancy

While there is clinical consensus that women with more than one previous VTE should receive antenatal thromboprophylaxis, the management of the woman with a single previous event is more controversial. This is because of the wide variation in reported risk, ranging from 1–13%.[25–29] The upper limit of this risk estimate has led many clinicians to use pharmacological prophylaxis with heparin or low molecular weight heparin (LMWH) during pregnancy and the puerperium. However, these studies have some limitations: objective testing was not used in all cases, some of the studies were retrospective and the prospective studies had relatively small sample sizes. Brill-Edwards *et al.*[30] recently provided valuable data for the management of these women. This was a prospective study of 125 pregnant women with a single previous objectively diagnosed VTE. No heparin was given antenatally but anticoagulant therapy, usually warfarin following an initial short course of heparin or LMWH, was given for four to six weeks postpartum. The overall antenatal recurrence rate was 2.4% (95% CI 0.2–6.9). However, there were no episodes of recurrent VTE in the 44 women (95% CI 0.0–8.0) who did not have an underlying thrombophilia and whose previous VTE had been associated with a temporary risk factor. This contrasted with women who were found to have an underlying thrombophilia or whose previous VTE was idiopathic. This group of women had an antepartum recurrence rate of 5.9% (95% CI 1.2–16.0%). These data suggest that women with a single previous event associated with a temporary risk factor and with no identifiable thrombophilia should not routinely receive heparin or LMWH antenatally. Nonetheless, given the wide confidence intervals and the implications of a further event, this decision should be discussed with the patient and her opinion should be taken into account. In women with an underlying thrombophilia or whose VTE was idiopathic, there is a much stronger case for pharmacological thromboprophylaxis.

Diagnosis of venous thromboembolism

The clinical features of DVT include leg pain or discomfort (especially on the left), swelling, tenderness, increased temperature and oedema, lower abdominal pain, mild pyrexia and elevated white cell count. Features suggestive of PTE include dyspnoea, collapse, chest pain, haemoptysis, faintness, raised jugular venous pressure, focal signs in chest, sometimes combined with the symptoms and signs of DVT. Just as in the non-pregnant, the clinical diagnosis of VTE during pregnancy is unreliable, particularly as problems such as leg-swelling and discomfort are common features of normal pregnancy. In a study of consecutive pregnant women presenting with a clinical suspicion of DVT, the diagnosis was confirmed in less than 10%.[29] This compares with around 25% of diagnoses being confirmed in the non-pregnant situation.[31,32,33] Around 30% of patients presenting with possible PTE outwith pregnancy have the diagnosis confirmed,[34,35] but the number of positive results following investigation appears to be substantially lower in pregnancy,[29] possibly because of a low threshold for investigation. Objective diagnosis of VTE in pregnancy is therefore essential, as failure to identify a VTE will endanger the mother, while unnecessary treatment will expose her to the hazards of therapeutic anticoagulation. Such treatment may also label her as having had a VTE, a factor that will significantly alter her future health care with regard to contraception, thromboprophylaxis in future pregnancies and hormone replacement therapy in later life.

Real time or Duplex ultrasound venography is the main diagnostic tool for DVT.[35] If DVT is confirmed, anticoagulant treatment should be commenced or continued. In non-pregnant subjects, the pre-test clinical probability of DVT modifies both the positive predictive value and the negative predictive value of objective diagnostic tests.[37,38] Applying this to pregnancy, a negative ultrasound result with a low level of clinical suspicion suggests that anticoagulant treatment can be discontinued or withheld. With a negative ultrasound report and a high level of clinical suspicion, the woman should be anticoagulated and ultrasound repeated in one week or alternative imaging techniques such as X-ray venography or magnetic resonance imaging (MRI) should be considered. If repeat testing is negative, anticoagulant treatment should be discontinued.[39]

Where PTE is suspected, both a ventilation/perfusion (V/Q) lung scan and bilateral duplex ultrasound leg examinations should ideally be performed. Outwith pregnancy, a normal perfusion scan has a negative predictive value of over 99% and a high-probability lung scan has a positive predictive value of over 85%. Where there is a strong clinical suspicion of PTE, the positive predictive value of a high probability lung scan increases to over 95% but with low clinical probability decreases to under 60%. The greatest diagnostic problem is when the V/Q scan is in the medium range. In practical terms, when the V/Q scan reports a 'medium' or 'high' probability of PTE or where there is a 'low' probability of PTE on V/Q scan but positive ultrasound for DVT anticoagulant treatment should be continued. When a V/Q scan reports a low risk of PTE and there are negative leg ultrasound examinations, yet there remains a high level of clinical suspicion, anticoagulant treatment should continue with repeat testing in one week (V/Q scan and leg ultrasound examination) or alternative imaging techniques such as pulmonary angiography or MRI or helical computerised tomography (CT) should be used.[39] Similarly, if the chest X-ray has abnormalities that lead to difficulties in the diagnosis of PTE using V/Q scanning, then alternative imaging techniques are warranted. Helical CT scanning is likely to be of particular value and as the test becomes more widely available will threaten the place of V/Q scans in the diagnosis of PTE. Helical CT can rapidly image the whole thorax within the time of a single breath hold with good visualisation of the pulmonary arterial tree down to the level of the segmental arteries. Technical advances are likely to allow even greater resolution and faster image acquisition times. It can sometimes be useful to employ echocardiography of the right heart, particularly when performed transoesophageally, where PTE is suspected. This may allow direct visualisation of thrombus in the pulmonary arteries or right heart. Indirect signs of PTE include a dilated hypokinetic right ventricle, tricuspid regurgitation and high pulmonary artery pressures as measured with Doppler ultrasound. It must be emphasised that the radiation dose from investigations such as V/Q scanning, chest X-ray, helical CT and even limited venography is modest[40] and considered to pose a negligible risk to the fetus, particularly when set in the context of the risk from PTE. Thus objective diagnostic testing should not be withheld because of concern regarding fetal radiation exposure.

D-dimer is now used as a screening test for VTE in non-pregnant women, where it has a high negative predictive value,[36] i.e. a low level of D-dimer suggests the absence of VTE and further objective tests are not performed, while an increased level of D-dimer leads to an objective diagnostic test for VTE. In pregnancy, D-dimer can be increased due to the physiological changes in the coagulation system and particularly if there is a concomitant problem such as pre-eclampsia. Thus, a 'positive' D-dimer test in pregnancy is not necessarily consistent with VTE and objective diagnostic testing is required. However, a low level of D-dimer in pregnancy is likely, as in the non-pregnant, to suggest that there is no VTE. Nonetheless, there is limited information on the efficacy and safety of D-dimer screening for VTE in pregnancy and, until more information is available, firm guidance cannot be given.

Thrombophilia screening at the time of presentation and before starting anticoagulant therapy can sometimes be useful in women with VTE.

- APTT, prothrombin time and thrombin time
- activated protein C resistance (NB genetic testing for factor V Leiden is only required where there is evidence of activated protein C resistance on the modified test for aPC resistance that predilutes the test sample with factor V deficient plasma)
- protein C deficiency
- protein S deficiency
- antithrombin deficiency
- prothrombin 20210A mutation
- lupus anticoagulant

- anticardiolipin antibodies (IgG and IgM).

This should include a family history of thrombosis. Although the results of a thrombophilia screen will not influence immediate management, they may influence the duration and intensity of anticoagulation, for example when antithrombin deficiency is identified. It is important to be aware of the effects of pregnancy and thrombus on the results of a thrombophilia screen. For example, protein S levels fall in normal pregnancy, making it extremely difficult to make a diagnosis of protein S deficiency during pregnancy. Activated protein C resistance occurs in around 40% of pregnancies and anticardiolipin antibodies can also influence the result of this test. Antithrombin may be reduced when thrombus is present. Genotyping for factor V Leiden and prothrombin G20210A will not be influenced by pregnancy or thrombosis. It is important therefore that thrombophilia screens be interpreted by clinicians with specific expertise in the area.

It is interesting that, although factor V Leiden is associated with an increase in risk of VTE, this is largely due to DVT. Outwith pregnancy, the prevalence of underlying factor V Leiden in PTE is around half of that for DVT.[41] This differs from other thrombophilias such as prothrombin G20210A, where there is no difference in the underlying prevalence between DVT and PTE. It has been proposed that factor V Leiden is associated with a more adherent and stable thrombus, possibly due to increased local thrombin generation reducing the likelihood of embolisation. Whether this applies in pregnancy is not yet established.

Antithrombotic therapy

Unfractionated heparin (UFH) and LMWH are the anticoagulants of choice in pregnancy due to the fetal hazards of coumarins.[42] Warfarin is not secreted in breast milk in clinically significant amounts and is safe to use during lactation but it does cross the placenta and is a teratogen. Warfarin embryopathy (midface hypoplasia, stippled chondral calcification, scoliosis, short proximal limbs and short phalanges) can occur in around 4% and 5%[42] of cases exposed between six and nine weeks of gestation. Substitution of heparin for warfarin during the first trimester can prevent this problem. The risk of embryopathy may be dose-dependent, with an increased risk when the dose of warfarin is greater than 5 mg/day.[43] In addition to warfarin embryopathy, there is the possibility of problems arising due to fetal bleeding. As the fetal liver is immature and levels of vitamin K-dependent coagulation factors low, maternal warfarin therapy maintained in the therapeutic range will be associated with excessive anticoagulation and therefore potential bleeding problems in the fetus. Warfarin should be avoided beyond 36 weeks of gestation[42,44] because of the excessive bleeding risk to both mother and fetus in the peripartum period.

In contrast to warfarin, neither UFH[45] nor LMWH crosses the placenta,[46,47] as determined by measuring heparin activity in fetal blood, and there is no evidence of teratogenesis or risk of fetal haemorrhage. These agents appear on a systematic review to be safe for the fetus.[48] Heparins are not secreted in breast milk and can be used during breastfeeding. Prolonged use of UFH can be associated with symptomatic osteoporosis (with around a 2% incidence of osteoporotic fractures), allergy and heparin-induced thrombocytopenia.[48] LMWHs appear to have substantially less risk of osteoporosis. One study has randomised women to UFH or dalteparin for thromboprophylaxis in pregnancy and measured bone mineral density in the lumbar spine for up to three years after delivery.[50] Bone density did not differ between healthy controls and the dalteparin group but was significantly lower in the UFH group than in both controls and dalteparin-treated women. Multiple logistic regression found that the type of heparin therapy was the only independent factor associated with reduced bone mass. Heparin-induced thrombocytopenia is a rare but life-threatening adverse effect. It is an idiosyncratic immune mediated reaction associated with extensive venous thrombosis that usually occurs between five and 15 days after the institution of heparin. The risk has been estimated at 1–3% with UFH and is substantially lower with LMWH.[51] Allergic reactions usually take the form of itchy, erythematous lesions at the injection sites. Switching heparin preparations may be helpful but a degree of cross-reactivity can still occur. Allergic reactions should be distinguished from faulty injection technique with associated bruising. LMWH is now the heparin of choice in pregnancy because of a better adverse-effect profile, a good safety record for mother and fetus and once-daily dosing.[48,52–57]

Dextran should be avoided in pregnancy and alternative thromboprophylactic measures taken because of the risk of maternal anaphylactoid reactions, which have been associated with uterine hypertonus, profound fetal distress and a high incidence of fetal death or severe neurological damage.[58]

Graduated elastic compression stockings are effective in the non-pregnant and, in view of the pregnancy-related changes in the venous system, could be of considerable value in pregnancy. They may act by preventing overdistension of veins, so preventing endothelial damage and exposure of subendothelial collagen.[59] They can also be used in acute DVT. Other mechanical techniques, such as intermittent pneumatic compression, are of value during caesarean section and immediately postpartum for prophylaxis.

Hirudin, a direct thrombin inhibitor, is used in the non-pregnant for treatment of heparin-induced thrombocytopenia and also for postoperative prophylaxis. As it crosses the placenta, it should not be used in pregnancy. It has been used in a lactating mother because of heparin-induced thrombocytopenia and hirudin was not detectable in breast milk.[60]

Aspirin has been found in meta-analysis to have a beneficial effect in the prevention of DVT. Its effectiveness in pregnancy, in comparison with heparin, remains to be established, but it is likely to offer some benefit. Its effectiveness is likely to be less than that of LMWH.[61] In women who are unable to take heparin or in whom the balance of risk is not considered sufficient to merit heparin, it may be useful. Low-dose (60–75 mg daily) aspirin is not associated with adverse pregnancy outcome in the second and third trimesters.[62,63]

Management of acute venous thromboembolism

When DVT or PTE are suspected clinically, treatment with UFH or LMWH should be given until the diagnosis is excluded by objective testing, unless anticoagulation is contraindicated. Thromboembolic deterrent stockings should also be used, together with leg elevation for DVT. Analgesia for pleuritic pain and oxygen are often required in PTE. Traditionally, UFH has been used in the initial management of VTE, where such treatment reduces the risk of further thromboembolism compared with no

Table 14.2. Regimen for the administration of enoxaparin in the immediate management of VTE in pregnancy at the Princess Royal Maternity Unit, Glasgow

Early pregnancy weight	Initial dose of enoxaparin
< 50 kg	40 mg twice daily
50–69 kg	60 mg twice daily
70–89 kg	80 mg twice daily
≥ 90 kg	100 mg twice daily

treatment.[64–67] Failure to achieve the lower limit of the target therapeutic range of the activated partial thromboplastin time (APTT) ratio is associated with a 10–15-fold increase in the risk of recurrent VTE.[68] When used to monitor UFH, the APTT is often poorly measured and is technically problematic, particularly in late pregnancy when an apparent heparin resistance occurs due to increased fibrinogen and factor VIII, which influence the APTT. This can lead to unnecessarily high doses of heparin being used, with subsequent haemorrhagic problems. Where such problems are considered to exist, it may be useful to determine the anti-Xa level as a measure of heparin dose (target range 0.35–0.7 u/ml).[64] Alternatively, LMWH could be used. Two meta-analyses of randomised controlled trials have compared LMWH to UFH in the initial treatment of DVT in non-pregnant subjects.[69,70] LMWH was found to be more effective than UFH and to have lower mortality. It was also associated with a lower risk of haemorrhagic complications. LMWH is as effective as UFH in the initial treatment of PTE in studies carried out in non-pregnant subjects.[71] LMWH has been used for the initial management of VTE in pregnancy[72,54] and has been recommended for this purpose.

Occasionally for life-threatening PTE or where a massive DVT threatens limb viability, thrombolytic therapy may be required. Experience is limited, and there is a risk of major haemorrhage if systemic thrombolysis is used around the time of delivery or postpartum.

UFH can be given by continuous intravenous infusion or by subcutaneous injection. UFH is preferred to LMWH by some authorities in the initial management of massive PTE because of its rapid effect and the extensive experience in this situation. The dose is adjusted by monitoring the APTT, with a therapeutic target ratio of 1.5–2.5 times the mean laboratory control value.[73] The APTT should be measured six hours after the loading dose, then on a daily basis. Protocols for heparin dose adjustment according to APTT ratio results can be useful[64,74] and each laboratory should standardise its own target range for the APTT ratio.[73,64] If anti-Xa measurements are used to monitor heparin, the target range for the anti-Xa level is 0.35–0.70 iu/ml. Subcutaneous UFH is an effective alternative to intravenous administration. In a meta-analysis of randomised controlled trials, 12-hourly subcutaneous UFH was as effective and at least as safe as intravenous unfractionated heparin (IVUFH) in the prevention of VTE in non-pregnant patients with acute DVT.[75] When administered subcutaneously, UFH is given in subcutaneous injections of 15 000–20 000 iu, 12-hourly after an initial intravenous bolus of 5000 iu. The dose should be adjusted to maintain the mid-interval APTT at 1.5–2.5 times the control.[73]

In non-pregnant patients, once-daily administration is recommended for acute treatment of VTE with LMWH (enoxaparin 1.5 mg/kg body weight once daily; dalteparin 10 000–18 000 units once daily depending on body weight; tinzaparin

175 units/kg body weight once daily). However, in view of the alterations in the pharmacokinetics of dalteparin and enoxaparin during pregnancy,[76,77] we recommend a twice-daily dosage regimen for these LMWHs in the treatment of VTE in pregnancy (enoxaparin 1 mg/kg twice daily; dalteparin 100 units/kg twice daily up to a maximum of 18 000 units/24 hours. These doses are also used to treat VTE outwith pregnancy). The regimen at the Princess Royal Maternity Unit, Glasgow, for the administration of a LMWH (enoxaparin) in the immediate management of VTE in pregnancy is shown in Table 14.2. The initial dose of enoxaparin is 1mg/kg twice daily, based on the early pregnancy weight, as LMWH does not cross the placenta. Enoxaparin is available in syringes of 40, 60, 80 100 and 120 mg. The dose closest to the patient's weight should be used and should be continued 12-hourly until objective testing has been performed. If the diagnosis of VTE is confirmed, treatment is continued. Peak anti-Xa activity (three hours post-injection) can be measured by a chromogenic substrate assay to confirm that an appropriate dose has been given. A suitable target therapeutic range is 0.6–1.2 u/ml. If the peak anti-Xa level is above the upper limit of the therapeutic target range, the LMWH dose should be reduced (e.g. for enoxaparin, 100 mg twice daily to 80 mg twice daily, and 80 mg twice daily to 60 mg twice daily) and peak anti-Xa activity reassessed. Our experience indicates that satisfactory anti-Xa levels are obtained using this regimen and monitoring of anti-Xa levels can be deferred until the next routine working day, for example if treatment is commenced at weekends.[72] Care must be taken in women with an extremely high BMI, where it is critical to ensure that an appropriate dose of heparin is used.[1]

With heparin therapy, the platelet count should be monitored four to eight days after treatment commences, then on around a monthly basis to detect heparin-induced thrombocytopenia. Pregnant women who develop heparin-induced thrombocytopenia and require continued anticoagulant therapy should be managed with the heparinoid,[78] danaparoid sodium or, if postpartum, be treated with warfarin.

As oral anticoagulation is contraindicated in pregnancy, subcutaneous LMWH is usually used for maintenance treatment of VTE for the remainder of the pregnancy.[72,79,80] Women can be taught to self-inject and can be managed as outpatients once the acute event has been dealt with. Arrangements should be made to allow safe disposal of needles and syringes. Outpatient follow-up should allow assessment of platelets and peak anti-Xa levels during treatment. There is evidence that therapeutic doses of heparin should be used for maintenance therapy, as a 47% recurrence rate of VTE has been reported in a prospective randomised controlled trial in non-pregnant patients, when thromboprophylactic doses of UFH (5000 iu every 12 hours) were used after initial management with IVUFH.[80] The duration of therapeutic anticoagulant treatment in the non-pregnant situation is usually six months. As pregnancy is associated with prothrombotic changes in the coagulation system and venous flow, it would appear logical to apply this duration of therapy to pregnancy. If the VTE occurs early in the pregnancy then, provided that there are no additional risk factors, the dose of LMWH could be reduced to prophylactic levels (40 mg enoxaparin once daily or 5000 iu dalteparin). Following delivery, treatment should continue for at least 6–12 weeks. Warfarin can be used following delivery. If the woman chooses to commence warfarin postpartum, this can usually be initiated on the second or third postnatal day. The international normalised ratio (INR) should be checked on day two and subsequent warfarin doses titrated to maintain the INR at 2.0–3.0.[81] Heparin treatment should be continued until the INR is greater than 2.0 on two successive days.

Labour and delivery

The patient on anticoagulants should be advised that once she is established in labour or thinks that she is in labour, she should not inject any further heparin until she has been assessed and further doses should be prescribed by medical staff on an individual basis. In general terms, where induction of labour is planned, the dose of heparin should be reduced to its thromboprophylactic dose on the day before delivery. The treatment dose (twice-daily administration) should be recommenced following delivery. Because of the small risk of epidural haematoma formation during spinal instrumentation in anticoagulated patients, epidural anaesthesia should be sited only after discussion with a senior anaesthetist. Clearly, there must be a degree of caution in the concomitant use of LMWH and neuraxial anaesthesia, with vigilance for signs of cord compression. The combination must be avoided in patients on therapeutic anticoagulation. In women on prophylactic doses of heparin and LMWH, neuraxial anaesthesia should be avoided around the time of peak heparin levels. Thus the timing of anaesthesia and/or heparin administration need to be adjusted. Generally, regional techniques are not used until at least 12 hours after the previous prophylactic dose of LMWH. When a woman presents while on a therapeutic regimen of LMWH (i.e. a twice-daily regimen), regional techniques should not be employed for at least 24 hours after the last dose of LMWH. LMWH should not be given for at least three hours after the epidural catheter has been removed and the cannula should not be removed within 10–12 hours of the most recent injection.[82,83]

For elective caesarean section, the woman should receive a thromboprophylactic dose of LMWH on the day before delivery and, on the day of delivery, the morning dose of enoxaparin should be omitted and the operation performed as soon as possible thereafter. Graduated elastic compression stockings can still be worn or mechanical methods used to provide some thromboprophylaxis intraoperatively. A thromboprophylactic dose of LMWH should be given by three hours postoperatively and after removal of the epidural catheter. The treatment dose should be recommenced that evening. Again, this reflects the general principles of management and individual management plans are often required with regard to anticoagulant treatment. There is an increased risk of wound haematoma following caesarean section with both UFH and LMWH of around 2%. Consideration should be given to the use of drains (abdominal and rectus sheath) at caesarean section and the skin incision should be closed with staples or interrupted sutures to allow drainage of any haematoma that develops.

If there is considered to be a high risk of haemorrhage where continued heparin treatment is considered essential, the patient should be managed with IVUFH until the risk factors for haemorrhage are resolved. This is because IVUFH has a short duration of action and anticoagulation will reverse soon after cessation of the infusion should a haemorrhagic problem occur. The risk factors that would lead to IVUFH use would include recent major antepartum haemorrhage or coagulopathy, progressive wound haematoma, suspected intra-abdominal bleeding and postpartum haemorrhage.

Thromboprophylaxis in pregnancy: practical issues

In the woman with a previous VTE that was not pregnancy-related and was associated with a risk factor that is no longer present and with no additional risk factor or underlying thrombophilia antenatal, LMWH should not be routinely prescribed, but this strategy must be discussed with the woman and her views taken into account. Graduated elastic compression stockings and or low-dose aspirin can be employed antenatally in these women. Postpartum, she should receive anticoagulant therapy for at least six weeks (e.g. 40 mg enoxaparin or 5000 iu dalteparin daily or warfarin, target INR 2.0–3.0) with LMWH overlap until the INR is ≥ 2.0 with or without graduated elastic compression stockings.

In those women with a single previous VTE and an underlying thrombophilia or where the VTE was idiopathic or where there are additional risk factors such as obesity or nephrotic syndrome, there is a stronger case for pharmacological prophylaxis antenatally, although this will depend in part on the severity of the event and the type of thrombophilia. Antenatally, these women should be considered for prophylactic doses of LMWH (e.g. 40 mg enoxaparin or 5000 iu dalteparin daily) with or without graduated elastic compression stockings. More intense LMWH therapy in the presence of antithrombin deficiency is usually prescribed, although many women with previous VTE and antithrombin deficiency will be on long-term anticoagulant therapy. Postpartum anticoagulant therapy for at least six weeks (e.g. 40 mg enoxaparin or 5000 iu dalteparin daily or warfarin (target INR 2.0–3.0) with LMWH overlap until the INR is ≥ 2.0), with or without the use of graduated elastic compression stockings, is recommended.

In the woman with multiple previous VTE and no identifiable thrombophilia who is not on long-term anticoagulant therapy, there is consensus that she should receive antenatal LMWH thromboprophylaxis and graduated elastic compression stockings. Postpartum, she should receive at least six weeks of pharmacological prophylaxis, either with LMWH or warfarin. If she is switched to warfarin postpartum, the target INR is 2.0–3.0 and LMWH should be continued until the INR is 2.0 or greater. A longer duration of postpartum prophylaxis may be required for women with additional risk factors.

The woman with previous episode(s) of VTE on long-term anticoagulants should switch from oral anticoagulants to LMWH (for example, dalteparin 50–100 u/kg every 12 hours or enoxaparin 0.5–1 mg/kg every 12 hours) by six weeks of gestation, and should be fitted with graduated elastic compression stockings. Postpartum, she should resume long-term anticoagulants with LMWH overlap until the INR is in the pre-pregnancy therapeutic range.

Where a woman has a heritable thrombophilia diagnosed on laboratory testing, such as because of a positive family history, but no prior VTE, surveillance or prophylactic LMWH with or without graduated elastic compression stockings can be used antenatally. However, in antithrombin-deficient women in particular there is a strong case for antenatal LMWH. Similarly, in strongly symptomatic kindred there is also a strong case for antenatal LMWH. Postpartum, these women should receive anticoagulant therapy for at least six weeks (e.g. 40 mg enoxaparin or 5000 iu dalteparin daily or warfarin (target INR 2.0–3.0) with LMWH overlap until the INR is ≥ 2.0.) with or without graduated elastic compression stockings.

Women undergoing caesarean section and vaginal delivery should also have a risk assessment for VTE.[33] In a patient undergoing caesarean section, thromboprophylaxis (e.g. 40 mg enoxaparin or 5000 iu dalteparin) should be prescribed if she has one or more additional risk factors, such as emergency section in labour, high BMI, or is aged over 35 years. In patients at high risk, graduated elastic compression stockings should be used. These can also be used if heparin is contraindicated. In women undergoing vaginal delivery, a similar strategy can be used, with LMWH being prescribed if there are two or more additional risk factors.[1]

Conclusion

VTE remains the major cause of maternal mortality and continues to be a source of morbidity for women in later life. If we wish to impact further upon the continuing problem of VTE in pregnancy, obstetricians must have an understanding of the risk factors for VTE, the appropriate use of prophylaxis, the need for objective diagnosis in women with suspected VTE and the appropriate use of anticoagulant therapy. In particular, attention must be given to the greater use of prophylaxis after vaginal delivery. As acute VTE is relatively uncommon, greater use of guideline documents[4] will also be of value in improving the management, but involvement of clinicians with expertise in the management of these cases is also critically important.

References

1. Drife J, Lewis G, editors. *Why Mothers Die: The Confidential Enquiries into Maternal Deaths in the United Kingdom 1997–1999*. London: RCOG Press; 2001.
2. Macklon NS, Greer IA. Venous thromboembolic disease in obstetrics and gynaecology: the Scottish experience. *Scott Med J* 1996;41:83–6.
3. Rutherford S, Montoro M, McGhee W, Strong T. Thromboembolic disease associated with pregnancy: an 11 year review. *Am Obstet Gynecol* 1991;164 Suppl:286.
4. Thomson AJ, Greer IA. *Thromboembolic Disease in Pregnancy and the Puerperium: Acute Management*. RCOG Guideline No 28. London: RCOG Press; 2001.
5. McColl M, Ramsay JE, Tait RC, Walker ID, McCall F, Conkie JA, et al. Risk factors for pregnancy associated venous thromboembolism. *Thromb Haemost* 1997;78:1183–8.
6. McColl M, Ellison J, Greer IA, Tait RC, Walker ID. Prevalence of the post-thrombotic syndrome in young women with previous venous thromboembolism. *Br J Haematol* 2000;108:272–4.
7. Clarke P, Brennand J, Conkie JA, McCall F, Greer IA, Walker ID. Activated protein C sensitivity, protein C, protein S and coagulation in normal pregnancy. *Thromb Haemost* 1998;79:1166–70.
8. Greer IA. Haemostasis and thrombosis in pregnancy. In: Bloom AL, Forbes CD, Thomas DP, Tuddenham EGD, editors. *Haemostasis and Thrombosis*. Edinburgh: Churchill Livingstone; 1994. p. 987–1015.
9. Macklon NS, Greer IA, Bowman AW. An ultrasound study of gestational and postural changes in the deep venous system of the leg in pregnancy. *Br J Obstet Gynaecol* 1997;104:191–7.
10. Lindhagen A, Bergqvist A, Bergqvist D, Hallbook T. Late venous function in the leg after deep venous thrombosis occurring in relation to pregnancy. *Br J Obstet Gynaecol* 1986;93:348–52.
11. Den Heijer M, Koster T, Blom HJ, Bos GMJ, Briet E, Reitsma PH, *et al.* Hyperhomocysteinemia as a risk factor for deep vein thrombosis. *N Engl J Med* 1998;334:759–62.
12. Greer IA. The challenge of thrombophilia in maternal-fetal medicine. *N Engl J Med* 2000;342:424–5.
13. Gerhardt A, Scharf RE, Beckman MW, Struve S, Bender HG, Pillny M, *et al.* Prothrombin and factor V mutations in women with thrombosis during pregnancy and the puerperium. *N Engl J Med* 2000;342:374–80.
14. McColl MD, Ellison J, Reid F, Tait RC, Walker ID, Greer IA. Prothrombin 20210 G–> A, MTHFR C677T mutations in women with venous thromboembolism associated with pregnancy. *BJOG* 2000;107:565–9.
15. Walker ID. Congenital thrombophilia. In: Greer IA, editor. *Bailliere's Clinical Obstetrics and Gynaecology – Thromboembolic Disease in Obstetrics and Gynaecology*. London. Bailliere Tindall; 1997. p. 431–45.
16. Zoller B, Holm J, Dahlback B. Resistance to activated protein C due to a Factor V gene mutation: the most common inherited risk factor of thrombosis. *Trends Cardiovasc Med* 1996;6:45–9.

17. Poort SR, Rosendaal FR, Reitsma PH, Bertina RM. A common genetic variation in the 3'untranslated region of the prothrombin gene is associated with elevated plasma prothrombin levels and an increase in venous thrombosis. *Blood* 1996;88:3698–703.
18. McColl MD, Walker ID, Greer IA. A mutation in the prothrombin gene contributing to venous thrombosis in pregnancy. *Br J Obstet Gynaecol* 1998;105:923–5.
19. Greer IA. Thrombosis in pregnancy: maternal and fetal issues. *Lancet* 1999;353:1258–65.
20. Rosendaal FR. Venous thrombosis: a multicausal disease. *Lancet* 1999;353:1167–73.
21. Conard J, Horellou MH, van Dreden P, Le Compte T, Samama M. Thrombosis in pregnancy and congenital deficiencies in AT III, Protein C or Protein S: study of 78 women. *Thromb Haemost* 1990;63:319–20.
22. Pabinger I, Schneider B. GTH Study Group on Natural Inhibitors. Thrombotic risk in hereditary antithrombin III, protein C or protein S deficiency. *Arterioscler Thromb Vasc Biol* 1996;16:742–8.
23. Bokarewa MI, Bremme K, Blomback M. Arg 506-Gln mutation in factor V and risk of thrombosis during pregnancy. *Br J Haematol* 1996;92:473–8.
24. Clark P, Twaddle S, Walker ID, Scott L, Greer IA. Cost-effectiveness of screening for the factor V Leiden mutation in pregnant women. *Lancet* 2002;359:1919–20.
25. De Swiet M, Floyd E, Letsky E. Low risk of recurrent thromboembolism in pregnancy. *Br J Hosp Med* 1987;38:264.
26. Howell R, Fidler J, Letsky E, De Swiet. The risk of antenatal subcutaneous heparin prophylaxis: a controlled trial. *Br J Obstet Gynaecol* 1983;90:1124–8.
27. Badaracco MA, Vessey M. Recurrent venous thromboembolic disease and use of oral contraceptives. *BMJ* 1974;1:215–17.
28. Tengborn L, Bergqvist D, Matzsch T, Bergqvist A, Hedner U. Recurrent thromboembolism in pregnancy and puerperium: is there a need for thromboprophylaxis? *Am J Obstet Gynecol* 1989;160:90–94.
29. Ginsberg J, Greer IA, Hirsh J. Sixth ACCP consensus conference on antithrombotic therapy. Use of antithrombotic agents during pregnancy. *Chest* 2001;119:1225–315.
30. Brill-Edwards P, Ginsberg JS. Safety of withholding antepartum heparin in women with a previous episode of venous thromboembolism. *N Engl J Med* 2000;343:1439–44.
31. Hull RD, Raskob GF, Carter CJ. Serial IPG in pregnancy patients with clinically suspected DVT. Clinical validity of negative findings. *Ann Intern Med* 1990;112:663–7.
32. Hull RD, Hirsh J, Sackett D, Powers P, Turpie A, Walker I. Diagnostic efficacy of IPG in suspected venous thrombosis: an alternative to venography. *N Engl J Med* 1977;296:1497–500.
33. Lensing AW, Prandoni P, Brandjes D, Huisman P, Vigo M, Tomasella G, *et al.* Detection of DVT by real-time B-mode ultrasonography. *N Engl J Med* 1989;320:342–5.
34. PIOPED Investigators. Value of the ventilation/perfusion scan in acute pulmonary embolism. Results of the prospective investigation of pulmonary embolism diagnosis (PIOPED). *JAMA* 1990;263:2753–9.
35. Hull RD, Hirsh J, Carter CJ, Raskob GE, Gill GJ, Jay RM, *et al.* Diagnostic value of ventilation-perfusion lung scanning in patients with suspected pulmonary embolism. *Chest* 1985;88:819–28.
36. Macklon NS. Diagnosis of deep venous thrombosis and pulmonary embolism. *Baillieres Best Pract Res Clin Obstet Gynaecol* 1997;11:463–77.
37. Wheeler HB, Hirsh J, Wells P, Anderson FA Jr. Diagnostic tests for deep vein thrombosis. Clinical usefulness depends on probability of disease. *Arch Intern Med* 1994;154:1921–8.
38. Wells PS, Anderson DR, Bormanis J, Guy F, Mitchell M, Gray L, *et al.* Value of assessment of pretest probability of deep-vein thrombosis in clinical management. *Lancet* 1997;350:1795–8.
39. Thomson AJ, Greer IA. Non-haemorrhagic obstetric shock. *Baillieres Best Pract Res Clin Obstet Gynaecol* 2000;14:19–41.
40. Ginsberg JS, Hirsh J, Rainbow AJ, Coates G. Risks to the fetus of radiological procedures used in the diagnosis of maternal venous thromboembolic disease. *Thromb Haemost* 1989;61:189–96.
41. Bounameaux H. Factor V Leiden paradox: risk of deep-vein thrombosis but not of pulmonary embolism. *Lancet* 2000;356:182–3.
42. Bates SM, Ginsberg JS. Anticoagulants in pregnancy: fetal effects. *Baillieres Best Pract Res Clin Obstet Gynaecol* 1997; 11:479–88.
43. Vitale N, De Feo M, De Santo LS, Pollice A, Tedesco N, Contrufo M. Dose-dependent fetal complications of warfarin in pregnant women with mechanical heart valves. *J Am Coll Cardiol* 1999;33:1642–5.
44. Letsky E. Peripartum prophylaxis of thromboembolism. *Baillieres Clin Obstet Gynaecol* 1997;11:523–43.
45. Flessa HC, Klapstrom AB, Glueck MJ, Will JJ. Placental transport of heparin. *Am J Obstet Gynecol* 1965;93:570–73.

46. Forestier F, Daffos F, Capella-Pavlovsky M. Low molecular weight heparin (PK 10169) does not cross the placenta during the second trimester of pregnancy by direct fetal blood sampling under ultrasound. *Thromb Res Suppl* 1984;34:557–60.
47. Forestier F, Daffos F, Rainaut M, Toulemonde F. Low molecular weight heparin (CY 216) does not cross the placenta during the third trimester of pregnancy. *Thromb Haemost* 1987;57:234.
48. Sanson BJ, Lensing AWA, Prins MH, Ginsberg JS, Barkagan ZS, Lavenne-Pardonge E, *et al.* Safety of low-molecular-weight heparin in pregnancy: a systematic review. *Thromb Haemost* 1999;81:668–72.
49. Nelson-Piercy C. Hazards of heparin: allergy, heparin-induced thrombocytopenia and osteoporosis. *Bailliere's Clin Obstet Gynaecol* 1997;11:489–509.
50. Pettila V, Leinonen P, Markkola A, Hiilesmaa V. Kaaja R. Postpartum bone mineral density in women treated for thromboprophylaxis with unfractionated heparin or LMW heparin. *Thromb Haemost* 2002;87:182–6.
51. Warkentin TE, Levine MN, Hirsh J, Horsewood P, Roberts RS, Gent M, *et al.* Heparin induced thrombocytopenia in patients treated with low molecular weight heparin or unfractionated heparin. *N Engl J Med* 1995;332:1330–35.
52. Nelson-Piercy C, Letsky EA, de Swiet M. Low-molecular-weight heparin for obstetric thromboprophylaxis: experience of sixty-nine pregnancies in sixty-one women at high risk. *Am J Obstet Gynecol* 1997;176:1062–8.
53. Greer IA. Epidemiology, risk factors and prophylaxis of venous thrombo-embolism in obstetrics and gynaecology. *Baillieres Clin Obstet Gynaecol* 1997;11:403–30.
54. Ellison J, Walker ID, Greer IA. Antifactor Xa profiles in pregnant women receiving antenatal thromboprophylaxis with enoxaparin for prevention and treatment of thromboembolism in pregnancy. *BJOG* 2000;107:1116–21.
55. Lepercq J, Conard J, Borel-Derlon A, Darmon JY, Boudignat O, Francoual C, *et al.* Venous thromboembolism during pregnancy: a retrospective study of enoxaparin safety in 624 pregnancies. *BJOG* 2001;108:1134–40.
56. Hunt BJ, Doughty HA, Majumdar G, Copplestone A, Kerslake S, Buchanan N, *et al.* Thromboprophylaxis with low molecular weight heparin (Fragmin) in high risk pregnancies. *Thromb Haemost* 1997;77:39–43.
57. Blomback M, Bremme K, Hellgren M, Siegbahn A, Lindberg H. Thromboprophylaxis with low molecular mass heparin, 'Fragmin' (dalteparin), during pregnancy – longitudinal safety study. *Blood Coagul Fibrinolysis* 1998;9:1–9.
58. Barbier P, Jongville AP, Autret TE, Coureau C. Fetal risks with dextran during delivery. *Drug Saf* 1992;7:71–3.
59. Macklon NS, Greer IA. Technical note: compression stockings and posture: a comparative study of their effects on the proximal deep veins in the leg at rest. *Br J Radiol* 1995;68:515–18.
60. Lindoff-Last E, Willeke A,Thalhammer C, Nowak G, Bauersachs R. Hirudin treatment in a breastfeeding woman. *Lancet* 2000;355:467–8.
61. Clagett GP, Anderson FA, Geerts W, Heit JA, Knudson M, Lieberman JR, *et al.* Prevention of venous thromboembolism. *Chest* 1998;114:521S–60S.
62. CLASP Collaborative Group. CLASP: a randomised trial of low dose aspirin for the prevention and treatment of pre-eclampsia among 9364 pregnant women. *Lancet* 1994;343:619–29.
63. Imperiale TF, Petrulis AS. A meta-analysis of low-dose aspirin for prevention of pregnancy-induced hypertensive disease. *JAMA* 1991;266:260–64.
64. Hirsh J. Heparin. *N Engl J Med* 1991;324:1565–74.
65. Barritt DV, Jordan SC. Anticoagulant drugs in the treatment of pulmonary embolism: a controlled trial. *Lancet* 1960;i:1309–12.
66. Kanis JA. Heparin in the treatment of pulmonary thromboembolism. *Thromb Diath Haemorrh* 1974;32:519–27.
67. Carson JL, Kelley MA, Duff A, Weg JG, Fulkerson WJ, Palevsky HI, *et al.* The clinical course of pulmonary embolism. *N Engl J Med* 1992;326:1240–45.
68. Hyers TM, Agnelli G, Hull RD, Weg JG, Morris TA, Samama M, *et al.* Antithrombotic therapy for venous thromboembolic disease. *Chest* 2001;119 Suppl 1:176–93.
69. Dolovich L, Ginsberg JS. Low molecular weight heparin in the treatment of venous thromboembolism: an updated meta-analysis. *Vessels* 1997;3:4–11.
70. Gould MK, Dembitzer AD, Doyle RL, Hastie TJ, Garber AM. Low molecular weight heparins compared with unfractionated heparin for treatment of acute deep venous thrombosis. A meta-analysis of randomized, controlled trials. *Ann Intern Med* 1999;130:800–9.
71. Simmoneau G, Sors H, Charbonnier B, Page Y, Laaban JP, Azarian R, *et al.* A comparison of low-

molecular weight heparin with unfractionated heparin for acute pulmonary embolism. *N Engl J Med* 1997;337:663–9.
72. Thomson AJ, Walker ID, Greer IA. Low-molecular-weight-heparin for the immediate management of thromboembolic disease in pregnancy. *Lancet* 1998;352:1904.
73. Lowe GDO. Treatment of venous thromboembolism. *Baillieres Clin Obstet Gynaecol* 1997;11:511–21.
74. Hirsh J, Raschke R, Warkentin TE, Dalen JE, Deykin D, Poller L. Heparin: mechanism of action, pharmacokinetics, dosing considerations, monitoring, efficacy, and safety. *Chest* 1995;108 Suppl 4:258–75.
75. Hommes DW, Bura A, Mazzolai L, Buller HR, ten Cate JW. Subcutaneous heparin compared with continuous intravenous heparin administration in the initial treatment of deep venous thrombosis. A meta-analysis. *Ann Intern Med* 1992;116:279–84.
76. Blomback M, Bremme K, Hellgren M, Lindberg H. A pharmacokinetic study of dalteparin (Fragmin) during late pregnancy. *Blood Coagul Fibrinolysis* 1998;9:343–50.
77. Casele HL, Laifer SA, Woelkers DA, Venkataramanan R. Changes in the pharmacokinetics of the low molecular weight heparin enoxaparin sodium during pregnancy. *Am J Obstet Gynecol* 1999;181:1113–17.
78. Magnani HN. Heparin-induced thrombocytopenia (HIT): an overview of 230 patients treated with Orgaran (Org 10172). *Thromb Haemost* 1993;70:554–61.
79. Monreal M. Long-term treatment of venous thromboembolism: the place of low molecular weight heparin. *Vessels* 1997;3:18–21.
80. Hull RD, Delmore T, Carter C, Hirsh J, Genton E, Gent M, *et al.* Adjusted subcutaneous heparin versus warfarin sodium in the long-term treatment of venous thrombosis. *N Engl J Med* 1982;306:189–94.
81. British Society for Haematology. Guidelines on oral anticoagulation. 3rd ed. *Br J Haematol* 1998;101:374–87.
82. Checketts MR, Wildsmith JAW. Central nerve block and thromboprophylaxis – is there a problem? *Br J Anaesth* 1999;82:164–7.
83. Horlocker TT, Wedel DJ. Spinal and epidural blockade and perioperative low molecular weight heparin: smooth sailing on the Titanic. *Anesth Analg* 1998;86:1153–6.

Chapter 15

Amniotic fluid embolism

Derek J. Tuffnell

Introduction

Although amniotic fluid embolism (AFE) is an uncommon condition, it is appropriate to include it in a discussion of maternal morbidity and mortality for two reasons. First, it is a leading cause of maternal death in the developed world. In the latest report on maternal mortality from the UK,[1] it was the fifth greatest cause of direct maternal deaths and was responsible for 7.5% of deaths. Over the last five triennia, AFE has been responsible for 8.4% of maternal deaths in the UK[1–5] and, in the USA and Australia, it is responsible for 7.5–10.0% of maternal deaths.[6,7] Second, there is increasing evidence that the outlook for women with AFE may no longer be as gloomy as it has been. A review[8] from 1979 suggested mortality of 86% and the national registry from the USA in 1995 suggested a mortality of 61%, but only 15% survived neurologically intact.[9] However, population-based surveys suggest mortality of less than 30%[7,10] and the UK register of cases for 1997–2000 showed a mortality of 16% (4 of 25) for reported cases. This changing mortality is probably a result of both better intensive care and a recognition of the fact that 'milder' cases do occur.[11]

Background

The first description of amniotic fluid entering the maternal circulation, by Meyer in 1926,[12] was followed by Steiner and Luschbaugh[13] reporting cases of unexpected death, together with the clinical features and the histopathological findings. Animal studies have been undertaken to try to understand the condition further but much of the current knowledge about the condition stems from reviews or clinical cases. The diagnostic and therapeutic knowledge also comes from small series or individual clinical cases and this chapter brings together some of that information.

Effects of amniotic fluid in the circulation

Steiner and Luschbaugh[13] demonstrated that rabbits and dogs could be killed by the infusion of human amniotic fluid and meconium. Clark[14] summarised the reports on experimental animals up to 1990 and found conflicting results in the outcome of the 15 studies. Most of the studies demonstrated adverse events, but the amniotic fluid infused was often more particulate than that in clinical cases, making its relevance to humans doubtful. In the primate studies, large volumes of amniotic fluid were needed before an adverse reaction occurred. Clark felt that investigators' over-reliance on animal models had led to an incorrect belief that the pathophysiology of AFE principally involved pulmonary hypertension secondary to occlusion or vasospastic changes in the pulmonary vasculature.

Studies by Clark[15,16] and Girard[17] in humans showed only mild to moderate elevations in pulmonary artery pressure but there was evidence of left ventricular dysfunction or failure. There is also *in vitro* evidence of decreased myometrial contractility in the presence of amniotic fluid,[18] which may affect the myocardium and possibly the myometrium. Clark[14] reconciled these two findings of both pulmonary hypertension and left ventricular failure by suggesting a biphasic model. Some patients would have a profound acute pulmonary hypertension and this could cause neurological damage and early fatalities, but this was not a sustained feature. The survivors would resolve the pulmonary hypertension and go on to develop left ventricular failure. In a more recent animal study, Hankins *et al.*[19] showed that in the pregnant goat there was an immediate marked increase in the systemic and pulmonary vascular resistance, but this was not sustained and only occurred in the presence of meconium. This suggested a possible humoral cause rather than an obstructive one.

The myocardial depressant effect of amniotic fluid may come from its constituents. High concentrations of endothelin have been found in amniotic fluid and in the lungs of women after AFE.[20,21] This is a powerful constrictor of the coronary and pulmonary arteries, as well as causing bronchoconstriction. However, a study looking at the effect of human amniotic fluid on the human omental artery did not demonstrate any pressor effect.[22] This led the authors to suggest that there was no direct effect of amniotic fluid on the circulation and that the features of AFE must be due to some secondary effect.

Leukotrienes seem to be produced in response to the infusion of amniotic fluid into the circulation and they may be generated from amniotic fluid surfactant.[23] Clark[14] observed that leukotrienes and prostaglandins could cause the haemodynamic changes in AFE. There is also evidence that inhibitors of leukotriene synthesis can prevent the fatal haemodynamic collapse of AFE in experimental studies.[24]

Coagulopathy is an important part of AFE. Amniotic fluid contains tissue factor[25] and has been shown to have direct factor X, activating property and thromboplastin-like effect.[26] These increase with gestational age. It has been postulated that, in addition to triggering a coagulopathy, effects in the pulmonary vasculature may also cause vasoconstriction. Studies have also demonstrated a direct effect on clotting, enhanced by the presence of meconium with reductions in platelet count, prolonged prothrombin index and reduced fibrinogen.[27]

Reviewing the national registry, Clark[9] suggested that 'The syndrome of peripartum cardiovascular collapse and coagulopathy is, from a clinical, haemodynamic and haematologic standpoint, similar to anaphylaxis and septic shock and suggests the possibility of a common underlying pathophysiologic mechanism'. It was suggested that, while material commonly passed from fetus to mother, it was a predisposition to react that created the clinical syndrome. Each of these studies suggests that the response to the stimulus of fetal material in the maternal circulation is dependent on the nature and quantity of the material and also the mother's susceptibility. It is plausible that the effect is sometimes occlusive, sometimes direct and 'toxic' and is sometimes a trigger to a cascade reaction. In some women the effects may progress through each element. This suggests that clinical management will be aimed at supportive therapy with an understanding that the patient will pass through different phases of the clinical presentation.

The issue of amniotic fluid in the circulation is important if intraoperative autologous blood transfusion is being considered. This has been discussed in relation to cell salvage, and leucocyte depletion filtering seems to reduce particulate contaminants to the level equivalent to maternal venous blood.[28] The safety of intraoperative autologous blood collection has been examined in a cohort study of 139 women and no demonstrable increase in complications was found.[29]

Clinical features

The clinical features of AFE are those of sudden maternal or fetal deterioration. Clark[9] established clinical criteria for cases to be considered in the national register in the USA. These were:

- acute hypotension or cardiac arrest
- acute hypoxia (dyspnoea, cyanosis or respiratory arrest)
- coagulopathy (laboratory evidence of intravascular coagulation or severe haemorrhage)
- onset of all of the above during labour or within 30 minutes of delivery
- no other clinical conditions or potential explanations for the symptoms and signs.

These have been taken up in the UK to develop a register of cases, using the same criteria, since 1997, to establish a further understanding of the condition. Also, difference in early treatments between deaths and survivors may allow a view on the advantages and disadvantages of the treatments to be taken.[30]

Cases seem to occur in older women. Only one death in the last 15 years from AFE has occurred in a woman under the age of 25 years in the UK[1–5] and only two women under 25 years have been reported to the national register. While, in a non-specific way, intervention or complications seem to be more common in women who go on to have an AFE, there is no specific trigger for a case to occur. Multiparity has been suggested as a risk factor but eight of the 25 women reported to the UK register had no previous pregnancies and one had had two miscarriages but no other pregnancies. Parity was not found to be a risk factor in the US register either.[9] While labour is seen as important in the aetiology of AFE, cases have been reported under other circumstances, in particular after caesarean section,[31] following blunt abdominal trauma,[32] amniocentesis,[33] ruptured uterus[34] and amnioinfusion in labour.[35]

While atypical presentations are reported, the presentations in larger series tend to present with a cluster of features. The early series from Morgan,[8] with a high mortality, had almost all cases with cardiorespiratory collapse. Breathlessness was the presenting feature in 51%. In the US series,[9] breathlessness was present in 27% and the most common presentation was fits, in 30%. Fits occurred in 10% of Morgan's series. In the UK register, 12 cases presented with hypotension and collapse (48%), with five of these (20%) having accompanying fits. Hypotension was the presenting feature of 13% of the US series and 27% in Morgan's series. Fetal distress did not feature in the Morgan series but was the presenting feature in the US series in 17% with bradycardia. In the UK series, nine cases (36%) presented with concern about the fetal heart-rate patterns. Coagulopathy and bleeding were uncommon presenting features in all three series, with 12% in Morgan's series, none in the US series and only one in the UK series.

Coagulopathy and massive haemorrhage seem to be features that develop later. However, it must be remembered that often the coagulopathy is present shortly after presentation, if looked for, but may become clinically apparent only with the passage of time.

The multiple clinical presentations fit the hypothesis that the early deaths are caused by the direct and 'toxic' effects of a bolus of fetal material or 'amniotic fluid' but that the women who survive that initial event then become exposed to the delayed or cascade-related problems that follow.

Diagnosis

The diagnosis of AFE is often one of exclusion or one made at postmortem. The differential diagnosis involves considering an exhaustive list of the causes of maternal collapse in the peripartum period. These include thrombotic embolus, air embolus, septic shock, acute myocardial infarction, peripartum cardiomyopathy, anaphylaxis, aspiration, placental abruption, transfusion reactions, local anaesthetic toxicity, pre-eclampsia or eclampsia, uterine rupture and postpartum haemorrhage (uterine atony).[30,34]

Only after exclusion of all the other causes can a diagnosis be confirmed clinically. The most useful diagnostic test to exclude a large proportion of the differential diagnosis is to do a clotting screen. This is often abnormal even before the haemorrhage becomes apparent. When haemorrhage is already present, the possibility that abnormal clotting could be secondary to the haemorrhage needs to be considered. However, for haemorrhage itself to cause coagulopathy, normally considerable blood loss with blood replacement needs to have occurred.

It is also important to perform an electrocardiogram to look for signs of myocardial damage. However, in AFE, bizarre cardiac rhythms can often be present and may make interpretation difficult. Arterial blood gases may be useful, in addition to the use of a pulse oximeter, but will not differentiate causes specifically. In a patient who becomes stable, a ventilation–perfusion scan of the lungs may demonstrate defects. However, occlusive change can occur in the pulmonary vessels with AFE, so defects do not exclude AFE as a diagnosis.

Zinc coproporphyrin has been analysed in patients with AFE and controls.[36] Levels were increased to a mean of 97 nmol/l (range 38–240 nmol/l) in women with AFE, with normal women having a mean of 26 nmol/l after delivery. A cut-off point of 35 nmol/l was suggested for diagnosis. This was felt to be a test that could rapidly be made available.[36]

Following a suggestion by Clark[14] that AFE may have an anaphylactoid component, the use of serum tryptase to help confirm the diagnosis has been suggested.[37] In a sample taken post mortem from a woman dying after AFE, the level of serum tryptase was found to be 4.7 ng/ml (with a normal result <1 ng/ml).[38] The difficulty with this test is that it will usually take a considerable time to obtain the result and it will not influence management. Pulmonary mast cell tryptase has been examined and is elevated in women with AFE but this is a postmortem test.[39] It was suggested that this finding supports an anaphylactoid response in AFE.

In one study, serum sialyl Tn antigen levels were elevated in women with meconium liquor (20.3 ± 15.4 u/ml) compared with those with clear liquor (11.8 ± 5.6 u/ml). Levels were significantly increased in women with an AFE (105.6 ± 59.0 u/ml; P <0.01).[40] Histologically, staining using antibody TKH-2, which is clearly directed to sialyl Tn and reacts to meconium and amniotic fluid-derived mucin-type glycoprotein, produced positive TKH-2 stainings clearly visible in the pulmonary vasculature.[41,42] However, a further study bringing together measurement of serum tryptase, urinary histamine, levels of fetal antigen (sialyl Tn) and complement (C3,C4) levels found no difference in histamine and tryptase in women with AFE. There was an increase in fetal antigen and there were abnormally low levels of complement.[43] This tends to suggest a role for complement activation rather than anaphylaxis.

The presence of squamous cells in the maternal circulation had been considered pathognomic for AFE. However, the presence of squamous cells has been reported by a number of authors in other conditions in pregnancy and even in non-pregnant women.[44–46] The pathology section of the Confidential Enquiry into Maternal Deaths[1] highlights the problem with squamous cells in the maternal circulation being relied on to make the diagnosis. With increasing survival, through intensive care, between the onset of symptoms and death, the squamous cells may have been washed out of the circulation making confirmation of the diagnosis difficult. In this situation, cytokeratin markers CAM5.2 and LP34 may show foci of cells not otherwise visible. The overall conclusion about making the diagnosis of AFE is that it remains, predominantly, a clinical diagnosis of exclusion. There are, as yet, no useful antemortem diagnostic tests to confirm the diagnosis. Also, careful pathological assessment is necessary post mortem to ensure that a case is not missed, particularly when the predominant feature clinically is haemorrhage and the diagnosis has not been considered prior to death.

Management

The management of AFE is supportive rather than specific, with current knowledge. As collapse is the predominant presentation, the initial management will be towards the basics of resuscitation – airway breathing and circulation. Maximal initial oxygenation is required, with early intubation and ventilation if there is concern. It is important to remember that it is part of the resuscitation of a woman who collapses undelivered to consider prompt delivery by rapid caesarean section if there is no response to cardiopulmonary resuscitation after five minutes.[47] This means that, as with any collapse, the early involvement of senior, experienced staff is required and that a multidisciplinary approach with obstetricians, anaesthetists, intensivists and haematologists is mandatory to give the best prospect of survival. Prompt transfusion of fluids will be necessary to replace blood loss. It is suggested that vasopressors such as phenylephrine may be useful in restoring aortic perfusion pressure.[34] The early consideration of clotting factor replacement with fresh frozen plasma, cryoprecipitate and platelets is important if there are signs of coagulopathy, such as haematuria or bleeding from the gums, even before massive blood loss is apparent. It is appropriate to start this before receiving the laboratory confirmation of coagulopathy. Indeed, it is suggested that cryoprecipitate may be of intrinsic value beyond its clotting factor components, as it contains fibronectin, which aids the reticuloendothelial system in the filtration of antigenic and toxic particulate matter.[34]

Cardiac dysrhythmias often occur in AFE. These may need specific treatment but myocardial suppression is more common, so inotropic support with dopamine is helpful. To guide therapy, the early use of pulmonary artery catheterisation is recommended.[14,30,34,48] This can be vital to ensure that fluid overload does not occur, as this can lead to worsening pulmonary oedema and subsequent acute respiratory distress syndrome.

The presentation of AFE can sometimes be acute fetal collapse, which is followed a little later by maternal deterioration. Consideration should be given to checking coagulation studies and monitoring pulse oximetry in women who have a sudden deterioration in fetal condition and where the baby is unexpectedly severely acidotic. Abnormalities could then provide the opportunity for earlier invasive monitoring.

A number of specific therapies have been used in AFE. In one case, an AFE was thought to be in progress as air bubbles and vernix were seen in the left uterine vein at caesarean section.[49] The infundibulopelvic ligament and uterine arteries were ligated and an area of Couvelaire uterus oversewn. Mild coagulopathy occurred, but no other problems were seen. Cardiopulmonary bypass and open pulmonary artery thromboembolectomy produced a good outcome in a single case, suggesting that AFE can have an occlusive element.[50] To replace pulmonary function, extracorporeal membrane oxygenation and intra-aortic balloon counterpulsation have also been used successfully.[51] Inhaled prostacyclin as a pulmonary vasodilator has been used[52] and inhaled nitric oxide suggested.[53] Given the anaphylactoid hypothesis put forward by Clark,[9] it has been suggested that high-dose hydrocortisone, 500 mg six-hourly, may be appropriate but no studies have yet examined this. More interestingly, several reports have suggested that haemofiltration or plasma exchange may be effective in clearing the plasma of the effects of the amniotic fluid and aiding recovery. In 1987, a report[54] detailed a successful outcome after two exchange transfusions for a probable AFE following amniocentesis. A further report in 2001 suggested that the effect of transfusing 1.5 times the patient's blood volume acted as an exchange transfusion.[55] This 'cleansing' process was used by continuous haemofiltration in a further case,[56] with a dramatic response in terms of improving clotting parameters. It seems that this approach may be one to take forward after women have been stabilised following the initial events.

Outcome

Causes of maternal death in population-based studies have similar rates. In the UK, the death rate from AFE has been 0.51/100 000 maternities from 1988–1999, accounting for 7.5% of the total direct deaths.[1] In Australia over 27 years the rate has been 0.90/100000 maternities but has fallen from 1.43 to 0.60/100 000.[7] It was the cause of 10% of direct deaths over the last 18 years and 7.5% over last 27 years. In Ireland from

1989–91, two of five direct deaths were due to AFE – a rate of 1.27/100 000 maternities.[57] In California in 1994–1995, mortality from AFE was also 1.27/100 000 maternities.[10]

The mortality in early series of AFE was 86%.[8] More recent series, particularly those on whole populations, have suggested that, with complete case ascertainment, mortality is likely to be lower (Table 15.1). The two series based on databases of whole populations have mortality rates under 30%.[7,10] The other series, including the UK register, tend to rely on case reporting. This may lead to an over-reporting of the more serious cases. This can be demonstrated by the fact that in the Weiwen series[58] 39% of women were dead within one hour of presentation and in the US register 36% were dead in one hour and 63% within five hours. Comparisons between series to consider whether a presentation can be related to outcome are difficult, as common terminology is not used (Table 15.2). However, there is no doubt that many of the women suffer morbidity even if they survive (Table 15.1).

Further analysis of the cases reported to the UK register shows that 76% of women needed intensive care and one of the women who died did not survive long enough to reach intensive care. Sixteen of 21 survivors went to intensive care and had a length of stay of 5.29 ± 9.76 days. Transfusion requirements were massive in these women. The four women who died had a total of 183 units of blood products. The 20 survivors, with information available, had an average of 33.65 units of blood products, range 2–106 units. Factors that may be important in improving outcome seem to be early consideration of the diagnosis and early involvement of anaesthetic staff. In the cases

Table 15.1 Outcome of amniotic fluid embolism

Source	Place	Year	Cases (n)	Mortality (%)	Other morbidity	Babies[a]
US register Clark[9]	USA	1988–93 (1995)[b]	46	61	Only 15% neurologically intact	22/28 survived; only 11 neurologically intact
Burrows and Khoo[7]	Brisbane	1984–93 (1995)[b]	9	22	2/9 had hysterectomy 1 long term disability	8/11 survived (2 twins)
Gilbert and Danielsen[10]	California	1994–95 (1999)[b]	57	28	5/39 survivors needed 'extra arrangements' on discharge	95% survived 72% normal discharge
Weiwen[58]	Suzhou, China	?1984–99 (2000)[b]	38	89	NR	NR
UK register	UK	1997–2000 (2001)[b]	25	16	4 survivors + 1 death – hysterectomy 1 internal iliac ligation and liver haematoma 2 renal failure – recovered 1 subglottic stenosis	3 perinatal deaths 5/15 survivors severely acidotic

[a] only from cases occurring before or at delivery; NR = not reported; [b] = year of publication

Table 15.2. Presentation of amniotic fluid embolism

Source	Primigravidae (%)	Shock/ collapse (%)	Dyspnoea/ cyanosis (%)	Fits (%)	Haemorrhage coagulopathy (%)	Fetal distress (%)	Presentation before or at delivery (%)
US register Clark[9]	39	100 (87% cardiac arrest)	83	48	83[a]	100	81
Burrows and Khoo[7]	33	88 (33% cardiac arrest)	100	0	55	NA	77
Gilbert and Danielsen[10]	NA	47	NA	NA	72	49	NA
Weiwen[58]	79	100	NA	16	42	NA	66
UK register	36	88 (40% cardiac arrest)	100	24	100	83	76

NA = not available; [a] others died before confirmation and live babies undelivered at presentation

where the time of first consideration of the diagnosis was recorded, the time from first symptom was 141.75 ± 110.8 minutes in women who died, whereas in survivors it was 44.4 ± 57.1 minutes ($P = 0.088$). There was little difference in the time that elapsed before survivors and women who died were seen by obstetricians. However, there was a trend to later involvement of anaesthetists in women who died. The time from first symptoms to being seen by anaesthetists in women who died was 108 ± 109 minutes, whereas in women who survived it was 41.5 ± 70 minutes ($P = 0.16$).

The outcomes for women in the UK register do not represent the outcomes of all women in the UK with an AFE. In the maternal mortality report[1] covering three of the four years of data, there are eight deaths from AFE. Therefore, only 50% of deaths were reported. One of these was in a woman undelivered with twins and the other three were sudden deaths surviving less than four hours. The feature of the deaths in this triennia is that seven of the eight were dead within seven hours of presentation. This means that efforts will need to be concentrated on the resuscitation and early treatment to improve survival. However, other treatments such as plasma exchange may be useful to reduce the morbidity. Unusual long-term morbidity has been reported, with one woman having occlusion of branch retinal arterioles leading to loss of vision in one eye.[59] One other woman presented three months after a stillbirth with a mass in the lung that histologically contained squamous cells and lanugo hair.[60] Further pregnancies have been reported in women with a successful outcome after AFE. There is a total of six cases with good fetal and maternal outcome.[61–64]

Conclusion

AFE is a rare condition but is responsible for 7–10% of maternal deaths in developed countries. Mortality from the condition is lower in population-based than in voluntary reporting systems and may be under 30%. Deaths now are generally in the women who do not survive the first few hours after collapse, but considerable morbidity occurs, with intensive care admission, major transfusion, hysterectomy and long-term neurological problems for both mother and baby. Early intervention with full intensive care support and early transfusion of clotting factor replacement, perhaps even exchange transfusion or haemofiltration, is appropriate. This requires early recognition and a heightened awareness of the condition should therefore be encouraged.

References

1. Drife J, Lewis G, editors. *Why Mothers Die, 1997–1999. The Confidential Enquiries into Maternal Deaths in the United Kingdom*. London: RCOG Press; 2001.
2. Drife J, Lewis G, editors. *Report on Confidential Enquiries into Maternal Deaths in the United Kingdom, 1985–87*. London: HMSO; 1991.
3. Department of Health, Welsh Office, Scottish Home and Health Department, Department of Health and Social Services, Northern Ireland. *Report on Confidential Enquiries into Maternal Death in the United Kingdom, 1988–90*. London: HMSO; 1994.
4. Department of Health, Welsh Office, Scottish Home and Health Department, Department of Health and Social Services, Northern Ireland. *Report on Confidential Enquiries into Maternal Death in the United Kingdom, 1991–93*. London: HMSO; 1996.
5. Department of Health, Welsh Office, Scottish Office Department of Health, Department of Health and Social Services, Northern Ireland. *Why Mothers Die. Report on Confidential Enquiries into Maternal Deaths in the United Kingdom, 1994–1996*. London: The Stationery Office; 1998.
6. Atrash HK, Koonin LM, Lawson HW, Franks AL, Smith JC. Maternal mortality in the United States,1979–1986. *Obstet Gynecol* 1990;76:1055–60.
7. Burrows A, Khoo SK. The amniotic fluid embolism syndrome: 10 years' experience at a major teaching hospital. *Aust N Z J Obstet Gynaecol* 1995;35:245–50.
8. Morgan M. Amniotic fluid embolism. *Anaesthesia* 1979;34:20–32.
9. Clark SL, Hankins GD, Dudley DA, Dildy GA, Porter TF. Amniotic fluid embolism: analysis of the national registry. *Am J Obstet Gynecol* 1995;172:1158–67.
10. Gilbert WM, Danielsen B. Amniotic fluid embolism: decreased mortality in a population-based study. *Obstet Gynecol* 1999;93:973–7.
11. Benson MD. Nonfatal amniotic fluid embolism. Three possible cases and a new clinical definition. *Arch Fam Med* 1993;2:989–94.
12. Meyer JR. *Brasilimedico* 1926;2:301.
13. Steiner PE, Lushbaugh CC. Maternal pulmonary embolism by amniotic fluid. *JAMA* 1941;117:1245–54, 1341–5.
14. Clark SL. New concepts of amniotic fluid embolism: a review. *Obstet Gynecol Surv* 1990;45:360–8.
15. Clark SL, Cotton DB, Gonik B, Greenspoon J, Phelan JP. Central hemodynamic alterations in amniotic fluid embolism. *Am J Obstet Gynecol* 1988;158:1124–6.
16. Clark SL, Montz FJ, Phelan JP. Haemodynamic alterations associated with amniotic fluid embolism: a reappraisal. *Am J Obstet Gynecol* 1985;151:617–21.
17. Girard P, Mal H, Laine JF, Petitpretz P, Rain B, Duroux P. Left heart failure in amniotic fluid embolism. *Anaesthesiology* 1986;64:262–5.
18. Courtney LD. Coagulation failure in pregnancy. *BMJ* 1970;1:691.
19. Hankins GD, Snyder RR, Clark SL, Schwartz L, Patterson WR, Butzin CA. Acute hemodynamic and respiratory effects of amniotic fluid embolism in the pregnant goat model. *Am J Obstet Gynecol* 1993;168:1113–29.
20. el Maradny E, Kanayama N, Halim A, Maehara K, Terao T. Endothelin has a role in early pathogenesis of amniotic fluid embolism. *Gynecol Obstet Invest* 1995:40:14–18.
21. Khong TY. Expression of endothelin-1 in amniotic fluid embolism and possible pathophysiological mechanism. *Br J Obstet Gynaecol* 1998;105:802–4.
22. Vedernikov YP, Saade GR, Zlatnik M, Martin E, Garfield RE, Hankins GD. The effect of amniotic fluid on the human omental artery *in vitro*. *Am J Obstet Gynecol* 1999;180:454–6.
23. Lee HC, Yamaguchi M, Ikenoue T, Miyakawa I, Mori N. Amniotic fluid embolism and leukotrienes

– the role of amniotic fluid surfactant in leukotriene production. *Prostaglandins Leukot Essent Fatty Acids* 1992;47:117–21.

24. Azegami M, Mori N. Amniotic fluid embolism and leukotrienes. *Am J Obstet Gynecol* 1986;155:1119–24.
25. Uszynski M, Zekanowska E, Uszynski W, Kuczynski J. Tissue factor (TF) and tissue factor pathway inhibitor (TFPI) in amniotic fluid and blood plasma: implications for the mechanism of amniotic fluid embolism. *Eur J Obstet Gynecol Reprod Biol* 2001;95:163–6.
26. Lockwood CJ, Bach R, Guha A, Zhou XD, Miller WA, Nemerson Y. Amniotic fluid contains tissue factor, a potent initiator of coagulation. *Am J Obstet Gynecol* 1991;165:1335–41.
27. Petroianu GA, Altmannsberger SH, Maleck WH, Assmus HP, Friedberg C, Bergler WF, *et al.* Meconium and amniotic fluid embolism: effects on coagulation in pregnant mini-pigs. *Crit Care Med* 1999;27:348–55.
28. Waters JH, Biscotti C, Potter PS, Phillipson E. Amniotic fluid removal during cell salvage in the cesarean section patient. *Anesthesiology* 2000;92:1531–6.
29. Rebarber A, Lonser R, Jackson S, Copel JA, Sipes S. The safety of intraoperative autologous blood collection and autotransfusion during cesarean section. *Am J Obstet Gynecol* 1998;179:715–20.
30. Tuffnell DJ. Johnson H. Amniotic fluid embolism: the UK Register. *Hosp Med* 2000;61:532–4.
31. Margarson MP. Delayed amniotic fluid embolism following caesarean section under spinal anaesthesia. *Anaesthesia* 1995;50:804–6.
32. Judich A, Kuriansky J, Engelberg I, Haik J, Shabtai M, Czerniak A. Amniotic fluid embolism following blunt abdominal trauma in pregnancy. *Injury* 1998;29:475–7.
33. Hasaart TH, Essed GG. Amniotic fluid embolism after transabdominal amniocentesis. *Eur J Obstet Gynecol Reprod Biol* 1983;16:25–30.
34. Davies S. Amniotic fluid embolus: a review of the literature. *Can J Anaesth* 2001;48:88–98.
35. Maher JE, Wenstrom KD, Hauth JC, Meis PJ. Amniotic fluid embolism after saline amnioinfusion: two cases and review of the literature. *Obstet Gynecol* 1994;83:851–4.
36. Kanayama N, Yamazaki T, Naruse H, Sumimoto K, Horiuchi K, Terao T. Determining zinc coproporphyrin in maternal plasma – a new method for diagnosing amniotic fluid embolism. *Clin Chem* 1992;38:526–9.
37. Benson MD, Lindberg RE. Amniotic fluid embolism, anaphylaxis, and tryptase. *Am J Obstet Gynecol* 1996;175:737.
38. Farrar SC, Gherman RB. Serum tryptase in a woman with amniotic fluid embolism. A case report. *J Reprod Med* 2001;46:926–8.
39. Fineschi V, Gambassi R, Gherardi M, Turillazzi E. The diagnosis of amniotic fluid embolism: an immunohistochemical study for the quantification of pulmonary mast cell tryptase. *Int J Legal Med* 1998;111:238–43.
40. Kobayashi H, Ohi H, Terao T. A simple, noninvasive, sensitive method for diagnosis of amniotic fluid embolism by monoclonal antibody TKH-2 that recognizes NeuAc alpha 2-6GalNAc. *Am J Obstet Gynecol* 1993;168:848–53.
41. Kobayashi H, Ooi H, Hayakawa H, Arai T, Matsuda Y, Gotoh K, *et al.* Histological diagnosis of amniotic fluid embolism by monoclonal antibody TKH-2 that recognizes NeuAc alpha 2-6GalNAc epitope. *Hum Pathol* 1997;28:428–33.
42. Oi H, Kobayashi H, Hirashima Y, Yamazaki T, Kobayashi T, Terao T. Serological and immunohistochemical diagnosis of amniotic fluid embolism. *Semin Thromb Hemost* 1998;24:479–84.
43. Benson MD, Kobayashi H, Silver RK, Oi H, Greenberger PA, Terao T. Immunologic studies in presumed amniotic fluid embolism. *Obstet Gynecol* 2001;97:510–4.
44. Giampaolo C, Schneider V, Kowalski BH, Bellaver LA. The cytologic diagnosis of amniotic fluid embolism: a critical reappraisal. *Diagn Cytopathol* 1987;3:126–8.
45. Lee W, Ginsburg KA, Cotton DB, Kaufman RH. Squamous and trophoblastic cells in the maternal pulmonary circulation identified by invasive hemodynamic monitoring during the peripartum period. *Am J Obstet Gynecol* 1986;155:999–1001.
46. Clark SL, Pavlova Z, Greenspoon J, Horenstein J, Phelan JP. Squamous cells in the maternal pulmonary circulation. *Am J Obstet Gynecol* 1986;154:104–6.
47. Grady K, Prasad BGR, Howell C. Cardiopulmonary resuscitation in the non-pregnant and pregnant patient. In: Johanson R, Cox C, Grady K, Howell C, editors. *Managing Obstetric Emergencies and Trauma. The MOET Course Manual*. London: RCOG Press; 2002.
48. Burrows A, Khoo SK. The amniotic fluid embolism syndrome: 10 years' experience at a major teaching hospital. *Aust N Z J Obstet Gynaecol* 1995;35:245–50.
49. Gogola J, Hankins GD. Amniotic fluid embolism in progress: a management dilemma! *Am J*

Perinatol 1998;15:491–3.
50. Esposito RA, Grossi EA, Coppa G, Giangola G, Ferri DP, Angelides EM, *et al*. Successful treatment of postpartum shock caused by amniotic fluid embolism with cardiopulmonary bypass and pulmonary artery thromboembolectomy. *Am J Obstet Gynecol* 1990;163:572–4.
51. Hsieh YY, Chang CC, Li PC, Tsai HD, Tsai CH. Successful application of extracorporeal membrane oxygenation and intra-aortic balloon counterpulsation as lifesaving therapy for a patient with amniotic fluid embolism. *Am J Obstet Gynecol* 2000;183:496–7.
52. Van Heerden PV, Webb SA, Hee G, Corkeron M, Thompson WR. Inhaled aerosolized prostacyclin as a selective pulmonary vasodilator for the treatment of severe hypoxaemia. *Anaesth Intensive Care* 1996;24:87–90.
53. Tanus-Santos JE, Moreno H Jr. Inhaled nitric oxide and amniotic fluid embolism. *Anesth Analg* 1999;88:691.
54. Dodgson J, Martin J, Boswell J, Goodall HB, Smith R. Probable amniotic fluid embolism precipitated by amniocentesis and treated by exchange transfusion. *BMJ* 1987;294:1322–3.
55. Awad IT, Shorten GD. Amniotic fluid embolism and isolated coagulopathy: atypical presentation of amniotic fluid embolism. *Eur J Anaesthesiol* 2001;18:410–3.
56. Kaneko Y, Ogihara T, Tajima H, Mochimaru F. Continuous hemodiafiltration for disseminated intravascular coagulation and shock due to amniotic fluid embolism: report of a dramatic response. *Intern Med* 2001;40:945–7.
57. Jenkins DM, Carr C, Stanley J, O'Dwyer T. Maternal mortality in the Irish Republic, 1989–1991. *Ir Med J* 1996:89:140–1.
58. Weiwen Y, Ningyu Z, Lanxiang Z, Yu L. Study of the diagnosis and management of amniotic fluid embolism: 38 cases of analysis. *Obstet Gynecol* 2000:95 Suppl 1:S38.
59. Kim IT, Choi JB. Occlusions of branch retinal arterioles following amniotic fluid embolism. *Ophthalmologica* 2000;214:305–8.
60. Kaptanoglu M, Dogan K, Onen A, Cevit R, Berkan O, Aker H. Lung mass due to amniotic fluid embolism – an intrathoracic complication of pregnancy. *Scand Cardiovasc J* 1999;33:117–9.
61. Clark SL. Successful pregnancy outcomes after amniotic fluid embolism. *Am J Obstet Gynecol* 1992;167:511–2.
62. Duffy BL. Does amniotic fluid embolism recur? *Anaesth Intensive Care* 1998;26:333.
63. Collier C. Recurring amniotic fluid embolism. *Anaesth Intensive Care* 1998:26:599–600.
64. Stiller RJ, Siddiqui D, Laifer SA, Tiakowski RL, Whetham JC. Successful pregnancy after suspected anaphylactoid syndrome of pregnancy (amniotic fluid embolus). A case report. *J Reprod Med* 2000;45:1007–9.

Chapter 16

Pre-eclampsia and eclampsia

Stephen Robson

Terminology and classification

Pre-eclampsia is a syndrome (a group of symptoms or signs) that can be recognised but not diagnosed because there is no specific diagnostic test. The presentation is highly variable and, although hypertension and proteinuria are the signs most easily detected, they are not central to the pathogenesis of the disorder. Other features that may aid recognition are shown in Table 16.1. Eclampsia is the occurrence of convulsions during pregnancy or in the first ten days after delivery in association with pre-eclampsia. Convulsive disorders have been recognised as a cause of maternal death since Roman times but it was not until the 19th century that the link with proteinuria and hypertension was recognised.[1] The features of severe pre-eclampsia are:

- severe hypertension (blood pressure ≥ 160 mmHg systolic or ≥ 110 mmHg diastolic on at least two occasions at least six hours apart)
- proteinuria (≥ 5 g/24 hours)
- oliguria (≤ 400 ml/24 hours)
- cerebral or visual disturbance
- epigastric pain
- pulmonary oedema or cyanosis
- thrombocytopenia
- impaired liver function.

Incidence

Data from North America indicate that pre-eclampsia complicates 2.6–3.2% of all births.[2,3] In Aberdeen, UK, the incidence of pre-eclampsia in first pregnancies is 5.3%

Table 16.1. Features of pre-eclampsia

Maternal syndrome	Fetal syndrome
Pregnancy-induced hypertension[a]	Fetal growth restriction
Proteinuria[b]	Abnormal fetal Doppler waveforms
Generalised oedema	Fetal hypoxaemia
Hyperuricaemia	
Thrombocytopenia	
Increased liver transaminases	
Hypocalciuria	
Increased haematocrit	
Abnormal uterine artery Doppler waveforms	

[a] one measurement of diastolic blood pressure (DBP) ≥ 110 mm Hg or two consecutive measurements ≥ 90 mm Hg four hours or more apart; this definition includes a significant number of women with chronic hypertension; this problem can be circumvented by incorporating in the definition an increase in DBP of ≥ 25 mm Hg;[b] 24-hour protein excretion ≥ 300 mg per day

compared with 1.4% in subsequent pregnancies.[4] There is no evidence in either population that the incidence of pre-eclampsia is falling. Accurate figures on the incidence of pre-eclampsia in developing countries are harder to find. Rates of 0.7–4.7% have been reported from Asia,[5] while a large study from Latin America has reported an incidence of 4.8%.[6] Severe pre-eclampsia[7] complicates 5–10% of cases, but higher figures have been reported from India, where 3.7% of all women were reported to have severe pre-eclampsia.[8]

The incidence of eclampsia in the UK has fallen from around 80/10 000 maternities in the 1920s[9] to 4.9/10 000 in 1992.[10] Locally collected data confirm this trend; at the Glasgow Royal Maternity Hospital the incidence of eclampsia fell from 74/10 000 deliveries between 1931 and 1940 to 7.2/10 000 between 1981 and 1990.[11] The incidence of eclampsia in the UK is similar to that in most other countries in north-western Europe and the USA,[12,13] although slightly higher than that reported in Scandinavia (2.4–2.7/10 000 deliveries).[14,15] In contrast, the rate of eclampsia is considerably higher in developing countries; in Bangladesh, a country with major social deprivation and few trained birth attendants, the rate of eclampsia has been reported to be as high as 300/10 000 deliveries.[16] Sawhney *et al.*[8] reported their experience in Chandigarh, India: the incidence of eclampsia increased from 94/10 000 deliveries between 1982 and 1989 to 220/10 000 between 1990 and 1998.

Pathophysiology

The multisystem disorder of pre-eclampsia is characterised by maternal endothelial cell dysfunction. This appears to be part of a more generalised maternal intravascular inflammatory response involving intravascular leucocytes, as well as the coagulation and complement systems.[17] The stimulus to this response is unknown but appears to be strongly linked to an underperfused placenta, secondary to failed trophoblast invasion of the maternal uterine spiral arteries, the generation of free radicals and a state of oxidative stress.[18]

The cause of eclamptic seizures is disputed. Two possible mechanisms have been proposed: cerebral vasoconstriction (and ischaemia) and hypertensive encephalopathy.

Cerebral vasoconstriction and ischaemia

Cerebral vasospasm has been described in eclampsia using computed tomography and digital subtraction angiography.[19,20] Vasoconstriction leads to ischaemia and cytotoxic oedema.

Hypertensive encephalopathy

Encephalopathy results from damage to the blood–brain barrier secondary to severe hypertension. This is usually associated with loss of cerebral autoregulation. Once perfusion pressure exceeds 140–150 mmHg, the autoregulatory mechanism fails, leading to passive overdistension of the cerebral resistance vessels and subsequent hyperperfusion.[21] In this scenario, disruption of the blood–brain barrier leads to pressure-driven extravasation of fluid (vasogenic oedema) and potentially fibrinoid necrosis of cerebral vessels.

Non-invasive studies of middle cerebral artery (MCA) Doppler have provided valuable insights into cerebral changes in pre-eclampsia/eclampsia. Estimated cerebral perfusion pressure (CPP) can be calculated from MCA velocity and blood pressure.[22] Belfort *et al.*[23] reported that women with mild pre-eclampsia are more likely to have a CPP below that of normal pregnant women, while women with severe pre-eclampsia with a headache have an increased CPP (Figure 16.1). These findings may explain the dual pathophysiology of eclamptic seizures; in women who have seizures with a normal or mildly elevated blood pressure, cerebral ischaemia is likely to be the major cause, whereas in women with severe hyperetension it is more likely that seizures are secondary to hypertensive encephalopathy and cerebral overperfusion.[23]

Mortality rates

Deaths from pre-eclampsia and eclampsia continue to fall in most developed countries. Data from the Confidential Enquiries into Maternal Deaths for England and Wales have shown that the death rate from hypertensive disorders of pregnancy per million maternities fell from 97.4 in 1952–4 to 11.5 in 1988–90.[24] Enquiry data for the UK were first published for the triennium 1985–87. Since then, deaths from pre-eclampsia have fallen from 6.7 to 5.2 per million maternities, while those from eclampsia have fallen to a greater extent – from 5.4 to 2.4 per million maternities (Figure 16.2).[25] Hypertensive disorders currently account for 14% (15/106) of direct maternal deaths, with eclampsia being a factor in 33% (5/15).[25] Mackay *et al.*[26] recently reported pregnancy-related mortality from hypertensive disorders for the USA between 1979 and 1992 based on data from the Centers for Disease Control and Prevention's Pregnancy Mortality Surveillance System. Pre-eclampsia and eclampsia accounted for 387/4024 (9.6%) of the pregnancy-related deaths after 20 or more weeks of gestation (mortality rate 1.5/100 000 livebirths), with eclampsia being a factor in 49% of the deaths.

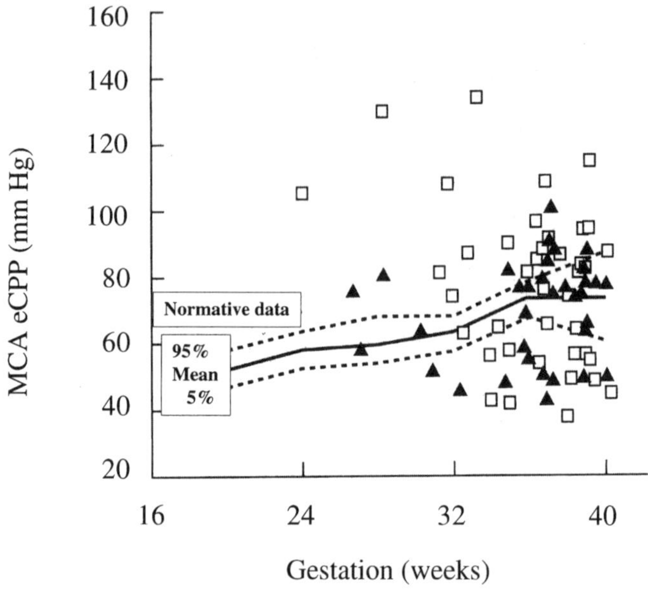

Figure 16.1 Relationship between middle cerebral artery estimated cerebral perfusion pressure (MCA eCPP), as determined by transcranial Doppler, and gestational age in women with pre-eclampsia (squares) and without (triangles) headache; normative curve with upper and lower 95% prediction limits derived from 63 longitudinally studied pregnant women is also plotted;[11] reproduced with permission from the *British Journal of Obstetrics and Gynaecology*

Mortality rates from hypertension in the developing world are much higher. Estimated maternal mortality from hypertensive disorders ranges from 10–150 per 100 000 live/total births, with the highest rates being found in West Africa, Central America and Middle/South Asia (The Gambia 150/10 000; Mexico 135/100 000; Pakistan 120/100 000).[27] Hypertensive disorders are responsible for around 15% of maternal deaths worldwide (50 000/year) but in many of the poorest developing countries this figure is around 30% and more than 90% of hypertensive deaths are associated with eclampsia.[27] These figures are even more horrifying in the context of incomplete recording of maternal deaths, which means that the mortality rate from hypertension/eclampsia may be underestimated by as much as 50%.[27]

An accurate assessment of the case fatality rate from eclampsia in the UK is available from the British Eclampsia Survey conducted in 1992.[10] In this series, seven of 382 (1.8%) cases died. Lower rates have been reported from single centres in the USA with extensive experience of managing women with eclampsia; Mattar and Sibai[28] documented only two deaths in 399 consecutive women with eclampsia managed in Memphis, Tennessee. This compares with data from the Collaborative Eclampsia Trial, where mortality in the different treatment groups varied from 2.6–5.2%.[29] Although the trial included cases from centres in Africa, South America and India, the fatality rates in many parts of the developing world are higher. Two large series from Mexico City and Chandigarh in India reported mortality rates of 13.9% and 6.9% respectively,[30,8] while one referral centre in Bangladesh is reported as having a mortality rate of over 20%.[31]

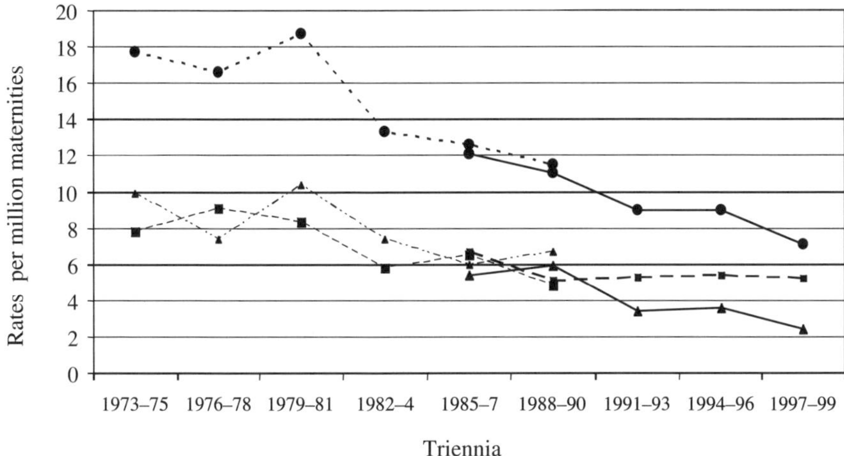

Figure 16.2 Maternal mortality rate (deaths per million maternities) from hypertensive disorders in the United Kingdom[25] (deaths from eclampsia (▲), pre-eclampsia (■) and total hypertensive deaths (●); Crown copyright material reproduced with permission of the Controller of HMSO and the Queen's Printer for Scotland

Case fatality rates for pre-eclampsia are much more difficult to determine, primarily because of the varying definitions of pre-eclampsia and severe pre-eclampsia. Data from the USA suggest an overall mortality rate from pre-eclampsia of 3.4/10 000 cases, much lower than that from eclampsia (71.6/10 000 cases).[26] No data are available for the UK but, assuming an incidence of pre-eclampsia of 3%,[4] mortality can be estimated as 2.3/10 000 cases.[25] Data from large referral centres suggest much higher rates in severe disease; Odendaal *et al.*[32] (1995) reported a mortality rate of 60/10 000 from Tygerberg (South Africa) and Sawhney *et al.*[8] a rate of 39/10 000 from Chandigarh (India). Case fatality rates are influenced by many factors, not least of which are the quality and accessibility of perinatal care. In developed countries, maternal age and gestational age appear to be the most important; in the large series from the USA, mortality increased from 1.1/100 000 livebirths in women aged 20–24 years to 6.0/100 000 in women aged 40–49 years (risk ratio 5.3, 95% CI 3.5–7.9).[26] A similar pattern was seen for hypertensive deaths in the UK.[25] Compared with women presenting at 37 weeks or more (mortality 0.5/10 000 livebirths), women with pre-eclampsia/eclampsia before 28 weeks (mortality 12.5/10 000 livebirths) had a risk ratio of 23.7 (95% CI 17.6–31.8).[26]

Cause of death

The exact cause of death may be difficult to determine in the presence of multisystem failure, especially if postmortem examination is not carried out. Cerebral haemorrhage is the principal cause of death in the UK and worldwide. Data from the UK Confidential Enquiries between 1985 and 1999 indicate that 44/110 deaths (40%) from

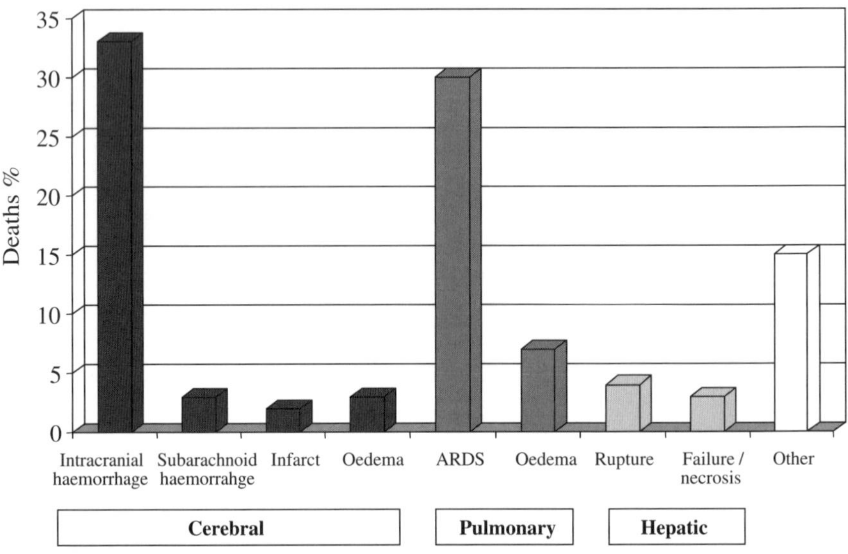

Figure 16.3 Causes of death due to eclampsia and pre-eclampsia in the UK 1985–1999; ARDS = acute respiratory distress syndrome;[25] Crown copyright material reproduced with permission of the Controller of HMSO and the Queen's Printer for Scotland

eclampsia/pre-eclampsia were ascribed to cerebral causes, of which 39 (89%) were secondary to haemorrhage (intracranial 36, subarachnoid 3). Cerebral infarction was recorded in two cases and isolated cerebral oedema in three.[25] The remaining deaths were ascribed to pulmonary (41/110 [37%]), hepatic (7/110 [6%]) and other (16/110 [15%]) causes (Figure 16.3).

Much larger numbers are available from the recent large study from the USA.[26] Thirty-eight percent of the 790 deaths attributed to pre-eclampsia and eclampsia were due to cerebrovascular events, of which 90% were cerebrovascular haemorrhage, 7% cerebral oedema and 3% cerebral embolus. Renal or hepatic failure accounted for 12.5% of deaths, HELLP (haemolysis, elevated liver enzymes, low platelets) syndrome 7%, 'Other complications of hypertension' 26% and 'Not specified hypertension' 16%. Disseminated intravascular coagulation (DIC) was reported as a contributing condition in 15% of hypertension deaths.[26] Generally the proportion of deaths from each cause was similar in pre-eclampsia and eclampsia. It is noteworthy that pulmonary deaths were much less common than in the UK. This may relate to the method of reporting; in a recent study of maternal deaths associated with HELLP syndrome collected from the membership of the American Society for Maternal-Fetal Medicine, adult respiratory distress syndrome (ARDS) was the fourth most common contributing factor (present in 28% of deaths) after cerebrovascular accidents (45%), cardiac arrest (40%) and DIC (34%).[33]

The pattern in developing countries is more difficult to determine; reliable data tend only to be available from specialist centres. Cerebrovascular accidents appear to be the

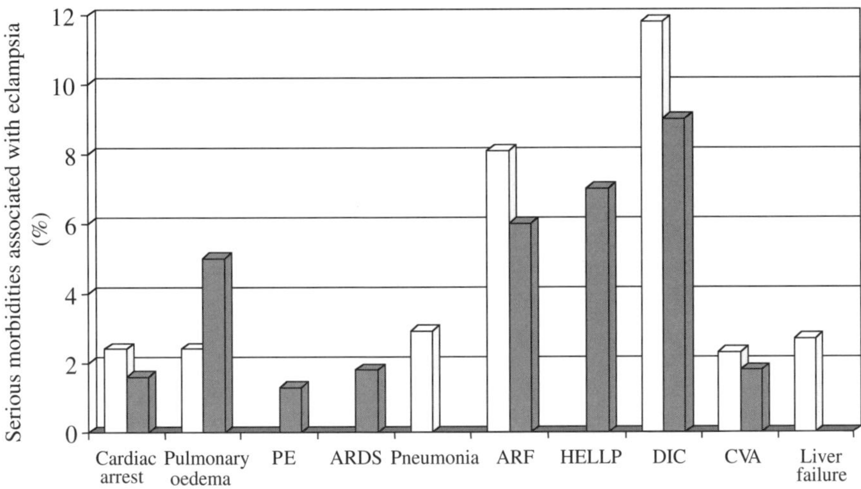

Figure 16.4 Incidence of serious morbidities associated with eclampsia in the Collaborative Eclampsia Trial (magnesium treated arms only)[25] (unshaded) and the British Eclampsia Survey[10] (shaded); ARDS = acute respiratory distress syndrome; ARF = acute renal failure; CVA = cerebrovascular accident; DIC = disseminated intravascular coagulation; HELLP = haemolysis, elevated liver enzymes and low platelet count; PE = pulmonary embolus; the incidence of PE, ARDS and HELLP was not reported in the Collaborative Eclampsia Trial[25]

leading cause of death, accounting for 72% of eclampsia-related deaths in Mexico City[34] and 35% in Chandigarh, India.[8] However, in this latter study, cerebrovascular accidents were the principal cause of 53% of deaths occurring within 24 hours of hospitalisation and cerebral pathology was present in 62% of postmortem examinations. The other major causes of death are respiratory failure (usually secondary to aspiration pneumonia or pulmonary oedema), renal failure and DIC/haemorrhage.

Morbidity

Associated morbidity in women recruited to the magnesium arm of the Collaborative Eclampsia Trial and the UK Eclampsia survey are shown in Figure 16.4.[10,29] Serious respiratory complications occur in up to 5% of women, with a further 7–8% experiencing respiratory depression.[29,35] This results in 10–23% of women with eclampsia requiring ventilation. Coagulation problems (including HELLP syndrome) and renal failure occur in 10–15% and 5–8% of eclamptics respectively.

The range of morbidity in pre-eclampsia is identical to that in eclampsia. Incidences vary with the severity of disease but in most series of severe pre-eclampsia, the rates of pulmonary, coagulation and renal complications are similar or slightly lower than those reported for eclampsia..[36,37] Data from the Yorkshire Regional Audit of severe pre-eclampsia confirm that pulmonary morbidity is frequent; between 1998 and 2000, 6% of cases had evidence of hypoxaemia and 2.9% had clinical pulmonary oedema.[38] Identical rates of pulmonary oedema were reported from Memphis, with 70% occurring postpartum, usually associated with excessive colloid and crystalloid infusions.[37] Renal failure has been reported in 1.7–2.1% of women with severe pre-eclampsia.[39,40] The majority of cases occur after delivery and are associated with postpartum haemorrhage and/or HELLP syndrome.[39] Dialysis rates vary from 10–50%;[39,40] this is consistent with the Yorkshire series, in which 0.8% of women with severe pre-eclampsia required dialysis.[38] Maternal morbidity is generally greater in women with HELLP syndrome; Martin *et al.*[36] reported that 38% of women with class I HELLP (platelet nadir ≤ 50 000 cells/μl) had morbidity in at least one system (haematological/coagulation, cardiopulmonary, central nervous system, renal and hepatic/gastrointestinal), compared with 19% in class II HELLP (platelet nadir > 50 000 and ≤ 100 000 cells/μl), 18% in class III HELLP (platelet nadir > 100 000 and ≤ 150 000 cells/μl), and 10% in severe pre-eclampsia. The rates for two- and three-system morbidity were 9%, 3%, 3% and 1% and 2.5%, 0.33%, 0% and 0%, respectively. Haddad *et al.*[41] compared outcome in women with HELLP syndrome and severe pre-eclampsia with onset prior to 28 weeks of gestation. They reported similar trends with respect to pulmonary, renal and coagulation problems, although the only statistically significant difference was a higher rate of transfusion of blood products in the HELLP group (25%) than in the severe pre-eclampsia group (3%).

Strategies to reduce maternal morbidity and mortality from pre-eclampsia/eclampsia

Early recognition of pre-eclampsia/eclampsia

Regular screening for hypertension, proteinuria and fetal size during antenatal care allows early recognition of the pre-eclampsia syndrome. The traditional frequency of antenatal visits (monthly to 28 weeks, twice weekly to 36 weeks and weekly thereafter) takes little account of a woman's risk of pre-eclampsia or of the impact of the syndrome on mother and fetus. Since it is the early-onset syndrome that is associated with the highest risk of maternal and fetal mortality (and morbidity), screening in high-risk women should be more frequent (twice weekly) between 24 and 30 weeks. A markedly reduced frequency of visits is appropriate in low-risk women.[42] Risk factors are as follows:

- primiparity
- extremes of age (over 35 years, less than 20 years)
- obesity
- multiple pregnancy
- pre-eclampsia/eclampsia in a previous pregnancy
- family history of pre-eclampsia/eclampsia

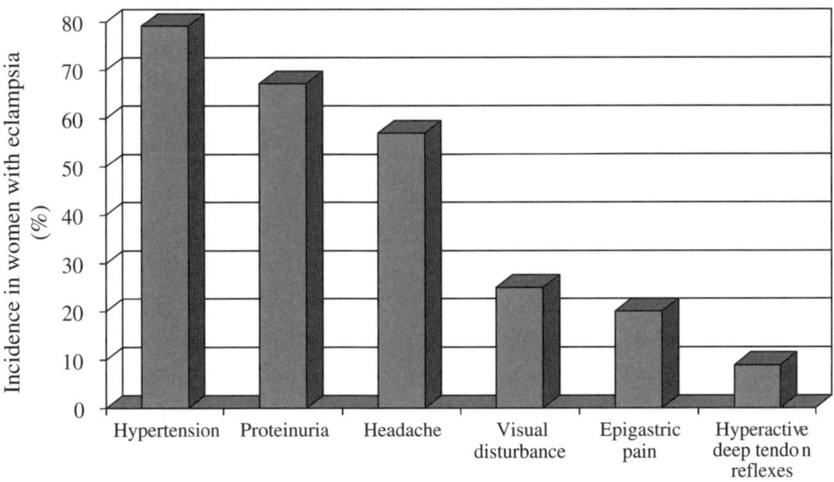

Figure 16.5 Premonitory signs and symptoms in women who develop eclampsia[10, 35,47,48]

- pre-existing hypertension/renal disease
- abnormal uterine artery Doppler waveforms.

The definition of pregnancy-induced hypertension (PIH) is controversial but there is evidence that the use of a combination of a maximum diastolic pressure of ≥ 90 mmHg (based on Korotkoff phase V), together with an increase in diastolic pressure of ≥ 25 mmHg, is more successful at identifying a group of women with features of pre-eclampsia than the absolute threshold alone.[43,44] Once a diagnosis of PIH or proteinuria is made, repeated multisystem screening for other features of the syndrome is required.[45] The most important factor determining progression from PIH to pre-eclampsia is the gestation at presentation; 42% of women with PIH presenting prior to 30 weeks develop pre-eclampsia, compared with 7% presenting at term.[46]

The risk of developing eclampsia in women with pre-eclampsia is 1.5–2%.[47] Seizure rates are higher in women with severe disease; Martin *et al.*[36] reported seizures in 5.2% of women with severe pre-eclampsia without HELLP syndrome and 9.2% of women with HELLP syndrome. This is comparable to the data from the Yorkshire Region Audit (1998–2000) where 50 of 649 (7.7%) women with severe pre-eclampsia developed eclampsia.[39] Although seizures generally develop in women with PIH and proteinuria, around 20% have no hypertension and a similar or slightly greater proportion have no proteinuria.[10,35] Premonitory symptoms occur in 60–70% of women developing eclampsia (Figure 16.5).[10,35,48,49] Based on an analysis of 445 consecutive women with severe pre-eclampsia, Witlin *et al.*[49] found that, of the clinical and haematological/biochemical indices investigated, only headache and hyperactive deep tendon reflexes were predictive of eclampsia. Thus symptomatic women with PIH or pre-eclampsia must be referred to an appropriate centre for further assessment.

Management of severe hypertension

In order to reduce death from cerebrovascular accidents, it is crucial that severe hypertension is treated aggressively. Under normal conditions, cerebral blood flow remains stable if mean arterial pressure (MAP) is between 60–140 mmHg. Above this level, there is cerebral hyperperfusion and the risks of arterial injury and cerebrovascular accident increases.[50] Breakthrough hyperperfusion occurs at higher MAPs in subjects with pre-existing hypertension. Blood pressures of 180/120 mmHg (MAP 140 mmHg) or more require urgent treatment and the aim should be to keep blood pressure below 170/110 mmHg.[45] There is no good evidence that one antihypertensive agent is better than another, with the exceptions of diazoxide, associated with profound hypotension, and ketanserin, which is less effective than hydralazine.[51] Intravenous hydralazine (5–10 mg), intravenous labetolol (20–40 mg) and oral nifedipine (5–10 mg) are effective; the choice of antihypertensive should depend on the experience and familiarity of the clinician (as well as the cost and availability of the drug).[51]

Although treatment of mild to moderate hypertension (diastolic pressures 90–109 mmHg) reduces the risk of severe hypertension (RR 0.52, 95% CI 0.41–0.64], there is no evidence that antihypertensives reduce the risk of subsequent pre-eclampsia (RR 0.99, 95% CI 0.84–1.18) or significant maternal morbidity.[52]

Use of magnesium sulphate in eclampsia

There is now clear evidence that magnesium sulphate is the anticonvulsant of choice in women with eclampsia.[53,54] Magnesium is associated with a substantial reduction in the recurrence of seizures, when compared with diazepam (RR 0.45, 95% CI 0.35–0.58)[53] and phenytoin (RR 0.30, 95% CI 0.20–0.46).[53] Magnesium also leads to reduced maternal morbidity (pneumonia, ventilation and intensive care admission) and a trend towards reduced mortality (RR 0.51, 95% CI 0.25–1.06) compared with phenytoin[54] while the reduction in maternal mortality relative to diazepam (RR 0.60, 95% CI 0.36–1.00) is of borderline significance. All women with an eclamptic seizure should therefore be given 4 g magnesium sulphate intravenously followed by either an intravenous infusion of 1 g hourly or 5 g intramuscularly every four hours.

Appropriate investigations in women with 'complex' eclampsia

Women with prior pre-eclampsia who present with typical tonic–clonic seizures rarely present a diagnostic problem. The differential diagnosis of unheralded postnatal seizures, especially if recurrent and/or associated with altered consciousness, includes cerebral infarction, cerebral haemorrhage, subarachnoid haemorrhage, cerebral venous thrombosis and cerebral oedema. All may occur as primary pathologies or as secondary complications of eclampsia.

Most cases of eclampsia, particularly those without focal neurological deficits (e.g. cortical blindness, aphasia and limb weakness), have normal imaging studies.[55] Patients with focal findings and atypical cases warrant investigation by cranial computed tomography (CT) and/or magnetic resonance imaging (MRI). CT is the optimum modality for excluding haemorrhage but is relatively insensitive compared with MRI

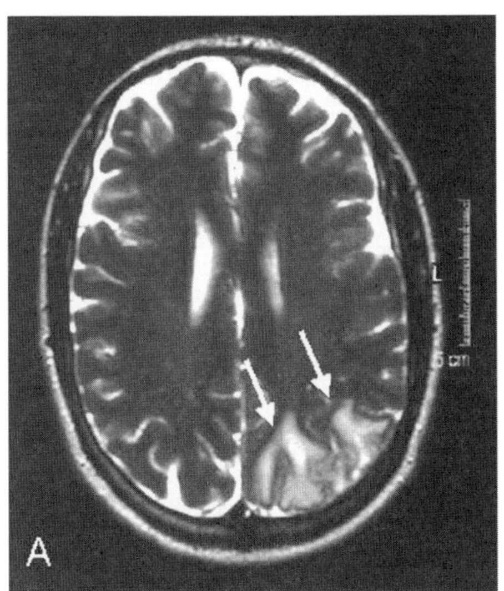

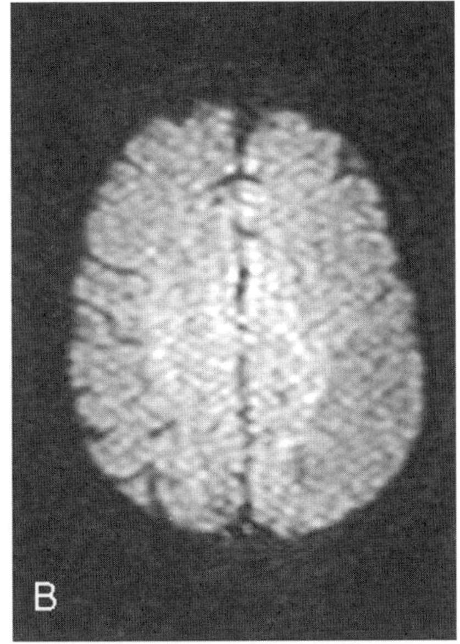

Figure 16.6 (A) Axial T2-weighted magnetic resonance image showing diffuse hyperintense signal abnormalities in the parieto-occipital subcortical white matter and adjacent grey matter (arrows); (B) axial diffusion-weighted magnetic resonance image showing no abnormal signal in the parieto-occipital region suggesting the hyperintensities on T2-weighted images were due to vasogenic oedema and not cerebral infarction

for acute ischaemia. Hypodensities on CT or hyperintensities on T2-weighted MRI images may indicate cerebral infarction or vasogenic oedema secondary to hypertensive encephalopathy. Diffusion-weighted MRI will differentiate between cytotoxic oedema (secondary to infarction) and vasogenic oedema (Figure 16.6), allowing appropriate management.[56]

Conclusion

Overall around 13% of maternal deaths worldwide are due to hypertensive disorders. All women should be screened for PIH and proteinuria at each antenatal visit, although the frequency of these visits should reflect the risk of the syndrome. The most common cause of death is intracranial haemorrhage; reducing deaths from this cause requires effective treatment of severe hypertension. A substantial proportion of deaths from pre-eclampsia, especially in the developing world, is associated with eclampsia. Magnesium sulphate has been shown to reduce the risk of recurrent seizures and may improve maternal mortality. Cranial imaging allows accurate diagnosis of cerebral pathology and should be undertaken in all women with atypical eclampsia and in those with focal signs. Substandard care is a recurrent finding in confidential enquiries into maternal deaths. All units should have clear written guidelines for the referral and management of women with severe pre-eclampsia and eclampsia.

References

1. Lever JCW. Cases of puerperal convulsions, with remarks. *Guy's Hosp Rep* 1843; 495–517.
2. Saftlas AF, Olson DR, Franks A, Atrash HK, Pokras R. Epidemiology of preeclampsia and eclampsia in the United States, 1979–1986. *Am J Obstet Gynecol* 1990;163:460–5.
3. Gofton EN, Capewell V, Natale R, Gratton RJ. Obstetrical intervention rates and maternal and neonatal outcomes of women with gestational hypertension. *Am J Obstet Gynecol* 2001;185:798–803.
4. Campbell DM, MacGillivray I. Preeclampsia in twin pregnancies: incidence and outcome. *Hypertens Pregnancy* 1999;18:197–207.
5. Hall MH, Campbell DM. Geographical epidemiology of hypertension in pregnancy. In: Sharp F, Symonds EM, editors. *Hypertension in Pregnancy*. New York: Perinatology Press; 1987. p. 33–46.
6. Conde-Agudelo A, Belizan JM. Risk factors for pre-eclampsia in a large cohort of Latin American and Caribbean women. *BJOG* 2000;107:75–83.
7. American College of Obstetricians and Gynecologists. *Hypertension in Pregnancy*. Technical Bulletin No. 219. Washington, DC: ACOG; 1996.
8. Sawhney H, Aggarwal N, Biswas R, Vasishta K, Gopalan S. Maternal mortality associated with eclampsia and severe preeclampsia of pregnancy. *J Obstet Gynaecol Res* 2000;26:351–6.
9. Eden TW. Eclampsia. *J Obstet Gynaecol Br Empire* 1922;29:386–401.
10. Douglas KA, Redman CWG. Eclampsia in the United Kingdom. *BMJ* 1994;1395–400.
11. Leitch CR, Cameron AD, Walker JJ. The changing pattern of eclampsia over a 60-year period. *Br J Obstet Gynaecol* 1997;104:917–22.
12. Saftlas AF, Olson DR, Franks AL, Atrash HK, Pokras R. Epidemiology of preeclampsia and eclampsia in the United States 1979–1986. *Am J Obstet Gynecol* 1990;163:460–5.
13. Geirsson RT, Arngrimsson R, Apalset E, Einarsson A, Snaedal G. Falling population incidence of eclampsia. *Acta Obstet Gynecol Scand* 1994;73:465–7.
14. Moller B, Lindmark G. Eclampsia in Sweden 1976–1980. *Acta Obstet Gynecol Scand* 1986;65:307–14.
15. Ekholm E, Salmi MM, Erkkola R. Eclampsia in Finland in 1990–1994. *Acta Obstet Gynecol Scand* 1999;78:877–82.
16. Eclampsia Working Group. Eclampsia in Bangladesh: a review and a guideline. *Bangladesh Journal of Obstetrics and Gynaecology* 1996;12:1–25.
17. Redman CW, Sacks GP, Sargent IL. Preeclampsia: an excessive maternal inflammatory response to pregnancy. *Am J Obstet Gynecol* 1999;180:499–506.
18. Hubel CA. Oxidative stress and preeclampsia. *Fetal and Maternal Medicine Review* 1997;9:73–101.
19. Will AD, Lewis KL, Hinshaw DB Jr, Jordan JK, Cousins LM, Hasso HN, *et al.* Cerebral vasoconstriction in toxaemia. *Neurology* 1987;37:1555–7.
20. Trommer BL, Homer D, Mikhael MA. Cerebral vasospasm and eclampsia. *Stroke* 1988;19:326–9.
21. Johansson B, Strandgaard S, Lassen NA. On the pathogenesis of hypertensive encephalopathy. *Circ Res* 1974;34 Suppl 1:167–71.
22. Belfort MA, Tooke-Miller C, Varner M, Saade G, Grunewald C, Nisell H, *et al.* Evaluation of a non-invasive transcranial Doppler and blood pressure-based method for the assessment of cerebral perfusion pressure in pregnant women. *Hypertens Pregnancy* 2000;19:331–40.
23. Belfort MA, Saade GR, Grunewald C, Dildy GA, Abedejos P, Herd JA, *et al.* Association of cerebral perfusion pressure with headache in women with pre-eclampsia. *Br J Obstet Gynaecol* 1999;106:814–21.
24. Department of Health, Welsh Office, Scottish Office Home and Health Department, Department of Health and Social Security, Northern Ireland. *Report into Maternal Deaths in the United Kingdom 1988–1990*. London: HMSO; 1994.
25. Drife J, Lewis G, editors. *Why Mothers Die 1997–1999. The Confidential Enquiries into Maternal Deaths in the United Kingdom*. London: RCOG Press; 2001.
26. Mackay AP, Berg CJ, Atrash HK. Pregnancy-related mortality from pre-eclampsia and eclampsia. *Obstet Gynecol* 2001;97:533–8.
27. Duley L. Maternal mortality associated with hypertensive disorders of pregnancy in Africa, Asia, Latin America and the Caribbean. *Br J Obstet Gynaecol* 1992;99:547–53.
28. Mattar F, Sibai BM. Eclampsia. VIII. Risk factors for maternal morbidity. *Am J Obstet Gynecol* 2000;182:307–12.
29. Eclampsia Trial Collaborative Group. Which anticonvulsant for women with eclampsia? Evidence from the Collaborative Eclampsia Trial. *Lancet* 1995;345:1455–63.
30. Lopez-Llera M. Main clinical types and subtypes of eclampsia. *Am J Obstet Gynecol* 1992;166:4–9.

31. Johanson R. Towards safer childbirth: an historical view of eclampsia. *The Obstetrician and Gynaecologist* 2001;3:97–9.
32. Odendaal HJ, Steyn DW, Norman K, Kirsten GF, Smith J, Theron GB. Improved perinatal mortality rate in 1001 patients with severe pre-eclampsia. *S Afr Med J* 1995;85:1071–6.
33. Isler CM, Rinehart BK, Terrone DA, Martin RW, Magann EF, Martin JN. Maternal mortality associated with HELLP (hemolysis, elevated liver enzymes, and low platelets) syndrome. *Am J Obstet Gynecol* 1999;181:924–8.
34. Lopez-Llera M. Complicated eclampsia – fifteen years experience in a referral medical centre. *Am J Obstet Gynecol* 1982;142:28–35.
35. Sibai BM. Eclampsia. VI. Maternal-perinatal outcome in 254 consecutive cases. *Am J Obstet Gynecol* 1990;163:1049–55.
36. Martin JN Jr, Rinehart BK, May WL, Magann EF, Terrone DA, Blake PG. The spectrum of severe preeclampsia: comparative analysis by HELLP (hemolysis, elevated liver enzyme levels, and low platelet count) syndrome classification. *Am J Obstet Gynecol* 1999;180:1373–84.
37. Sibai BM, Mabie BC, Harvey RN, Gonzalez AR. Pulmonary edema in severe preeclampsia-eclampsia: analysis of thirty-seven consecutive cases. *Am J Obstet Gynecol* 1987;156:1174–9.
38. D Tuffnell, personal communication.
39. Sibai BM, Villar MA, Mabie BC. Acute renal failure in hypertensive disorders of pregnancy. Pregnancy outcome and remote prognosis in thirty-one consecutive cases. *Am J Obstet Gynecol* 1990;162:777–83.
40. Drakeley AJ, Le Roux PA, Anthony J, Penny J. Acute renal failure complicating severe preeclampsia requiring admission to an obstetric intensive care unit. *Am J Obstet Gynecol* 2002;186:253–6.
41. Haddad B, Barton JR, Livingstone JC, Chahine R, Sibai BM. HELLP (hemolysis, elevated liver enzyme levels, and low platelet count) syndrome versus severe preeclampsia: onset at ≤ 28.0 weeks' gestation. *Am J Obstet Gynecol* 2000;183:1475–9.
42. Carroli G, Villar J, Piaggio G, Khan-Neelofur D, Gulmezoglu M, Mugford M, *et al.* WHO systematic review of randomised controlled trials of routine antenatal care. *Lancet* 2001;357:1565–70.
43. Redman CWG, Jeffries M. Revised definition of pre-eclampsia. *Lancet* 1988;1:809–12.
44. Shennan A, Gupta M, Halligan A, Taylor D, de Swiet M. Lack of reproducibility in pregnancy of Korotkoff phase IV as measured by mercury sphygmomanometry. *Lancet* 1996;347:139–42.
45. Robson SC. Hypertension and renal disease in pregnancy. In: Edmonds DK, editor. *Dewhurst's Textbook of Obstetrics and Gynaecology for Postgraduates*. 6th ed. Oxford: Blackwell Science; 1999. p.166–85.
46. Saudan P, Brown MA, Buddle ML, Jones M. Does gestational hypertension become pre-eclampsia? *Br J Obstet Gynaecol* 1998;105:1177–84.
47. Duley, L. Gulmezoglu, AM. Henderson-Smart, DJ. Anticonvulsants for women with pre-eclampsia. *Cochrane Database Syst Rev* 2002;(1).
48. Ekholm E, Salmi MM, Erkkola R. Eclampsia in Finland in 1990-1994. *Acta Obstet Gynecol Scand* 1999;78:877–82.
49. Witlin AG, Saade GR, Mattar F, Sibai BM. Risk factors for abruptio placentae and eclampsia: analysis of 445 consecutively managed women with severe preeclampsia and eclampsia. *Am J Obstet Gynecol* 1999;180:1322–9.
50. Paulson OB, Strandgaard S, Edvinsson L. Cerebral autoregulation. *Cerebrovasc Brain Metab Rev* 1990;2:161–92.
51. Duley L, Henderson-Smart DJ. Drugs for the rapid treatment of very high blood pressure during pregnancy. *Cochrane Database Syst Rev* 2002;(1).
52. Abalos E, Duley L, Steyn DW, Henderson-Smart DJ. Antihypertensive drug therapy for mild to moderate hypertension during pregnancy. *Cochrane Database Syst Rev* 2002;(1).
53. Duley L, Henderson-Smart D. Magnesium sulphate versus diazepam for eclampsia. *Cochrane Database Syst Rev* 2002;(1):CD 000127.
54. Duley L, Henderson-Smart D. Magnesium sulphate versus phenytoin for eclampsia. *Cochrane Database Syst Rev* 2002;(1):CD 000128.
55. Sibai BM, Spinnato JA, Watson DL, Levis JA, Anderson GD. Eclampsia IV. Neurological findings and future outcome. *Am J Obstet Gynecol* 1985;152:184–92.
56. Kanki T, Tsukimori K, Mihara F, Nakano H. Diffusion-weighted images and vasogenic edema in eclampsia. *Obstet Gynecol* 1999;93:821–3.

Chapter 17

Early pregnancy deaths

James P Neilson

Introduction

The concept of monitoring maternal mortality as a tool to improve public health is not a new one. In the Department of Obstetrics and Gynaecology at Liverpool University is a letter written by Florence Nightingale in 1869 to the superintendent of the lying-in department of the Liverpool Workhouse commending the staff for 'having achieved ... a very enviable notoriety for the absence of puerperal disease' and seeking data about the number of maternal deaths in the previous four years. It has not been possible to discover if this information was provided and whether this was pooled with data from other cities to provide a larger picture of maternal deaths in mid-Victorian England. From other documents, it is clear that in the following year, 1870, there was a particularly serious outbreak of puerperal sepsis, linked to a virulent outbreak of scarlatina.

Florence Nightingale was well equipped to undertake such a mission. In 1858, she had produced for the government of the day what was essentially a confidential enquiry into deaths among the British Army at war in the Crimea. She was the first woman to be elected as a Fellow of the Royal Statistical Society and she achieved recognition for her use of graphics in her reports. She is sometimes credited with being the inventor of the 'pie chart'. In fact, the first known pie chart was used in a document written by William Playfair in 1801 to illustrate that the British paid more tax than anyone else. However, Florence Nightingale was probably the inventor of a more sophisticated graphic that she described a 'bat's wing', which included the use of wedges as in a pie chart. The image clearly showed that illness was a greater cause of death among soldiers in the Crimea than wounds and illustrated the improved mortality rates resulting from improvements in sanitation.[1]

A pie chart illustrates the major direct causes of maternal death in the latest UK Confidential Enquiry into Maternal Deaths (CEMD 1997–1999)[2] to show the continuing importance of deaths from early pregnancy complications (Figure 17.1). In this chapter, this and the previous report (CEMD 1994–1996)[3] are used to highlight some themes that have emerged that seem to be important to practice and policy. The vignettes that describe the case histories of women who died are not replicated here, as these may be read in the CEMD reports.

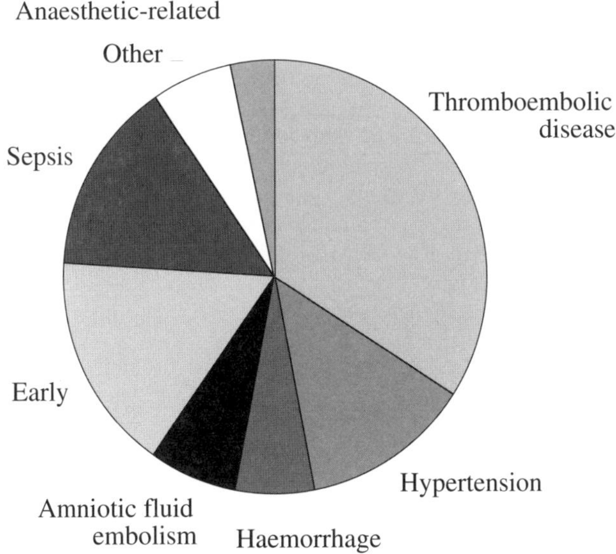

Figure 17.1 The major direct causes of maternal death; Confidential Enquiries into Maternal Deaths 1997–99[2]

What place 'evidence' and the Confidential Enquiry into Maternal Deaths?

The CEMD project is so well-established and generally carries such authority that it could easily become fossilised through a lack of self-reflection. The most recent report[2] has taken a quantum leap forward in obtaining important demographic and denominator data that have, for example, highlighted the importance of social exclusion in heightening the maternal hazards associated with pregnancy. This is discussed elsewhere in these proceedings.

There is still a need to move onwards from dichotomising assessments of the quality of care into 'sub-standard' and 'not sub-standard'. This is analogous to use of a *P* value of 0.05 in statistical analysis to prove 'effect' or 'no effect'. While the quality of clinical care in some cases of maternal death is manifestly poor, in many there are shades of suboptimal care that are perhaps better illustrated by narrative than binary classification.

It has been argued that the CEMD is not 'evidence-based'. To a large extent, this is an unfair criticism. There is certainly a danger that general recommendations for clinical care based on a single case of maternal death may conflict with good evidence. Best evidence of clinical effectiveness comes from systematic reviews of randomised controlled trials (RCTs). Recent CEMD reports have highlighted such reviews in supporting recommendations – notably antibiotic prophylaxis before caesarean section[4] and the use of magnesium sulphate for eclampsia.[5,6] However, many problems tackled in successive reports have not been addressed by RCTs, including prevention of thromboembolic disease and treatment of amniotic fluid embolism and of massive obstetric haemorrhage.

Further, few large RCTs (or meta-analyses that pool the results of several trials) have sufficient power to measure the incidence of rare but important complications of treatment – i.e. effectiveness is more easily assessed than safety. The CEMDs have the capability, because of their comprehensive cover in the UK, to identify rare, fatal complications of treatment. The CEMDs thus have an important complementary role in evidence-based clinical practice.

Many causes of maternal death are extremely rare (e.g. cervical pregnancy) and treatment options for these may never be subjected to formal scientific study. Inevitably, recommendations for care to avoid such deaths in the future rely on lesser levels of evidence and frequently on 'expert opinion'. This does not mean that the report is not evidence-based, merely that there is a lack of solid available evidence.

Early pregnancy deaths

Deaths from early pregnancy complications in recent triennia are shown in Table 17.1. Numerically, ectopic pregnancy is the most important.

Ectopic pregnancy

The incidence of ectopic pregnancy has been rising in many countries – although there is evidence of a plateau effect.[7] Table 17.2 shows that this rate is rising in the UK and that the rate of deaths from ectopic pregnancies has not declined, and still represents an increase on the rates described for 1991–93. This is in contrast to some other direct obstetric causes of maternal death, such as pre-eclampsia or antepartum/postpartum haemorrhage, of which the incidence has steadily decreased.

Table 17.1. Causes of deaths in early pregnancy 1985–99, UK[2]; until the 1994–6 CEMD report, early pregnancy deaths were defined as occurring before 20 weeks of pregnancy, whereas since then, 24 weeks has been used as the upper gestational limit, which may make direct comparisons with data from previous triennia inappropriate

Triennium	Ectopic pregnancies (*n*)	Miscarriages (*n*)	Terminations of pregnancy (*n*)	Total (*n*)
1985–87	11	1	4	16
1988–90	15	6	3	24
1991–93	9	3	5	17
1994–96	12	2	1	15
1997–99	13	7	2	22

Table 17.2. Deaths from ectopic pregnancies and rates per 1000 estimated pregnancies; England and Wales 1988–90 and the UK 1991–99[2]

Triennium	Total estimated pregnancies (*n*)	Total estimated ectopic pregnancies (*n*)	Ectopic pregnancies per 1000 pregnancies (*n*)	Deaths from ectopic pregnancies (*n*)	Death rate per 1000 estimated ectopic pregnancies
England and Wales					
1988–90	2 886900	24 775	9.6	15	0.5
UK					
1991–93	3 139 500	30 160	9.6	9	0.3
1994–96	2 914 900	33 550	11.5	12	0.4
1997–99	2 873 300	31 946	11.1	13	0.4

Women dying from ectopic pregnancies in the last two triennia fall into the following four groups:

- failure to diagnose ectopic pregnancy despite self referral to clinical services ($n = 12$)
- complications of treatment after correct diagnosis ($n = 6$)
- sudden death without engagement of clinical services ($n = 5$)
- non-tubal ectopic pregnancies ($n = 2$).

Failure to diagnose ectopic pregnancy

In theory, establishing the diagnosis of ectopic pregnancy has never been easier. A combination of quantitative β human chorionic gonadotrophin (βhCG) testing and transvaginal ultrasound allows sensitivities and specificities for the diagnosis of ectopic pregnancy approaching 100%.[8]

There are now commercially available dipstick tests for hCG that are sensitive to values as low as 25 miu/ml, are simple to use and provide reliable results in three minutes. These alone do not diagnose ectopic pregnancy, but they do diagnose early pregnancy reliably. The site of the pregnancy relies on ultrasound. These dipstick tests should be made readily available in general practices and accident and emergency departments, as well as in specialist units in hospitals. They should lower the threshold for testing and improve the diagnosis of ectopic pregnancy.

However, the single major problem identified in the CEMD report was a failure to suspect the possibility of ectopic pregnancy in the first place and, therefore, to perform an appropriate investigation. In a minority of cases, women presented with classic symptoms of ectopic pregnancy and they should have been referred for specialist assessment and further investigation and treatment. However, it is striking that a majority of the women who died from ruptured tubal pregnancies and were known to have sought medical advice before death had symptoms suggestive of gastrointestinal or urinary tract disease. Presumably, clinical presentation with more typical gynaecological symptoms (including amenorrhoea and vaginal bleeding, as well as abdominal pain) is more likely to suggest the correct diagnosis and trigger the correct investigations and treatment. In the last triennium, five women who died presented with symptoms that suggested gastrointestinal disorder. The authors have been unable to identify any published report that systematically records gastrointestinal-type symptoms in a cohort of women presenting with ectopic pregnancies. The overall incidence is uncertain.

There is a clear need to highlight the reality of atypical clinical presentation of women with tubal pregnancies to undergraduate medical and nursing students and postgraduate trainees in relevant specialties, including primary care, emergency medicine, general surgery, and obstetrics and gynaecology.

The CEMD report 1997–99 recommended hCG testing for all women of reproductive age with unexplained abdominal pain. It is recognised that a small minority of women who present with abdominal pain and diarrhoea to primary-care physicians will have ectopic pregnancies, but it is difficult to see how progress will be made otherwise.

Complications of treatment

Six women died while under the care of gynaecologists in hospital. In four cases, deaths were associated with use of the laparoscope either for diagnostic or therapeutic purposes. A systematic review of treatments of ectopic pregnancies[9] has identified 39 RCTs – mainly small trials that assessed medical treatments such as local or systemic methotrexate. Only three surgical trials were found – comparing laparoscopic salpingostomy with open conservative surgery. All 228 women had small unruptured tubal pregnancies, were haemodynamically stable and had hCG levels of less than 3000 iu/l. Elimination of tubal trophoblast was more effective with open surgery, but there was no clear difference in the subsequent incidence of intrauterine and ectopic pregnancies. Laparoscopic surgery was associated with reduced operating time, blood loss, stay in hospital, analgesic needs and costs. A Royal College of Obstetricians and Gynaecologists Guideline[10] has stressed the importance of adequate training before surgeons undertake laparoscopic surgery, as well as the potential hazards in the presence of haemodynamic instability (supported by a case in CEMD 1994–96).

A further recommendation comes from CEMD 1997–99 that such surgery is best avoided in the haemodynamically stable patient during the night, when senior support is less immediate than during the day.

Sudden death

In each triennium, there are reports of women found dead at home with ruptured ectopic pregnancies. In each case, there was nothing to suggest that the woman knew that she was pregnant or that she had made any contact with the medical services. We simply do not know if these women had had symptoms or not. It is therefore impossible to know if greater public awareness of the symptoms of ectopic pregnancy might help to avoid these tragedies.

Non-tubal ectopic pregnancies

In the past six years, there was one death from an abdominal and one from a cervical pregnancy. Because these cases are so unusual, the vignettes in the CEMD reports have the potential to educate clinicians should they encounter a similar problem.

Miscarriage

In the two most recent CEMD reports, deaths from miscarriage have been split between early pregnancy and sepsis chapters, but they have been considered together here. Themes that have emerged include the need to consider the patient's needs before discharge from hospital and to recognise the rapidity of clinical deterioration that occurs with fulminating infection. The most recent CEMD report contains the summary of a particularly harrowing story of a homeless teenager discharged from hospital after surgical evacuation of the uterus after miscarriage, without apparent engagement of the social services. She was found, some time later, dead under a duvet in someone's front garden in freezing conditions. There is also evidence of failure to recognise the rapidity of clinical deterioration that occurs with fulminating infection, especially by junior medical staff unaccustomed to dealing with serious sepsis. Too often, treatment was too little too late, with absent or delayed input by senior clinicians, including consultant obstetricians and gynaecologists, and intensive-care specialists. After taking microbiological advice, the CEMD 1994–96 report recommended that surgical evacuation should optimally be performed about one hour after parenteral antibiotic treatment in cases of recognised septic miscarriage. In some such cases there was long delay, with the operation being performed by a junior doctor on an 'emergency list'. The aim of initial antibiotic therapy is to ensure adequate systemic tissue levels before further dissemination of bacteria at surgical evacuation. Antibiotics are unlikely to penetrate necrotic tissue in the uterine cavity to a significant degree.

In the latest CEMD report, fatal infection occurred in a woman with cervical sutures that were not removed after spontaneous rupture of membranes. Similar deaths have been described previously. One fatal case of infection following amniocentesis was described in the latest CEMD report and another will appear in the next report. A death was also reported in the previous triennium after invasive treatment for twin–twin transfusion syndrome. In the latter case, the precise cause and possible link to infection was less clear. However, these cases do illustrate that techniques of prenatal diagnosis and treatment are not necessarily innocuous.

Termination of pregnancy

Soon, there will be no obstetricians or gynaecologists in the UK who practised before the 1967 Abortion Act and have experience of the consequences of unsafe and illegal abortion. A recent account of the last woman to die in Edinburgh under such circumstances conveys the horrors of the circumstances that drove women to such desperate measures.[11] In this case, a woman living in a tenement flat in what was then a severely deprived area of the city got her sister to inject a solution of antiseptic through her cervix. The consequent acute renal failure with hyperkalaemia proved fatal after 11 days, in what were then pre-dialysis days.

The consequences of the availability of safe facilities for legal termination of pregnancy in the UK have been dramatic and are illustrated by successive CEMD reports. Sadly, in many parts of the world, unsafe abortion remains a major cause of maternal death. The solution appears simple – access to effective contraception and safe abortion facilities. The issue is, however, complicated by cultural, religious and political attitudes, not to mention funding restraints.

Additionally, the South African confidential enquiry into maternal death[12] has shown that a change in the law to permit legal pregnancy termination is insufficient in itself. There is also a need to publicise facilities and ensure access to them, to avoid further deaths from septic induced abortion or from the use of life-threatening abortifacient agents.

References

1. Small H. Florence Nightingale's statistical diagrams. 1998 [http://www.florence-nightingale.co.uk/small.htm].
2. Lewis G, Drife J, editors. *Why Mothers Die 1997–1999. The Confidential Enquiries into Maternal Deaths in the United Kingdom.* London: RCOG Press; 2001.
3. Department of Health, Welsh Office, Scottish Home and Health Department, Department of Health and Social Services, Northern Ireland. *Report on Confidential Enquiries into Maternal Death in the United Kingdom, 1994–96.* London: The Stationery Office; 1998.
4. Smaill F, Hofmeyr GJ. Antibiotic prophylaxis for caesarean section. *Cochrane Database Syst Rev* 2000;(2):CD000933.
5. Duley L, Henderson-Smart D. Magnesium sulphate versus diazepam for eclampsia. *Cochrane Database Syst Rev* 2000;(2):CD000127.
6. Duley L, Henderson-Smart D. Magnesium sulphate versus phenytoin for eclampsia. *Cochrane Database Syst Rev* 2000;(2):CD000128.
7. Boufous S, Quartararo M, Mohsin M, Parker J. Trends in the incidence of ectopic pregnancy in New South Wales between 1990–1998. *Aust N Z J Obstet Gynaecol Suppl* 2001;41:436–8.
8. Ankum WA. Diagnosing suspected ectopic pregnancy. *BMJ* 2000;321:1235–6.
9. Hajenius PJ, Mol BW, Bossuyt PM, Ankum WM, Van der Veen F. Interventions for tubal ectopic pregnancy. *Cochrane Database Syst Rev* 2000;(2): CD 000324.
10. Royal College of Obstetricians and Gynaecologists. *The Management of Tubal Pregnancies.* Guideline No. 21. London: RCOG Press; 1999.
11. P Myerscough, personal communication. Oral presentation, Edinburgh, January 2002.
12. Department of Health. *Saving Mothers. Report on Confidential Enquiries into Maternal Deaths in South Africa 1998.* Pretoria: Department of Health; 1999.

Chapter 18

Specific problems of mortality and morbidity I

Discussion

Discussion following the papers by Professor Greer, Mr Tuffnell, Professor Robson and Professor Neilson

De Swiet: Forgive me if I have asked you this before, but it is so important that it needs to be said again. When you were talking about whether or not to give prophylaxis to somebody with asymptomatic thrombophilia, you said something about 'when do we start in pregnancy?' The data from the Confidential Enquiry would show that your risk is horrendously high in the early part of pregnancy, and I am sure you do not really mean that, do you? If you need it at all, you need it all the way through pregnancy.

Greer: The short answer is that I personally start as soon as I see the patient. That was not true in the past, as you know, because we had some concerns about heparin and we were trying to minimise the time that patients were on it. Both of us were delaying treatment until the end of the first trimester, or even mid-pregnancy. Certainly, with the large amount of rapidly accumulating safety data on low molecular weight heparin (LMWH), I feel that that risk has now gone. I now start any patient who I think really needs it, as soon as I see them in the first trimester.

I do not think that patients with asymptomatic factor V Leiden, or asymptomatic prothrombin gene variant, should necessarily be treated, although I would discuss it with them. Antithrombin-deficient patients should be treated, whether or not they come from symptomatic kindred, and I treat them as soon as I see them.

Drife: Amniotic fluid embolism is the one example of where we have looked for morbidity, or suggested a morbidity survey, in the report. It is good to see that starting.

Is there anything specific and practical that we could do to improve the reporting to the Register? I was just wondering, while you were speaking, whether we should insert a report card with your address in every pack that went out from the Royal College of Obstetricians and Gynaecologists in its mailing.

Tuffnell: After the register was incorporated in the Confidential Enquiry report, I got a surge of reporting. A large part of it is about awareness, and an awareness at the time that it happens, I guess. The more informed people can be about it, the more likely they are to report.

Drife: There would be some messages, as opposed to the bleak review of the people who died, which did not give us any clues.

Greer: A large part of the problem lies in the failure to recognise when pre-eclampsia is severe. You referred a good deal to severe pre-eclampsia, but you did not tell us what you thought 'severe' was. This is a fulminating condition and quite often these mistakes happen because of a failure to appreciate the severity of a condition. How would you define 'severe'?

Robson: The definition of severe pre-eclampsia is fairly standard. The American College of Obstetricians and Gynecologists' definition of severe eclampsia relates to the level of blood pressure and the level of proteinuria or multi-system involvement, and this is fairly widely used and accepted. Clearly, this identifies the group of women who are likely to die or to experience morbidity. By and large, that is between five and ten percent of women with pre-eclampsia. That is quite well accepted worldwide. I have set out some definitions of severe pre-eclampsia that are reasonably standard and widely accepted in Chapter 16.

Oates: Professor Greer, what is the role of antipsychotic drugs in raising the risk of thromboembolism in this group of people?

Greer: We do not know specifically for pregnancy, so we have to extrapolate from the non-pregnant situation. Many people may not know that antipsychotic drugs are associated with an increased risk of venous thromboembolism (VTE). We do not encounter them too often in pregnancy, to obtain the data, but I would certainly regard them as a significant risk factor when combined with the prothrombotic stresses of pregnancy. This is something that needs more publicity for the small number of women who have that combination.

Oates: There were three cases in this enquiry. Do you think it is the fact that they are postpartum and on antipsychotic drugs that does it, or is there another factor that could perhaps enable us to increase our proactive study? Is there any way you can help me to know which of my patients I should put into thromboembolic deterrent stockings?

Greer: Perhaps all of them. VTE is not usually caused by a single factor – that is extremely rare. The only exception to this would be antithrombin deficiency, which is probably the only factor that would cause it alone. The vast majority are due to multiple factors, so that there is an interaction between pregnancy, obesity, antipsychotic drugs and immobility, and therefore you have to be aware of a variety of risk factors coming together.

Most of the common risk factors include age, obesity and suchlike. If you take account of those, appreciating that there is a threshold effect, and you start to see one or two of these risk factors coming together, you should be thinking about thromboprophylaxis – particularly after delivery, which I guess is when most antipsychotic drugs are used for puerperal psychosis or depression.

Bewley: I will make two quick points. First, thinking about the safety net and the issue of primary care, I understand from some GPs that the reason why pregnancy-testing is not offered is because it comes out of their partnership profits. If we want to engage women who are pregnant, either because they will develop a complication of early pregnancy, terminate or need booking, one of the innovations we should be considering is free, nurse-led pregnancy-testing in general practice.

My second point about general practice is the issue about women with symptoms. We know that there are very unusual presentations of severe pre-eclampsia and we should raise women's awareness that with any unusual symptoms they should go and see their GP because, even with weekly visits, they can fulminate in between. Second, if you see a pregnant woman, test her blood pressure and urine because she could have HELLP (haemolysis, elevated liver enzymes, low platelets) syndrome if she has neck or abdominal pain. We should re-emphasise the old lessons of symptoms, blood pressure and protein.

Drife: If women are advised to obtain a pregnancy test from a chemist's, do you know how much that costs?

Bewley: They will cost much more in a chemist's than through bulk-buying by the NHS. The issue is that some GPs do carry out pregnancy-testing and some do not. There is a financial disincentive to obtain access to care through pregnancy-testing. I do not know what the cost would be, but we will not think of the complications of pregnancy if we do not know they are pregnant. You will never get GPs to carry out beta-hCG testing on young women with abdominal pain because it is not free.

Nelson-Piercy: I have another question for Professor Greer, which is to challenge the recommendation about screening women with adverse pregnancy outcome for thrombophilia, other than for antiphospholipid antibody syndrome (AAS). You made the mistake of also showing that you do not know what to do with them, so what is the point of screening them, unless they have had a thrombosis, and for defects other than AAS?

Greer: You are absolutely correct that if you are trying to prevent a pregnancy complication, apart from an AAS, we do not know what to do. However, often, the fact that a patient has had a pregnancy complication can identify that she has a thrombophilia, as you would agree, and that thrombophilia puts her at risk of venous disease.

It depends how you regard a symptomatic thrombophilia. If you regard symptomatic thrombophilia as simply being restricted to venous disease, then you are absolutely right. If you think that symptoms can reflect either a pregnancy complication – such as a stillbirth, severe pre-eclampsia, growth restriction or venous disease, and all of these are manifestations, the argument would still hold, because it then becomes valuable to know because you can prevent the venous disease.

For AAS, the parallel to which you alluded, we call that a syndrome when there is a clinical expression. That clinical expression can be recurrent miscarriage, pre-eclampsia, venous disease or arterial thrombosis. I would argue that we should apply that to all the thrombophilias.

I do not think we should be hung-up on what a thrombophilia is. There are far too many of them and it is all confused. The take-home message is that it is all very complicated and, if you really want to know, it probably does not matter what you have. The bottom line is that you clot a great deal – the reason you do so is probably completely irrelevant, but let us find those who clot a lot and have an underlying reason for it, then we can all treat them, perhaps even generically.

Nelson-Piercy: Could I just come back on that? We are talking about maternal mortality and morbidity and we are straying to the fetus – I hope the rest of you will forgive us. That is fine, and I agree, provided the enoxaparin or dalteparin is not then given or recommended, with the rider that 'I am going to give you this because it may improve your pregnancy outcome'. My problem is with the extrapolation from your very sensible practice to the general *mêleé* of obstetricians who will start dishing out

LMWH with the thought and true belief that it is improving outcome. With that rider, I agree with you.

Van den Broek: I have a question and a comment for Professor Robson about eclampsia and data from developing countries. I am well aware that in many countries there are no facilities to measure proteinuria in pregnancy in antenatal clinics. In one way, I am quite pleased that you are still recommending that all women should have their blood pressure taken, because that is usually available, and also a urine test for protein. On the other hand, I have just been talking to my students about evidence-based medicine, and there is no good evidence to show that, if you do those two things, you will pick up most of your pre-eclampsias. Can you enlighten me on that?

Second, if you know that most of these tests are not taking place in developing countries, then it is with caution that you should interpret their data about eclampsia and pre-eclampsia. We basically do not see them at the pre-eclampsia stage – we see them fitting, which is when we hope that they get to the hospital.

Robson: The issue about proteinuria is fairly well proven. The presence of proteinuria is not just a marker of pre-eclampsia but it is a marker of bad pregnancy outcome as a whole. Proteinuria, *per se*, increases your perinatal mortality three-fold, even in the absence of hypertension. It can be viewed as an effective screen for pregnancy-related disease, the top of which list would be pre-eclampsia.

To say that women can have access to measurement of blood pressure but not to proteinuria is a cost issue that I do not think is based on evidence. I would accept all the problems of testing for proteinuria but, by and large, it is the presence of proteinuria that is the one single, simple test that predicts mortality. We must not lose sight of that.

SECTION 5

ANTEPARTUM AND POSTPARTUM HAEMORRHAGE

Chapter 19

Antepartum haemorrhage

Marion H Hall and Prabhath Wagaarachchi

Definitions

Antepartum haemorrhage (APH) is uterine bleeding during pregnancy after viability (the current legal definition of viability in the UK is 24 or more weeks of gestation). Vaginal bleeding due to cervical and vaginal lesions is not considered here. APH is usually divided into three categories:

- Abruption of the placenta: separation of part or all of a normally sited placenta. Bleeding may be revealed and/or concealed and is usually accompanied by constant pain.
- Placenta praevia: bleeding from a placenta that is sited partly or wholly in the lower segment of the uterus (in a small proportion of cases bleeding does not occur). In most cases, bleeding occurs only when uterine contractions and cervical dilatation are present and it is usually painless.
- Antepartum haemorrhage of unknown origin (APHUO): any uterine bleeding that is not included above.

These definitions are not absolutely exclusive and it is often useful to analyse all three together to take account of possible variations in classification or coding. However, because of the more serious implications of abruption and placenta praevia for the mother and the baby, these two conditions are discussed in this chapter.

It should be noted that, although there may be some genuine geographical variation in the incidence of the different types of APH, it is likely that much of the published variation is due to differences in interpretation of the above definitions and also to use of hospital-based rather than population-based data. This has an impact upon the rates of maternal and perinatal mortality and morbidity, which will tend to be lower if the denominator is 'diluted' by less severe types of APH.

Incidence

Singleton pregnancy

Recent reports of the incidence of abruption in singleton pregnancy vary between 0.51%,[1] 0.59%,[2] 0.62%,[3] 0.64%[4] and 1.1%.[5] This variation may be due to differing definitions: for example, the report of the higher incidence of 1.1%[5] used a definition that had to include only two of the four clinical features and did not need to include either haemorrhage or retroplacental clot. An increase in the rate over time has been described.[6,7] In case this was due to classification differences, the authors performed an analysis over time in Aberdeen City District,[8] where abruption has been strictly defined (retroplacental clot must be recorded) over many years. It is analysed together with APHUO in case of coding variation (Table 19.1). There does seem to be an increase in the rate at which abruption has occurred during the last 35 years that is not accounted for by a decrease in the rate of APHUO, which has also risen. However, because APHUO is at least ten times more common than abruption, the possibility of a coding change is not excluded. The recent rise in abruption and APHUO may be accounted for partly by the change in the UK definition of viability from 28 to 24 weeks in October 1992, which means that some bleeds previously categorised as threatened miscarriage became APH.

The incidence of placenta praevia is reported[9] as 0.36% from 1966–74, 0.37% from 1975–84 and 0.48% from 1985–95. This rise is attributed by the authors to the more widespread use of ultrasonography for detecting placenta praevia but, since most cases present with bleeding, this seems unlikely and it is possible that it is being overdiagnosed. Another possible explanation is the increase in the general caesarean section rate (see below).

In the Aberdeen City District,[8] Table 19.2 shows that the recent incidence is much lower, and no such rise in placenta praevia has occurred, although there has certainly been an increase in the use of ultrasound and in the caesarean section rate. In fact, the placenta praevia rate fell between 1966 and 1990. This may be accounted for partly by the lower incidence of multiparity.

Table 19.1. Incidence of abruption and antepartum haemorrhage of unknown origin in Aberdeen City District from 1966–2000

Years	Total	Abruption		APHUO	
	(*n*)	(*n*)	(%)	(*n*)	(%)
1966–70	13123	19	0.14	542	4.13
1971–75	10570	25	0.24	477	4.51
1976–80	14115	24	0.17	896	6.34
1981–85	15342	35	0.23	1196	7.80
1986–90	15651	48	0.31	1168	7.46
1991–95	15659	47	0.30	1348	8.61
1996–00	13282	57	0.43	1480	11.14

Table 19.2. Incidence of placenta praevia in Aberdeen City District 1966–2000

Years	Total (*n*)	Placenta praevia (*n*)	Placenta praevia (%)
1966–70	13123	67	0.51
1971–75	10570	34	0.32
1976–80	14115	24	0.17
1981–85	15342	37	0.24
1986–90	15651	15	0.10
1991–95	15659	15	0.10
1996–00	13282	15	0.11

Twin pregnancy

The incidence of abruption in 193 266 twin pregnancies in the USA was reported[2] as twice as high as in 7 465 858 singleton pregnancies (1.22% compared with 0.59%) with different risk profiles.

In Aberdeen City District,[10] the relative risk is similar (2.02 [95% CI 1.23–3.33]), although the incidences are a little lower (0.47% in 71 851 singletons and 0.94% in 1694 twins) between 1976 and 1999. The population-attributable risk of multiple pregnancy for abruption is low, but may become more significant if assisted reproduction results in more multiple pregnancies. In the Aberdeen study, placenta praevia was actually less common in twins than in singletons, although not significantly so.

Maternal mortality

There were 20 maternal deaths from abruption in the UK during the years 1985–1999, while there were 11 290 200 births.[11–24] No data are available about the number of pregnancies in which abruption occurred but, using the typical abruption incidence of 0.7%,[3] there would be around 79 031 cases of abruption, giving a case–fatality rate of 0.25/1000 (about five times the overall direct death rate during this period). Abruption accounted for about 3.5% of UK maternal direct deaths between 1985 and 1999.

There were 15 maternal deaths from placenta praevia in the UK between 1985 and 1999. Using the typical praevia incidence of 0.48%,[9] there would be about 54 192 cases of placenta praevia, giving a case–fatality rate of 0.28/1000 (about 5.6 times the overall direct death rate of 0.05/1000). Placenta praevia accounted for about 2.7% of UK maternal deaths in this period. Maternal death from APHUO has not been reported in the UK since 1985.

It should be noted that the above calculations are based on the primary cause of death as attributed by the assessors, and there may well have been a few more cases in which abruption or placenta praevia were major contributory factors; thus, the case–fatality rate may have been slightly but not greatly underestimated.

Maternal morbidity

Incidence

Because there are now so few maternal deaths, studies of severe maternal morbidity (near-misses) may give useful evidence about the aetiology of death.[25] Of the recent studies published, two[26,27] found that 4–11% of the pregnant women admitted to intensive therapy units had experienced APH and, in a system-based study[28] in Pretoria, 9.5% of the near-misses had APH. Thus, APH is associated with a bigger proportion of all near-misses than of all deaths. This suggests that successful treatment is often possible.

Mode of delivery

Delivery by caesarean section is particularly likely for placenta praevia (100% in Aberdeen City District 1996–2000)[8] in a setting with a low incidence of placenta praevia and is also common in abruption (45.8% in Aberdeen City District 1966–2000).[8] Caesarean section is associated with a higher overall maternal mortality than vaginal birth[29] but, in the case of placenta praevia, it is almost certain that maternal mortality would be higher if it were not performed, since it is carried out primarily for maternal reasons. In the case of abruption, caesarean section is performed primarily for fetal reasons but it may benefit the mother also. The caesarean section rate for APHUO is also elevated (16.0% for APHUO, compared with 10.6% for those without APHUO) in Aberdeen City District 1966–2000,[8] presumably for a mixture of fetal and maternal indications.

However, APH accounts for only a small proportion of all caesarean sections in developed countries. In a recent UK study,[30] abruption was the primary indication for 1.25% of all caesarean section and placenta praevia was the primary indication for 3.28% of all caesarean sections, so APH was the indication for 4.5% overall. In developing countries, where caesarean section is usually performed only for absolute maternal indications and obstetric need is to some extent unmet, APH is the primary indication for about 10–15% of all caesarean sections.[31]

Blood loss at delivery

Obviously, blood loss at delivery is postpartum rather than antepartum haemorrhage, but the latter may predispose to the former by impairing blood clotting and uterine tone. Furthermore, both abruption and placenta praevia often lead to caesarean section, which itself increases blood loss at delivery. The reported blood loss at delivery in Aberdeen City District by type of APH is shown in Table 19.3.[8]

Women with an abruption have a relative risk of 3.0 of losing 500–999 ml and a relative risk of 9.2 of losing more than 1000 ml. For placenta praevia, the relative risk for 500–999 ml is 6.2 and for ≥ 1000 ml it is 11.1. For APHUO, the relative risk for 500–999 ml is only 1.4 and for ≥ 1000 ml it is 2.67. It is clear that even when the problem is recognised well in advance (as is usually the case for placenta praevia, although not for abruption), excessive blood loss cannot be avoided in many cases.

Table 19.3. Blood loss at delivery by type of antepartum haemorrhage (APH), Aberdeen City District 1976–2000

APH type	Total	Blood loss (ml)			
		500–999		1000 +	
		(*n*)	%	(*n*)	%
None	40160	3909	9.7	715	1.8
Abruption	150	44	29.3	25	16.6
Placenta praevia	45	27	60.0	9	20.0
APHUO	3959	532	13.4	191	4.8

APHUO = antepartum haemorrhage of unknown origin

This is usually due to coagulopathy in the case of abruption and to large vessels in the lower uterine segment in the case of placenta praevia. The fact that the relative risk for severe haemorrhage (≥ 1000 ml) is greater than for moderate haemorrhage suggests that prompt treatment is helpful.

Blood transfusion

Blood transfusion can be life-saving but it also carries some risk of transmitting infection and of inducing antibody formation, so can be seen as morbidity. The rates of blood transfusion by type of APH for Aberdeen City District (1976–2000) are shown in Table 19.4. The overall rate of transfusion is low but it is more common in all types of haemorrhage, especially abruption and placenta praevia, where the relative risk is around 10.0. However, it should be noted that the vast majority of transfusions are given (presumably for postpartum haemorrhage) to women who have not experienced an APH. Thus, the population-attributable risk of APH for transfusion is low. It is also worth noting that, although blood loss at delivery is higher in placenta praevia than in abruption (Table 19.3), the rate of transfusion is identical. Presumably this is because delivery in placenta praevia is usually elective, with preparation made. Also, coagulopathy is less common in placenta praevia than in abruption.

Table 19.4 Blood transfusion by type of antepartum haemorrhage (APH), Aberdeen City District 1976–2000

APH type	Total	Blood transfusion	
		(*n*)	(%)
None	40160	958	2.4
Abruption	150	34	22.7
Placenta praevia	45	10	22.2
APHUO	3959	224	5.7

APHUO = antepartum haemorrhage of unknown origin

Table 19.5 Perinatal mortality in abruption in Aberdeen City District 1971–2000

	Abruptions (*n*)	Perinatal deaths	
		(*n*)	(%)
1971–80	49	22	44.9
1981–90	83	23	27.7
1991–00	104	21	20.2

Perinatal mortality

In the USA,[2] the incidence of perinatal death in abruption is 11.9%, compared with 0.82% for all other births. In Sweden[1] in 1987–93, the singleton perinatal mortality rate in cases of abruption was 10.6% (with smoking, severe pre-eclampsia and smallness for gestational age being more strongly associated with perinatal deaths due to abruption than in pregnancies without abruption). In Norway,[6] the perinatal case–fatality rate decreased from 47.1% in 1967–71 to 21.7% in 1987–91. Perinatal mortality rates in Aberdeen City District are shown in Table 19.5. While perinatal mortality has declined, it is still higher than in some other centres. Possible reasons may be a tighter definition of abruption, a less healthy population and higher smoking rates.

Perinatal mortality in cases of placenta praevia, on the other hand, seems to be virtually non-existent now in developed countries. There have been no perinatal deaths in cases of placenta praevia in Aberdeen City District since 1976.

The perinatal mortality rate in APHUO in Aberdeen City District[8] was 2.28% from 1971–2000, compared with 1.0% for the whole singleton population in the same period. The reasons for this are not known.

Perinatal morbidity

Gestational age at delivery

In general, not only perinatal mortality but also handicap rates are proportional to the rate of delivery preterm. Many analyses have been made of gestation-specific abruption rates and perinatal mortality rates[2,6] but these analyses usually beg the question as to the direction of the causal effect. It is obvious in clinical practice that abruption almost always antedates the onset of labour – in fact, labour often has to be induced to expedite delivery. It is certainly true that abruption often occurs preterm and, of course, the perinatal outcome is worse, the earlier the gestation at which it occurs.

In Aberdeen City District,[8] the distribution of gestation at delivery in various types of APH is shown in Figure 19.1. It is clear that the usual distribution of gestational age (almost 'normal' around 40 weeks, but with a long tail to the left) applies to those without APH, those with placenta praevia and those with APHUO, but for abruption, delivery can occur at any time. This makes intervention planning more difficult.

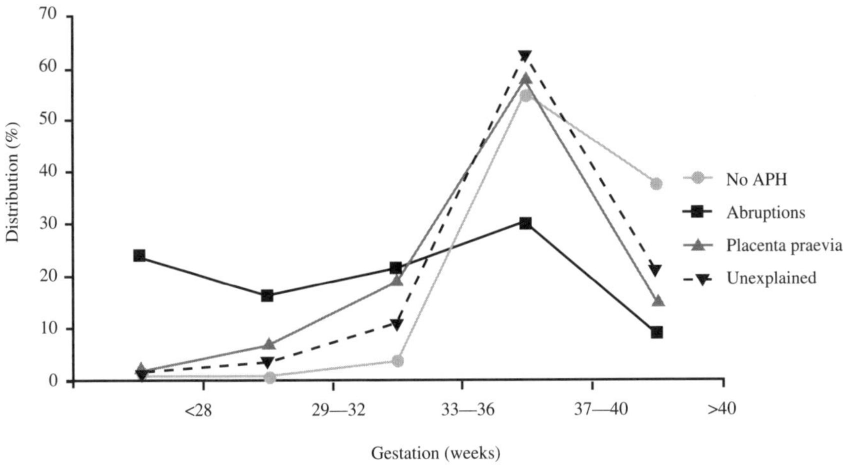

Figure 19.1. Percentage distribution of gestation at delivery by type of antepartum haemorrhage (APH), Aberdeen City District 1951–2000

Apgar scores

Apgar scores do not correlate well with ultimate outcome for the child, but are informative about the condition of the neonate at birth. In Norway,[6] the proportion of Apgar scores of less than 7 after five minutes was 13.0% in cases of abruption, compared with only 1.1% in the total population. After standardisation for gestational age, the relative risk was 7.8 (95% CI 7.7–7.9) and was stable during the years of the study (1978–91). A similar relative risk was found in Aberdeen City District 1976–2000.

Cerebral palsy

In a long-term follow-up study considering the antecedents of cerebral palsy for children born in Aberdeen City District in the years 1974–91,[32] 23.4% of the cerebral palsy cases had experienced an APH, compared with only 7.8% of the total population (relative risk 3.01). However, these are unadjusted rates.

Antecedents

APH in singleton pregnancy is associated with a number of demographic, obstetric and pathological factors, few of which are independent of each other.

Table 19.6. Different types of antepartum haemorrhage (APH) by social class, Aberdeen City District 1966–2000

Social class	Total	Type of APH					
		Abruption		Placental praevia		APHUO	
		(*n*)	%	(*n*)	%	(*n*)	%
I-III non-manual	25769	59	0.2	32	0.1	1759	6.8
III manual	19350	48	0.2	35	0.2	1516	7.8
IV & V	17795	56	0.3	34	0.2	1511	8.5
Missing	21733	73	0.3	39	0.2	1780	8.2

APHUO = antepartum haemorrhage of unknown origin

Demographic factors

Some large population-based studies report on a small increase in abruption in older mothers[2,5,6] but others do not.[7,33] No such risk was noted in Aberdeen City District. Placenta praevia, however, is consistently more common in older mothers. APHUO has no consistent pattern.[9]

Primiparity is associated with a higher risk of abruption.[6] Multiparity is difficult to study in developed countries but is clearly a risk factor for placenta praevia[33] and may be associated with abruption.[33] APHUO has no consistent pattern.

Various aspects of deprivation have been studied: non-cohabitation with the baby's father, lower education level and smoking are all associated with an increased abruption rate.[1,5,7] There did not seem to be a clinically significant social class gradient for abruption, placenta praevia or APHUO (Table 19.6) in Aberdeen City District.[8]

Obstetric factors

In the index pregnancy, threatened miscarriage (bleeding before viability) is more common in association with APH, but this may be an early manifestation of the APH rather than a risk factor. The increase in the proportion with threatened miscarriage was between two- and three-fold, highest for abruption (Table 19.7) in Aberdeen City District.[8] Again, the predictive value of threatened miscarriage for APH is extremely low.

A meta-analysis[3] of studies analysing the association of abruption with prolonged rupture of the membranes reported on a three-fold higher risk, especially in American case–control studies and those with a high reported incidence of abruption.

Previous obstetric history is obviously informative only for parous women. The adjusted recurrence risk after one abruption was 6.4 in the Norwegian registry-based study[4] – the ideal study design for looking at recurrence – and there may also be a 'dose-response' effect. In the same study, previous preterm delivery, smallness for gestational age in the baby, pre-eclampsia and caesarean delivery were associated with increased risk of abruption, which suggests that 'placental dysfunction' is an

Table 19.7. Threatened miscarriage by type of antepartum haemorrhage (APH), Aberdeen City District 1951–2000

	Total	Threatened miscarriage	
		(*n*)	(%)
None	136843	16169	11.8
Abruption	263	84	31.9
Placenta praevia	370	83	22.4
APHUO	8456	2172	25.7

APHUO = antepartum haemorrhage of unknown origin

underlying factor. The recurrence risk for placenta praevia is complicated by the fact that women are almost always delivered by caesarean section and hence it may really be caesarean section as a risk factor that is being studied. This may be because the previously incised lower segment is denuded of decidua. In any event, a prior caesarean section is associated with a 2.4-fold risk of placenta praevia in the 1997 meta-analysis,[9] with a clear 'dose-response' effect in the studies reporting on multiple prior caesarean section. Prior miscarriage and prior pregnancy termination were also associated with an approximately 1.7-fold increased risk of placenta praevia. Infertility (unspecified type but clearly relative) has been reported as a risk factor for abruption in Sweden.[1]

Pathological factors

An association between cocaine use and abruption has been described.[34] It was postulated that the mechanism might be the hypertensive effect of cocaine or its effect on uterine vasoconstriction. Whether this is a major problem depends on how common cocaine use currently is, which is difficult to establish, particularly since it may be associated with use of other substances.

The question of whether hypertension and pre-eclampsia predispose to abruption is complicated by the variable natural history of pre-eclampsia – sometimes slowly progressive and sometimes fulminating. Women are not usually under constant observation, so when signs of pre-eclampsia (hypertension and proteinuria) seem to be antedated by the abruption, it is rarely possible to be sure which came first. However, the data are most consistent with pre-eclampsia being a risk factor and there is also a strong reported association between chronic hypertension and abruption.[1,3,5] The relative risks reported are between 1.9 and 5.6.

The association between folate status and abruption, which was investigated 30 years ago with inconclusive results, has been revisited with current interest in homocysteine metabolism. A recent meta-analysis[35] has examined folate 'deficiency', hyperhomocysteinaemia, methionine loading and homozygosity for methylenetetrahydrofolate reductase. However, because the studies were observational and the data heterogenous, and because of the rarity of abruption, firm conclusions are not possible.

It must be emphasised that all of the antecedents discussed above have an extremely low population-attributable risk.

Management

Identification of risk factors or antecedents is theoretically valuable in risk reduction. However, there are several problems. First, the associations may not be causal. If the risk is known to the obstetrician or midwife, they make take action that will modify outcome, which makes estimating the risk more difficult. For example, if an obstetrician believes that there is a recurrence risk for abruption and delivers the woman before term, this may forestall any recurrence and lead to underestimation of the recurrence risk. However, harmful intervention such as very premature delivery might do more harm than good and lead to overestimation of the risk.

The majority of the risk factors identified above (e.g. age, parity, deprivation, infertility, previous obstetric history) cannot be changed in the short term. In the long term,[4] it might be possible to reduce overall caesarean section rates to reduce the rate of subsequent placenta praevia, although few hospitals or countries have been successful in reducing caesarean section rates and it has not been shown that it does lead to a reduction in placenta praevia.

There is a lack of evidence as to what useful action should be taken when increased risk is detected. Increased surveillance is usually implemented, but there is no good evidence as to whether this is beneficial at all and how intensive it should be. Highly intensive surveillance (sometimes including admission) involves significant costs for the service and for pregnant women and their families.

Modification of antecedents

It has been claimed[36] that since women who stop smoking have a lower risk of abruption than those who do not, abruption could be substantially reduced if women stopped smoking. Although this may be true, the study design (observational, albeit prospective) does not permit this conclusion, since women who stop smoking may have many other favourable characteristics and behaviours. Randomised controlled trials of smoking cessation initiatives are usually underpowered for study of rare outcomes such as abruption and, in any event, actual smoking cessation will not be randomly distributed between participants.

The arguments for lowering current caesarean section rates are many: prevention of placenta praevia (and its most severe variation – placenta accreta) would almost certainly be a benefit, but not a highly visible one, as placental praevia is so uncommon. The apparent modest increase in risk of placenta praevia in women with a prior pregnancy termination is not preventable by criminalising termination, since all the evidence suggests that termination would then occur illegally, converting a relatively safe procedure into a more dangerous one. Increasing use of medical (as opposed to surgical) termination may reduce the risk but, as yet, there are no data to support this.

Recommendations from Confidential Enquiries into Maternal Death

One of the most valued audits in the world, the Confidential Enquiries into Maternal Deaths (CEMD)[11–24] for England and Wales (1955–84) and the UK (1985–99) has

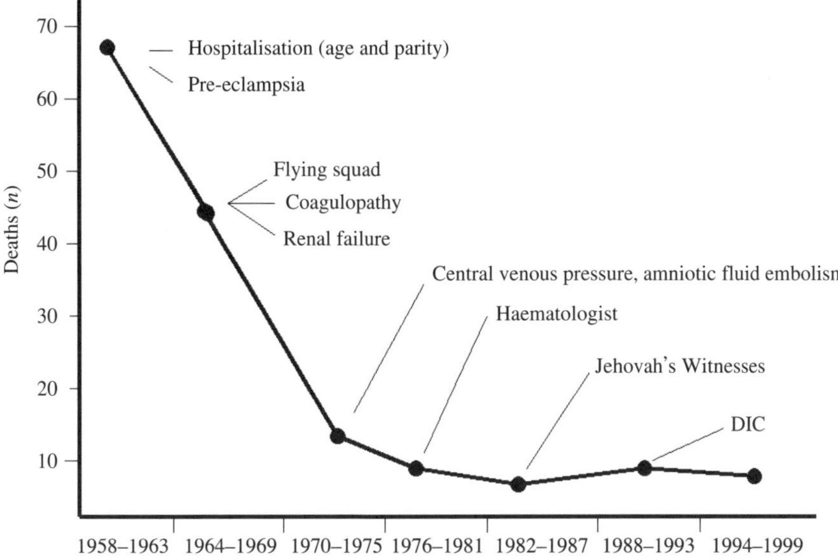

Figure 19.2. UK maternal deaths from abruption and recommendations made in Confidential Enquiries into Maternal Deaths reports[11–24]; DIC = disseminated intravascular coagulation; Crown copyright material reproduced with permission of the Controller of HMSO and the Queen's Printer for Scotland

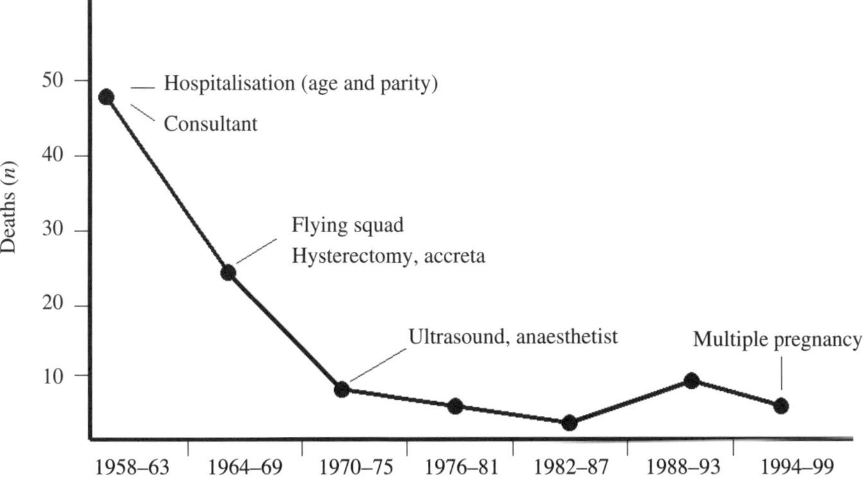

Figure 19.3. UK maternal deaths for placenta praevia and recommendations made in Confidential Enquiries into Maternal Deaths reports[11–24]; Crown copyright material reproduced with permission of the Controller of HMSO and the Queen's Printer for Scotland

always made recommendations on booking for confinement, protocols for massive haemorrhage and so on. These are summarised in Figure 19.2 and Figure 19.3. There may be many reasons for the reduction in numbers of deaths from abruption and placenta praevia between 1958 and 1975 but the recommendations for more hospital confinements for older women, those of high parity and those with other risk factors and for use of the Flying Squad may have helped. However, it is less clear that there have been further improvements between 1975 and 1999, in spite of many useful exhortations and initiatives. For abruption, these include vigilance for coagulopathy – disseminated intravascular coagulation (DIC), enlisting the aid of a haematologist and special protocols for religious groups who refuse transfusion. For placenta praevia, the importance of a senior anaesthetist is emphasised, as is the risk of multiple pregnancy, although this may not be soundly based (see under 'Incidence' in 'Twin pregnancy'). It is certainly true that some recommendations (such as the need for a consultant to be present during surgery for placenta praevia) are often ignored. More research is necessary on how staff behaviour may be influenced but also on how the evidence base for change could be improved.

Criterion-based clinical audit

In this type of audit, standards are set, practice is audited, feedback (information about performance, education) is given and then practice is re-audited. This procedure has been widely used in developed countries but has been shown to improve performance in managing haemorrhage in district hospitals in two developing countries.[37] This was not specifically in APH but in all obstetric haemorrhage.

Evidence-based management

Two Cochrane reviews (one completed[38] and one projected on 'interventions for placental abruption') indicate the paucity of evidence about what best practice in the management of APH would be. This is probably explained, especially for abruption, by the difficulty of recruiting women to trials when they are desperately ill and when urgent surgery to save the baby is considered necessary. This is less of a problem for placenta praevia, where intervention is usually elective, but the rarity of the condition means that trials into suitable questions, such as whether cerclage or hospital admission are beneficial, would have to be multicentred.

Conclusions

Abruption has a typical incidence of 0.7% but may be becoming more common. Maternal death is five times more common than overall, and morbidity is also increased. Perinatal death is high (10–20%) and morbidity is increased. Antecedents include primigravidity, multiple pregnancy, smoking and other social factors, threatened miscarriage, pre-eclampsia and previous abruption. None of the above accounts for more than a small proportion of the incidence.

Placenta praevia has a typical incidence of less than 0.5%. Maternal death is five times more common than overall and morbidity is also increased. Antecedents include increased maternal age, multiparity, threatened miscarriage, previous caesarean section and previous placenta praevia, but the population-attributable at risk is low.

APHUO has an incidence of 5–10%. Maternal morbidity and perinatal mortality and morbidity are modestly increased. Few antecedents have been identified, except for threatened miscarriage.

Acknowledgements

We are indebted to Mrs Linda Murdoch for data extraction from Aberdeen Maternity and Neonatal Databank, to Dr Doris Campbell for advice and to Mrs Elaine Stirton for preparing the manuscript.

References

1. Kyrklund-Blomberg NB, Gennser G, Cnattingius S. Placental abruption and perinatal death. *Paediatr Perinat Epidemiol* 2001;15:290–7.
2. Ananth CV, Smulian JC, Demissie K, Vintzileos AM, Knuppel RA. Placental abruption among singleton and twin births in the United States: risk factor profiles. *Am J Epidemiol* 2001;153:771–8.
3. Ananth CV, Savitz DA, Williams MA. Placental abruption and its association with hypertension and prolonged rupture of membranes: a methodologic review and meta-analysis. *Obstet Gynecol* 1996;88:309–18.
4. Rasmussen S, Irgens LM, Dalaker K. The effect on the likelihood of further pregnancy of placental abruption and the rate of its recurrence. *Br J Obstet Gynaecol* 1997;104:1292–5.
5. Kramer MS, Usher RH, Pollack R, Boyd M, Usher S. Etiologic determinants of abruptio placentae. *Obstet Gynecol* 1997;89:221–6.
6. Rasmussen S, Irgens LM, Bergsjø P, Dalaker K. The occurrence of placental abruption in Norway 1967–91. *Acta Obstet Gynecol Scand* 1996;75:222–8.
7. Saftlas AF, Olson DR, Atrash HK, Rochat R, Rowley D. National trends in the incidence of abruptio placentae, 1979–87. *Obstet Gynecol* 1991;78:1081–6.
8. Aberdeen Maternity and Neonatal Databank 2002. Analyses of population-based data carried out for this chapter.
9. Ananth CV, Smulian JC, Vintzileos AM. The association of placenta previa with history of cesarean delivery and abortion: a metaanalysis. *Am J Obstet Gynecol* 1997;177:1071–8.
10. DM Campbell, personal communication.
11. Ministry of Health. *Report on Confidential Enquiries into Maternal Death in England and Wales, 1958–60. Reports on Public Health and Medical Subjects.* No. 108. London: HMSO; 1963.
12. Ministry of Health. *Report on Confidential Enquiries into Maternal Death in England and Wales, 1961–63. Reports on Public Health and Medical Subjects.* No. 115. London: HMSO; 1966.
13. Ministry of Health. *Report on Confidential Enquiries into Maternal Death in England and Wales, 1964–66. Reports on Public Health and Medical Subjects.* No. 119. London: HMSO; 1969.
14. Department of Health and Social Security. *Report on Confidential Enquiries into Maternal Death in England and Wales, 1967–69. Reports on Health and Social Subjects.* No. 1. London: HMSO; 1972.
15. Department of Health and Social Security. *Report on Confidential Enquiries into Maternal Death in England and Wales, 1970–72. Reports on Health and Social Subjects.* No. 11. London: HMSO; 1975.
16. Department of Health and Social Security. *Report on Confidential Enquiries into Maternal Death in England and Wales, 1973–75. Reports on Health and Social Subjects.* No. 14. London: HMSO, 1979.
17. Department of Health and Social Security. *Report on Confidential Enquiries into Maternal Death in England and Wales, 1976–78. Reports on Health and Social Subjects.* No. 26. London: HMSO; 1982.
18. Department of Health and Social Security. *Report on Confidential Enquiries into Maternal Death in England and Wales, 1979–81. Reports on Health and Social Subjects.* No. 29. London: HMSO; 1986.
19. Department of Health and Social Security. *Report on Confidential Enquiries into Maternal Death in England and Wales, 1982–84. Reports on Health and Social Subjects.* No. 34. London: HMSO; 1989.

20. Department of Health, Welsh Office, Scottish Home and Health Department, Department of Health and Social Services, Northern Ireland. *Report on Confidential Enquiries into Maternal Death in the United Kingdom, 1985–87.* London: HMSO; 1991.
21. Department of Health, Welsh Office, Scottish Home and Health Department, Department of Health and Social Services, Northern Ireland. *Report on Confidential Enquiries into Maternal Death in the United Kingdom, 1988–90.* London: HMSO; 1994.
22. Department of Health, Welsh Office, Scottish Home and Health Department, Department of Health and Social Services, Northern Ireland. *Report on Confidential Enquiries into Maternal Death in the United Kingdom, 1991–93.* London: HMSO; 1996.
23. Department of Health, Welsh Office, Scottish Home and Health Department, Department of Health and Social Services, Northern Ireland. *Why Mothers Die. The Confidential Enquiries into Maternal Death in the United Kingdom, 1994–96.* London: The Stationery Office; 1998.
24. Lewis G, Drife J, editors. *Why Mothers Die 1997–1999. The Confidential Enquiries into Maternal Deaths in the United Kingdom.* London: RCOG Press; 2001.
25. Hall MH. Near misses and severe maternal morbidity. In: Drife J, Lewis G, editors. *Why Mothers Die 1997–1999. The Confidential Enquiries into Maternal Deaths in the United Kingdom.* London: RCOG Press; 2001. p. 323–4.
26. Bouvier-Colle MH, Salanave B, Ancel PY, Varnoux N, Fernandez H, Papiernik E, *et al.* Obstetric patients treated in intensive care units and maternal mortality. *Eur J Obstet Gynecol Reprod Biol* 1996;65:121–5.
27. Baskett TF, Sternadel J. Maternal intensive care and near-miss mortality in obstetrics. *Br J Obstet Gynaecol* 1998;105:981–4.
28. Mantel GD, Buchmann E, Rees H, Pattinson RC. Severe acute maternal morbidity: a pilot study of a definition for a near miss. *Br J Obstet Gynaecol* 1998;105:985–90.
29. Hall MH. Caesarean section. In Lewis G, Drife J, editors. *Why Mothers Die 1997–1999. The Confidential Enquiries into Maternal Deaths in the United Kingdom.* London: RCOG Press; 2001. p. 317–22.
30. Royal College of Obstetricians and Gynaecologists Clinical Effectiveness Support Unit. *The National Sentinel Caesarean Section Audit Report.* London: RCOG Press; 2001.
31. Dumont A, Bernis L, Bouvier-Colle MH, Breart G. Estimate of expected caesarean section rate for maternal indications in sub-Saharan Africa: a systematic review. *Lancet* 2001;358:1328–33.
32. Campbell DM, MacGillivray I. Obstetric antecedents of cerebral palsy in singleton pregnancies in Aberdeen and Avon. Presented at the Summer Meeting of the Neonatal Society and the Blair Bell Research Society, 1995.
33. Ananth CV, Wilcox AJ, Savitz DA, Bowes WA Jr, Luther ER. Effect of maternal age and parity on the risk of uteroplacental bleeding disorders in pregnancy. *Obstet Gynecol* 1996;88:511–16.
34. Plessinger MA, Woods JR. Maternal, placental, and fetal pathophysiology of cocaine exposure during pregnancy. *Clin Obstet Gynecol* 1993;36:267–78.
35. Ray JG, Laskin CA. Folic acid and homocyst(e)ine metabolic defects and the risk of placental abruption, pre-eclampsia and spontaneous pregnancy loss: a systematic review. *Placenta* 1999;20:519–29.
36. Naeye RL. Abruptio placentae and placenta previa: frequency, perinatal mortality, and cigarette smoking. *Obstet Gynecol* 1980;55:701–4.
37. Wagaarachchi PT, Graham WJ, Penney GC, McCaw-Binns A, Yeboah Antwi K, Hall MH. Holding up a mirror: changing obstetric practice through criterion-based clinical audit in developing countries. *Int J Gynaecol Obstet* 2001;74:119–30.
38. Neilson JP. Interventions for suspected placenta praevia *Cochrane Database Syst Rev* 2002;(2):CD001998.

Chapter 20

Prevention and treatment of postpartum haemorrhage

A Metin Gülmezoglu and G Justus Hofmeyr

Introduction

Excessive blood loss after childbirth is a major cause of morbidity and mortality in both developing[1] and developed countries.[2,3] In rural communities, in which the majority of the world's population lives, lack of access to skilled birth attendants able to administer parenteral uterotonics, high incidence of anaemia in pregnancy, unavailability of safe blood transfusion services and lack of refrigeration for storing uterotonics worsen the outcome of postpartum haemorrhage (PPH). A community-based study of causes of maternal mortality in rural Zimbabwe described PPH as the leading cause of death (40/100 000).[4] In developed countries, the magnitude of the problem is smaller. Overall rates of maternal mortality in the USA are below 10/100 000 but, of these, PPH is one of the leading causes.[2] In the UK between 1991 and 1993, maternal mortality from PPH was about 1/100 000 births.[5] The difference in absolute mortality rates from PPH between developing and developed countries underscores the effectiveness of medical care in the reduction of mortality from this cause and the need to improve this care further, as well as to find low-cost, implementable methods of reducing the problem in environments with limited medical facilities.

Assessment of blood loss after delivery

The conventional definition of PPH is an arbitrary, clinical one, based on visual estimation of blood loss of 500 ml or more. Visual estimation of blood loss after delivery is subjective and has been shown to underestimate true blood loss.[6] The use of visual estimation is a drawback of several of the randomised trials of active management of labour and comparisons of different uterotonics. The wide range of incidence of PPH in different trials may be due in part to differences in the estimation of blood loss.

A new method has been developed for directly measuring blood loss in order to measure it more objectively without interfering too much with routine care.[7] After delivery of the baby, the amniotic fluid is allowed to drain away and amniotic fluid-soaked bed-linen is covered with a dry disposable 'linen-saver'. A low-profile, wedge-shaped plastic 'fracture bedpan' is slipped under the woman's buttocks and left in place to collect blood loss over the next hour. Blood and clots from the bedpan are decanted into a measuring cylinder. Blood-soaked swabs and linen-savers are weighed, the known dry weight is subtracted and the calculated volume added to that from the bedpan.

In most cases, the great majority of the blood loss is retained in the bedpan and the method is not unduly uncomfortable for the women. Suturing of perineal tears is easily achieved while the bedpan is in place. Most importantly, the measurement is objective. This method is recommended for use in future studies of PPH. Because measured blood loss is considerably greater than that estimated, the threshold for clinically meaningful excessive blood loss should be set at 1000 ml rather than 500 ml.[8]

Strategies to reduce postpartum blood loss

Active management of the third stage of labour

One of the primary objectives of management of the third stage of labour is prevention of PPH. In clinical trials where blood loss was measured, the proportion of women losing 1000 ml or more varied from 0.0–12.5%. It is important to remember that even under experimental trial situations, where women are likely to receive closer attention, approximately 3% will have blood loss of 1000 ml or more. Although practices vary between countries and between units, broadly the third stage of labour can be managed actively or expectantly.[10–13]

Active management of the third stage of labour is usually implemented as a 'package' including early uterotonic administration (with delivery of the anterior shoulder or shortly after delivery of the baby), early cord clamping and placental delivery by controlled cord traction following signs of placental separation.

In expectant, conservative or physiological management, the above interventions are avoided. Usually signs of placental separation are awaited and the placenta is allowed to deliver spontaneously, aided by maternal effort and sometimes gravity.[14]

Active management of the third stage of labour is associated with meaningful reductions in clinically important outcomes, including PPH (blood loss ≥ 500 ml) and severe PPH (blood loss ≥ 1000 ml), postpartum anaemia and the need for blood transfusion during the puerperium, as well as with a reduced risk of prolonged third stage of labour and a reduction in the use of therapeutic uterotonic drugs.[15] Adverse effects of active management include an increase in nausea, vomiting, headache and hypertension when ergometrine is used. Manual removal of the placenta and secondary PPH were more common after active management in one trial in which ergometrine was administered intravenously. Neonatal outcomes were similar, but the rate of breastfeeding at hospital discharge and at six weeks was higher in the active group. Other adverse effects that have been ascribed to uterotonics administered in the third stage of labour include postpartum eclampsia, intracerebral haemorrhage, myocardial infarction, cardiac arrest, pulmonary oedema and inadvertent administration of the parenteral oxytocic to the neonate, causing neonatal convulsion.[15,16] Most of these effects have been attributed to ergot alkaloids that are used either alone or in combination with oxytocin.

Which uterotonic?

Ergometrine or oxytocin

Randomised trials comparing oxytocin with ergometrine or oxytocin-ergometrine combination have been systematically reviewed.[17] There is a significant reduction in the risk of postpartum blood loss of 500 ml or more for women receiving the combination drug ergometrine and oxytocin (Syntometrine®, Alliance Pharmaceuticals) when compared with oxytocin 5 iu. The advantage is smaller but still significant for those receiving the higher oxytocin dose of 10 iu. No statistically significant difference was observed between Syntometrine and either 5 iu or 10 iu oxytocin in terms of blood loss of 1000 ml or more, retained placenta and/or manual removal of the placental, nor for blood transfusion. However, Syntometrine increases the risk of hypertension and vomiting. There were no significant differences in neonatal outcome or the rate of full breastfeeding at the time of discharge from hospital.

For Syntometrine versus oxytocin 10 units, there is a trade-off between greater adverse effects and somewhat fewer women, with blood loss exceeding 500 ml when using Syntometrine. The choice will depend on the relative importance attached to these outcomes. The trade-off between oxytocin and Syntometrine use can be summarised in terms of absolute risk of benefits or harm. The main results of the review can then be as expressed as follows: when 100 women are treated with oxytocin plus ergometrine rather than oxytocin alone, three additional episodes of blood loss of 500 ml or more will be prevented, while one additional case of high blood pressure and ten additional cases of vomiting will occur.[18] Oral ergometrine has not proved as effective as parenteral therapy.[19]

Prostaglandins other than misoprostol

Prostaglandins have strong uterotonic properties and are used widely in obstetric practice. Prostaglandin preparations are available in injectable, tablet or gel forms according to their intended use. Because these agents do not cause hypertension, they can be used in hypertensive women. In the management of the third stage of labour, prostaglandins have been mainly used for intractable PPH as a last resort when other measures have failed. To date, the main disadvantages of prostaglandins have been their cost and availability. The main adverse effects of prostaglandins are nausea, vomiting and diarrhoea.

Systematic review of randomised trials in which intramuscular prostaglandins were used showed modestly decreased blood loss and shorter third stage of labour with prostaglandins compared with other uterotonics (methylergometrine, oxytocin + ergometrine and oxytocin).[20] PPH of 1000 ml or more was also lower in groups receiving prostaglandins, although the numbers were small and the difference was not statistically significant. Vomiting, diarrhoea and abdominal pain were more common in the prostaglandin group. One study was stopped prematurely by the supplier because of case reports of coronary spasm and myocardial infarction in women treated with sulprostone and mifepristone.[21]

The results of this review suggest that injectable prostaglandins may be superior to uterotonics in current use in decreasing blood loss after delivery. However, data on their safety are inadequate to allow recommendation of these agents for routine management.

Misoprostol

Misoprostol is a prostaglandin E_1 analogue that is affordable, easily stored at room temperature and possesses a shelf-life of several years.[22,23] There is considerable experience with misoprostol use, both for peptic ulcer disease and as a uterotonic in obstetrics and gynaecology, and the drug seems to be generally safe.[24] Misoprostol stimulates the myometrium of the pregnant uterus[25] by selectively binding to EP-2/EP-3 prostanoid receptors[26] and is clinically proven to be a uterotonic agent when administered orally and vaginally for induction of labour.[27–29] Measurement of the uterotonic effect on the postpartum uterus has also been documented.[30] Adverse effects of oral misoprostol are mainly gastrointestinal and are dose-dependent.[31] Clinically insignificant hypotensive effects of a high oral dose of misoprostol have been documented,[32] a property that can be an advantage over the ergot, which contains uterotonics that cause blood pressure to increase.

A case of pyrexia of 41.9°C that continued for three hours after postpartum administration of 800 μg of misoprostol has been reported.[30]

To quantify the adverse effects in relation to dosage, the WHO Collaborative Trial of Misoprostol in the Management of the Third Stage of Labour Group conducted a double-blind, double-placebo, randomised comparison of oral misoprostol 600 μg, 400 μg and oxytocin 10 units administered in the third stage of labour.[33] Shivering was more prevalent in the misoprostol 600 μg group and a clear dose-effect relationship was observed.

Following this dose-finding study, the same group conducted a large multicentre trial to evaluate whether misoprostol 600 μg orally was clinically equivalent to intramuscular or intravenously administered 10 iu of oxytocin without an unacceptable level of adverse effects.[34] The relative risk (RR) of blood loss of 1000 ml or more was 1.39 (95% CI 1.19–1.63). The number of women who need to receive oxytocin rather than misoprostol to prevent one extra case of blood loss of 1000 ml or more is 89 (95% CI 61–167) and to prevent one extra case of the use of additional uterotonics is 23 (95% CI 19–30). Shivering and high body temperature were relatively common with misoprostol. The effectiveness of different doses of misoprostol on blood loss of 1000 ml or more and in the use of additional uterotonics are shown in Figure 20.1 and Figure 20.2, respectively. Other trials comparing misoprostol to conventional uterotonics have results similar to the results of the WHO trial, although this is not always obvious because of the small sizes of those trials[20] (Figures 20.1, 20.2).

The results of trials comparing misoprostol (used orally or rectally) to placebo/no treatment are somewhat equivocal. In three trials,[35–37] misoprostol seemed to reduce the blood loss, while in one trial[38] misoprostol was less effective than placebo/no uterotonic at both 400 μg and 600 μg doses.

Although misoprostol is a potent uterotonic drug, its pharmacokinetic properties

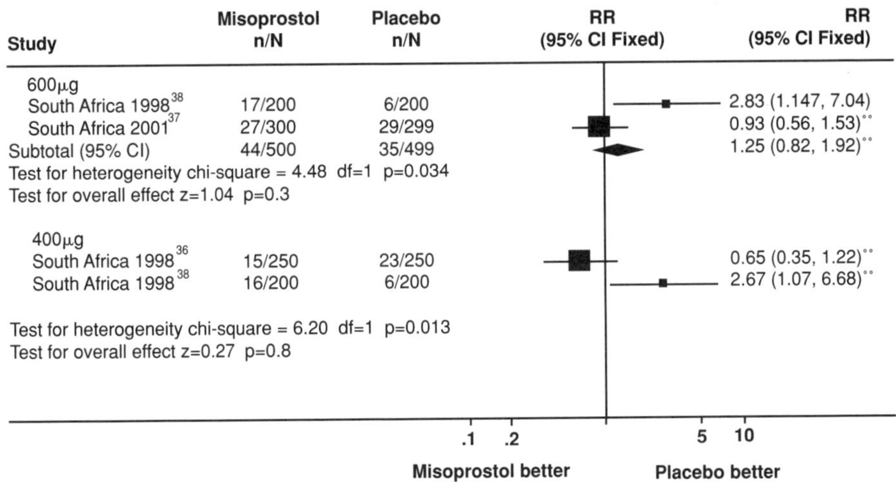

Figure 20.1. Effectiveness of oral misoprostol compared with placebo on blood loss ≥ 1000 ml; the size of the relative risk boxes reflects the weight of each trial in each meta-analysis

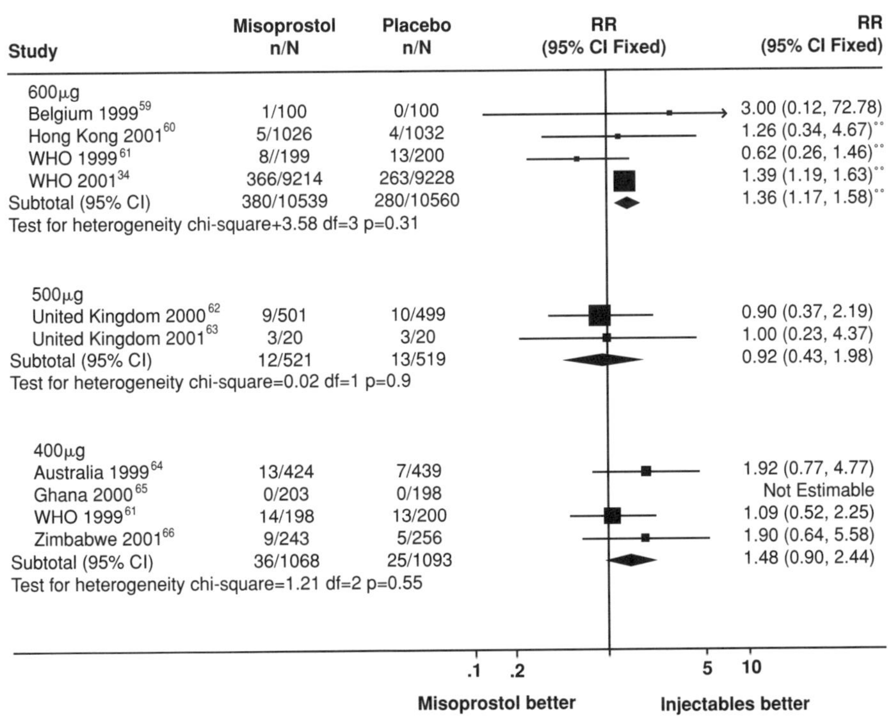

Figure 20.2. Effectiveness of oral misoprostol compared with injectable uterotonics on the use of additional uterotonics; the size of the relative risk boxes reflects the weight of each trial in each meta-analysis

after oral administration may explain these disappointing results. The third stage of labour is completed on average seven to eight minutes after delivery, while the peak blood levels of misoprostol are reached only after 20–30 minutes.

Randomised controlled trials evaluating misoprostol by the rectal route have been inconclusive but a large effect seems unlikely.

Restrictive use of episiotomy

Bleeding from episiotomies may contribute to PPH. In one randomised study of routine versus selective episiotomy, in which blood loss was evaluated after delivery, significantly less blood loss occurred in women allocated to a restrictive episiotomy policy.[39] Moreover, systematic review of randomised trials shows that the restrictive use of episiotomy is associated with a lower risk of clinically relevant morbidities, including posterior perineal trauma (RR 0.88; 95% CI 0.84–0.92), need for suturing perineal trauma (RR 0.74; 95% CI 0.71–0.77) and healing complications at seven days (RR 0.69; 95% CI 0.56–0.85). No difference is shown in the incidence of major outcomes such as severe vaginal or perineal trauma nor in pain, dyspareunia or urinary incontinence. The only disadvantage shown in the restrictive use of episiotomy is an increased risk of anterior vagina lacerations (RR 1.79; 95% CI 1.55–2.07). Avoidance of unnecessary episiotomies may contribute to the reduction in blood loss after delivery.

Umbilical vein injection for retained placenta

Retained placenta is a potentially life-threatening complication of the third stage of labour. If left untreated, there is a high risk of maternal death from haemorrhage or infection. The current standard management of retained placenta, manual removal, aims to prevent these problems but it is unsatisfactory. Manual removal usually requires general or regional anaesthesia in hospital. It is an invasive procedure with its own serious complications of haemorrhage, infection or genital tract trauma. Any management simple and safe enough to be performed at the place of delivery, which reduced the need for manual removal of placenta, could be of major benefit to women worldwide. The injection into the umbilical vein of fluid alone or fluid with a uterotonic drug seems a promising intervention, being simple and apparently safe. The suggested beneficial effect of the umbilical vein injection is that it may reduce the need for manual removal of the placenta by facilitating placental separation.[40]

Mojon and Asdrubali[41] first described umbilical vein injection for the management of retained placenta in 1826. In the early 20th century, various authors reported on the use of umbilical vein injection of saline at differing volumes. The possible benefits and risks of the use of umbilical vein injection versus expectant management for retained placenta were evaluated in a systematic review.[42] The review also included comparisons of different uterotonics and fluids administered through the umbilical vein. Twelve trials of variable quality were included in the review. In comparison to expectant management, umbilical vein injection of saline solution alone did not show any significant difference in the rate of manual removal of the placenta. Saline solution plus oxytocin compared with expectant management showed a clinically but not statistically significant reduction in manual removal. Saline solution with oxytocin compared with saline solution alone showed a significant reduction in manual removal of the placenta (number needed to treat 10, 95% CI 6–37). There was no difference in length of the third stage of labour, blood loss, haemorrhage, haemoglobin, blood transfusion, curettage, infection, hospital stay, fever, abdominal pain and oxytocin augmentation. Saline solution plus prostaglandin, in comparison to saline solution alone, was associated with a statistically significant lower incidence in manual removal of the placenta, but no difference in blood loss, fever, abdominal pain and oxytocin augmentation. There was no significant difference between saline solution plus prostaglandin and saline solution plus oxytocin. The results indicate that umbilical vein injection of saline solution plus oxytocin appears to reduce the need for manual removal of the placenta. Saline solution alone does not appear be more effective than expectant management. Further research into umbilical vein injection of oxytocin or prostaglandins is warranted. It may be worthwhile to include in the research ultrasound measurement of the myometrial thickness adjacent to the placenta as a method of assessing persistent placental attachment.[43]

Other measures aimed at reducing PPH that have been subjected to evaluation but not shown to be effective include early suckling and nipple stimulation.[44]

Management of postpartum haemorrhage

Non-operative measures

PPH is an acute life-threatening event. An indication of the problems experienced by clinicians faced with its management is given by the multitude of strategies reported, mostly as case reports or uncontrolled series. There is little in the way of systematic evaluation of interventions used in the treatment of PPH. Essential elements of its management include:

- treating shock
- ascertaining the origin of the bleeding
- controlling lower genital tract bleeding
- ensuring uterine contraction
- removing the placenta.

Immediate emergency measures include compression of the aorta against the sacral promontary[45] and bimanual uterine compression, the hand in the vagina elevating the uterus to keep the uterine arteries on 'stretch'.[46]

Uterine contraction is usually stimulated by uterine massage and the injection of oxytocin with or without ergometrine intravenously as a bolus injection or oxytocin as a continuous infusion at up to 100 iu per minute. When these methods fail, prostaglandin F2α has been administered intramuscularly or intramyometrially.[47,48] Risks of these methods have not been adequately evaluated. Prostaglandin F2α may be dangerous if inadvertently injected intravenously. In theory, small doses in dilution, injected in several intramyometrial sites after aspiration to check for intravascular position of the needle, may reduce such risks. Intrauterine administration of two gemeprost pessaries has also been described.[49]

Rectal administration of a large dose of misoprostol has been described in 14 women with PPH unresponsive to conventional therapy, with apparently good effect but with no control group for comparison.[50] In a randomised controlled trial in South Africa, 64 women with PPH were randomly allocated to 800 μg rectal misoprostol or intramuscular syntometrine plus 10 iu oxytocin infusion. The authors suggest that misoprostol was more effective. However, the endpoints used in this trial were subjective and open to bias.[51] The effectiveness of high-dose rectal misoprostol for the treatment of PPH needs to be confirmed with appropriately designed and conducted trials.

The use of intravenous tranexamic acid has also been reported.[52] It is interesting that this antifibrinolytic agent, for which good evidence of effectiveness for menorrhagia exists, has not been systematically studied in PPH.

Surgical measures

The usual approach to the management of PPH that is unresponsive to non-operative measures has been a sequence of surgical procedures of increasing invasiveness. Under general anaesthesia, the woman is examined vaginally to determine the source of bleeding. Good lighting and assistance with broad retractors to retract the vaginal walls are essential. If adequate retractors are not available, obstetric forceps with the curvature facing outwards may be used. If there is active bleeding from tears of the vagina or cervix, it is controlled by placement of haemostatic sutures. If bleeding is from the uterine cavity, manual examination for uterine tears or retained products of conception is carried out. Any retained products of conception are removed manually or with ovum forceps or a large-diameter curette. Packing the uterine cavity with gauze packs or abdominal swabs has enjoyed a resurgence of interest. Alternative methods suggested are the use of a Sengstaken–Blakemore tube,[53] a Foley catheter with a large bulb[54] or a silicone water-filled balloon.[55] These methods have not been systematically evaluated.

If uterine bleeding continues, laparotomy is usually performed. If the cause of the bleeding is uterine rupture, this may be repaired, or hysterectomy may be performed. Blood flow to the uterus may be reduced by ligating the anterior branches of the internal iliac arteries, or stepwise ligation of the uterine and ovarian arteries.[56] When all else has failed, the usual approach has been total hysterectomy. Direct compression of uterine bleeding sites has been achieved in five reported cases by means of a 'brace' suture incorporating the full thickness of the intact uterus.[57] Another conservative surgical method is the use of full thickness 'square' sutures to compress the anterior against the posterior uterine wall.

Uterine artery embolisation has been reported to be a life-saving procedure when appropriate radiological expertise and equipment is available.[58]

The management of PPH is an emergency situation that requires swift action and a systematic approach. It is striking that the various methods used to manage PPH have not been evaluated by means of randomised trials. There is clearly a need for trials to assess the effectiveness of the various treatment options to allow a logical, evidence-informed approach to this most dangerous and terrifying obstetric complication.

Conclusion

We have highlighted the evidence from recent systematic reviews of the literature that has established the effectiveness of active management of the third stage of labour in preventing PPH; the relative effectiveness and complications of various pharmacological options; the evidence regarding other methods of reducing blood loss after delivery; new surgical approaches; and the need for further research to determine the effectiveness of misoprostol, as well as the various strategies used to manage PPH once it occurs.

References

1. Kwast BE. Postpartum haemorrhage: its contribution to maternal mortality. *Midwifery* 1991;7:64–70.
2. Berg CI, Atrash HK, Koonin, LM, Tucker M. Pregnancy-related mortality in the United States, 1987–1990. *Obstet Gynecol* 1996;88:161–7.
3. Grimes DA. The morbidity and mortality of pregnancy: still risky business. *Am J Obstet Gynecol* 1994;170:1489–94.
4. Fawcus S, Mbizvo MT, Lindmark G, Nystrom L. A community based investigation of causes of maternal mortality in rural and urban Zimbabwe. *Cent Afr J Med* 1995;41:105–13.
5. Department of Health, Welsh Office, Scottish Home and Health Department, Department of Health and Social Services, Northern Ireland. *Report on Confidential Enquiries into Maternal Deaths in the United Kingdom 1991–1993.* London: HMSO; 1996.
6. Pritchard JA, Baldwin RM, Dickey JC, Wiggins KM. Blood volume changes in pregnancy and the puerperium. *Am J Obstet Gynecol* 1962;84:1–72.
7. Bamigboye AA, Merrell DA, Hofmeyr GJ, Mitchell R. Randomised comparison of rectal misoprostol with syntometrine for management of third stage of labor. *Acta Obstet Gynecol Scand* 1998;77:178–81.
8. Jouppila P. Postpartum haemorrhage. *Curr Opin Obstet Gynecol* 1995;7:446–50.
9. Stones RW, Paterson CM, Saunders NJ. Risk factors for major obstetric haemorrhage. *Eur J Obstet Gynecol Reprod Biol* 1993;48:15–18.
10. Elbourne D. Care in the third stage of labour. In: Robinson S, Thomson AM, editors. *Midwives, Research and Childbirth.* Vol. 4. London: Chapman & Hall; 1995. p. 192–207.
11. Gyte G. The significance of blood loss at delivery. *MIDIRS Midwifery Digest* 1992;2:88–92.
12. Prendiville WJ. The prevention of postpartum haemorrhage: optimising routine management of the third stage of labour. *Eur J Obstet Gynecol Reprod Biol* 1996;69:19–24.
13. Prendiville WJ, Elbourne DR. Care during the third stage of labour. In: Chalmers I, Enkin M, Keirse MJN, editors. *Effective Care in Pregnancy and Childbirth.* Oxford: Oxford University Press; 1989. p. 1145–69.
14. Gyte GML. Evaluation of the meta-analyses on the effects, on both mother and baby, of the various components of 'active' management of the third stage of labour. *Midwifery* 1994;10:183–99.
15. Prendiville WJ, Elbourne DR, McDonald S. Active versus expectant management of the third stage of labour. *Cochrane Database Syst Rev* 2000;(2):CD000007.
16. McDonald SJ, Prendiville WJ, Blair E. Randomised controlled trial of oxytocin alone versus oxytocin and ergometrine in active management of third stage of labour. *BMJ* 1993;307:1167–71.
17. McDonald S, Prendiville WJ, Elbourne D. Prophylactic syntometrine versus oxytocin for delivery of the placenta. *Cochrane Database Syst Rev* 2000;(2):CD000201.
18. Carroli G. RHL practical aspects. Oxytocin or Oxytocin Ergot Alkaloids in Active Management of Labour. WHO Reproductive Health Library, No. 5. Geneva: WHO. WHO/RHR/02.01.2002.
19. De Groot ANJA, van Roosmalen J, van Dongen PWJ, Borm GF. A placebo-controlled trial of oral ergometrine to reduce postpartum haemorrhage. *Acta Obstet Gynecol Scand* 1996;75:464–8.
20. Gulmezoglu AM, Forna F, Villar J, Hofmeyr GJ. Prostaglandins for prevention of postpartum haemorrhage. *Cochrane Database Syst Rev* 2001;(4):CD000494.
21. Van Selm M, Kanhai HHH, Keirse MJNC. Preventing the recurrence of atonic postpartum haemorrhage, a double-blind trial. *Acta Obstet Gynecol Scand* 1995;74:270–4.

22. Kararli TT, Catalano T, Needham TE, Finnegan PM. Mechanism of misoprostol stabilisation in hydroxypropyl methlycellulose. *Adv Exp Med Biol* 1991;302:275–89.
23. Toledo-Velasquez D, Gaud HT, Connors KA. Misoprostol dehydration kinetics in aqueous solution in the presence of hydroxypropyl methylcellulose. *J Pharm Sci* 1992;81:145–8.
24. Collins PW. Misoprostol: discovery, development and clinical applications. *Med Res Rev* 1990;10:149–72.
25. Norman JE, Thong KJ, Baird DT. Uterine contractility and induction of abortion in early pregnancy by misoprostol and mifepristone. *Lancet* 1991;338:1233–6.
26. Senior J, Marshall K, Sangha R, Clayton JK. *In vitro* characterisation of prostanoid receptors on human myometrium at term pregnancy. *Br J Pharmacol* 1993;108:501–6.
27. Fletcher H, Mitchell S, Fredrick J, Simeon D, Brown D. Intravaginal misoprostol versus dinoprostone as cervical ripening and labour inducing agents. *Obstet Gynecol* 1994;83:244–7.
28. Hofmeyr GJ, Gülmezoglu AM. Vaginal misoprostol for cervical ripening and labour induction in late pregnancy. *Cochrane Database Syst Rev* 2000;(2):CD000941.
29. Alfirevic Z, Howarth G, Gausamann A. Oral misoprostol for induction of labour with a viable fetus. *Cochrane Database Syst Rev* 2000;(2):CD001338.
30. Chong YS, Chua S, El-Refaey H, Choo WL, Chanrachakul B, Tai BC, *et al.* Postpartum intrauterine pressure studies of the utrotonic effect of oral misoprostol and intramuscular syntometrine. *BJOG* 2001;108:41–7.
31. Inman WHW. Report on current PEM studies: drugs for peptic ulcer or reflux. *Prescription Event Monitoring News* 1991;7:32–4.
32. Brecht T. Effects of misoprostol on human circulation. *Prostaglandins* 1987;33 Suppl:51–9.
33. Lumbiganon P, Hofmeyr, GJ, Gülmezoglu AM, Pinol A, Villar J. Misoprostol dose-related shivering and pyrexia in the third stage of labour. *Br J Obstet Gynaecol* 1999;106:304–8.
34. Gülmezoglu AM, Villar J, Ngoc NN, Piaggio G, Carroli G, Adetoro L, *et al.* WHO multicentre double-blind randomized controlled trial to evaluate the use of misoprostol in the management of the third stage of labour. *Lancet* 2001;358:689–95.
35. Bamigboye AA, Hofmeyr GJ, Merrell DA. Rectal misoprostol in the prevention of postpartum haemorrhage: a placebo-controlled trial. *Am J Obstet Gynecol* 1998;179:1043–6.
36. Hofmeyr GJ, Nikodem VC, de Jager M, Gelbart BR. A randomised controlled trial of oral misoprostol in the third stage of labour. *Br J Obstet Gynaecol* 1998;105:971–5.
37. Hofmeyr GJ, Nikodem VC, de Jager M, Drakely A. Side–effects of oral misoprostol in the third stage of labour: a randomised placebo controlled trial. *S Afr Med J* 2001;91:432–5.
38. Hofmeyr GJ, Nikodem C, de Jager M, Drakely A, Gilbart B. Oral Misoprostol for labour third stage management: randomised assessment of side-effects (part 2). Proceedings of the 17th Conference on Priorities in Perinatal Care, South Africa 1998:53–4.
39. House MJ, Cario G, Jones MH. Episiotomy and the perineum: a random controlled trial. *J Obstet Gynecol* 1986;7:107–10.
40. Carroli G. Management of retained placenta by umbilical vein injection. *Br J Obstet Gynaecol* 1991;98:348–50.
41. Jarcho A. Management of retained placenta. *Surgery, Gynecology and Obstetrics* 1928;46:265–72.
42. Carroli G, Bergel E. Umbilical vein injection for management of retained placenta. *Cochrane Database Syst Rev* 2001;(2):CD001337.
43. Herman A, Weinraub Z, Bukovsky I, Arieli S, Zabow P, Caspi E, *et al.* Dynamic ultrasonographic imaging of the third stage of labour: new perspectives into third-stage mechanisms. *Am J Obstet Gynecol* 1993;168:1496–9.
44. Bullough CHW, Msuku RS, Karonde L. Early suckling and postpartum haemorrhage: controlled trial in deliveries by traditional birth attendants. *Lancet* 1989;2:522–5.
45. Roberts WE. Emergency obstetric management of postpartum haemorrhage. *Obstet Gynecol Clin North Am* 1995;22:283–302.
46. Drife J. Management of primary postpartum haemorrhage. *Br J Obstet Gynaecol* 1997;104:275–7.
47. Bigrigg A, Chui D, Chisslell S, Read MD. Use of intramyometrial 15-methyl prostaglandin F2 alpha to control atonic postpartum haemorrhage following vaginal delivery and failure of conventional therapy. *Br J Obstet Gynaecol* 1991;98:734–6.
48. Jacobs M, Arias F. Intramyometrial prostaglandin F2 in the treatment of severe postpartum hemorrhage. *Obstet Gynecol* 1980;55:665–6.
49. El-Lakany N, Harlow RA. The use of gemeprost pessaries to arrest postpartum haemorrhage. *Br J Obstet Gynaecol* 1994;101:277.
50. O'Brien P, El-Refaey H, Gordon A, Geary M, Rodeck CH. Rectally administered misoprostol for the treatment of postpartum haemorrhage unresponsive to oxytocin and ergometrine: a descriptive study.

Obstet Gynecol 1998;92:212–14.

51. Lokugamage AU, Sullivan KR, Niculescu I, Tigere P, Onyangunga F, El-Refaey H, *et al.* A randomized study comparing rectally administered misoprostol versus Syntometrine combined with an oxytocin infusion for the cessation of primary postpartum hemorrhage. *Acta Obstet Gynecol Scand* 2001;80:835–9.
52. As AK, Hagen P, Webb JB. Tranexamic acid in the management of postpartum haemorrhage. *Br J Obstet Gynaecol* 1996;103:1250–1251.
53. Katesmark M, Brown R, Raju KS. Successful use of a Sengstaken–Blakemore tube to control massive postpartum haemorrhage. *Br J Obstet Gynaecol* 1994;101:259–60.
54. Gilstrap LC III, Ramin SM. Postpartum hemorrhage. *Clin Obstet Gynecol* 1994;37:824–30.
55. Bakri YN, Amri A, Abdul Jabbar F. Tamponade-balloon for obstetrical bleeding. *Int J Gynecol Obstet* 2001;74:139–42 .
56. AbdRabbo SA. Stepwise uterine devascularisation: a novel technique for management of uncontrollable postpartum hemorrhage with preservation of the uterus. *Am J Obstet Gynecol* 1994;171:694–700.
57. B-Lynch C, Coker A, Lawal AH, Abu J, Cowen MJ. The B-Lynch surgical technique for the control of massive postpartum haemorrhage: an alternative to hysterectomy? Five cases reported. *Br J Obstet Gynaecol* 1997;104:372–5.
58. Deux JF, Bazot M, Le Blanche AF, Tassart M, Khalil A, Berkane N, *et al.* Is selective embolization of uterine arteries a safe alternative to hysterectomy in patients with postpartum hemorrhage? *Am J Roentgenol* 2001;177:145–9.
59. Amant F, Spitz B, Timmerman D, Corremans A, Van Assche FA. Misoprostol compared with methylergometrine for the prevention of postpartum haemorrhage: a double-blind randomised trial. *Br J Obstet Gynaecol* 1999;106:1066–70.
60. Ng PS, Chan ASM, Sin WK, Tang LCH, Cheung KB, Yuen PM. A multicentre randomized controlled trial of oral misoprostol and i.m. syntometrine in the management of the third stage of labour. *Hum Reprod* 2001;16:31–5.
61. Lumbiganon P, Hofmeyr J, Gülmezoglu AM, Pinol A, Villar J. Misoprostol dose-related shivering and pyrexia in the third stage of labour. *Br J Obstet Gynaecol* 1999;106:304–8.
62. El-Refaey H, Nooh R, O'Brien P, Abdalla M, Geary M, Walder J, *et al.* The misoprostol third stage of labour study: a randomised controlled comparison between orally administered misoprostol and standard management. *BJOG* 2000;107:1104-10.
63. Lokugamage A, Paine M, Bassaw-Balroop K, Sullivan K, El-Refaey H, Rodeck C. Active management of the third stage at caesarean section: a randomised controlled trial of misoprostol versus syntocinon. *Aust N Z J Obstet Gynaecol* 2001;41:411-4.
64. Cook C, Spurrett B, Murray H. A randomized clinical trial comparing oral misoprostol with synthetic oxytocin or syntometrine in the third stage of labour. *Aust N Z J Obstet Gynaecol* 1999;39:414–9.
65. Walley RL, Wilson JB, Crane JM, Matthews K, Sawyer E, Hutchens R. A double-blind placebo controlled randomised trial of misoprostol and oxytocin in the management of the third stage of labour. *BJOG* 2000;107:1111–5.
66. Kundodyiwa TW, Majoko F, Rusakaniko S. Misoprostol versus oxytocin in the third stage of labor. *Int J Gynecol Obstet* 2001;75:235–41.

Chapter 21

Antepartum and postpartum haemorrhage

Discussion

Discussion following the papers by Dr Hall and Dr Gülmezoglu

Yentis: I have a question relating to anaesthetics. If there is no major haemodynamic instability, it is often the fear of a coagulopathy that pushes us towards a general anaesthetic rather than a regional one. I personally suspect that we are doing many more general anaesthetics than we need to. Do your figures suggest the actual incidence of coagulopathy in these relatively small groups?

Hall: No, I cannot give you any information about that. It is not very well documented. My own feeling, which I know not every anaesthetist shares, is that if there is a major risk of hypovolaemia, I would prefer a general anaesthetic, both as a patient and when operating.

Yentis: I am surprised to hear that there are people who would consider a regional anaesthetic in those situations.

Robson: I was interested that the rate of placenta praevia that you commented on is relatively low compared to the literature and I was fascinated by the fact that you have a 100% caesarean section rate in placenta praevia. Are you just talking about major praevia, where you would expect a 100% caesarean section rate, or are you including minor praevia as well?

Hall: I suppose this is a self-fulfilling prophecy, that we are not including people who are able to be delivered vaginally. I am old enough to remember the days when you diagnosed placenta praevia by whether the head touched the pelvis when you pushed it into the pelvis. There were certainly false positives and false negatives then. Now, there are lots of false positives in early pregnancy – at the 20-week scan there are many false positives for placenta praevia, but there are no false positives later on in pregnancy.

If a patient did not bleed at all, but the scan detected some placenta praevia, and an examination suggested it was possible to go on with the delivery, we would conclude that that was not placenta praevia. Obviously, if you are prepared to say that any encroachment in the lower segment – which of course cannot necessarily be seen on the scan anyway – constitutes a placenta praevia, you would have a higher incidence. So I agree that it is rather arbitrary.

Robson: But that, presumably, accounts for rate being much lower than that of the published literature.

Hall: Yes.

Robinson: I would like to ask one of the awkward consumer questions but not about major problems such as placenta praevia. We were intrigued by a study[1] carried out at Northwick Park Hospital by a senior midwife about eight years ago that examined haemorrhage rates according to which senior registrar did the delivery. I seem to remember that there was an 11-fold variation that, so far as she could see, correlated with personality. She also did not have sufficient data but found the same trend in midwives.

It has seemed to me ever since that this is something that people looking at haemorrhage rates ought to be considering a little more, and it certainly seems to come into some of the suggestions from people who contact us. Of course, they are very skewed data and I am sure that we are biased, but we would like to put that on the table and ask people to keep an eye on it, or think about it.

Hall: It would be very difficult to set up a study that had anything like adequate power. You would also have to be extremely careful not to attribute higher rates to the people who were called in when everyone else was in trouble, which is a problem with all sorts of government outcome indicators and league tables. It would be a very difficult study to do properly, although there could be a grain of truth in it. There are some manually unskilled people practising both midwifery and obstetrics.

Neilson: And estimates of blood loss may relate to personality traits as well!

MacLean: Dr Hall, could you comment on management? When I was a junior, once you bled, you stayed in hospital until you delivered. However, because of pressure on beds, increasingly, if a patient stops bleeding and there is not a major praevia, they are sent home. I know that some of our patients return, sometimes after quite brisk bleeds. Do you have any comments on morbidity? I suspect there is not a contribution to mortality, although one of these days there will be, from our current policy of keeping patients six hours, 24 hours or a week after they have stopped bleeding, and then letting them go home.

Hall: This question is eminently suitable for a trial, as Professor Neilson showed in his review. We do not have evidence at the moment. Our practice is conservative and if we have diagnosed placenta praevia we keep them in, but this is eminently suitable for a trial.

Bewley: I would agree that it is eminently suitable for a trial. I was slightly concerned that the Royal College of Obstetricians and Gynaecologists, in the absence of evidence, gave a recommendation that people should stick to conservative management, because we have the problem that none of our consultant obstetricians agrees with that. I should say that we live in London and we are not that far from medical help, and we feel that there is incredible morbidity in keeping women in hospital, which has nothing to do with pressure on the beds. It is very bad for their thromboembolism, mental health state and so on, so I think we should get on with it. Interestingly, a vote was taken last week at the British Maternal and Fetal Medicine Society, showing that we have enough equipoise. It came out three to one in favour of outpatient rather than inpatient management.

MacLean: Could I just draw people's attention to the fact that in London the interval between dialling for an ambulance and it arriving can be frighteningly long? Although if you live in London you tend to think you have ready access to the hospital, that is not always true. Yes, if you have a car parked on the drive with petrol in the tank, you could probably get to hospital, but not everyone has this, which may contribute to some of the risk.

Bewley: We do have the proviso that patients should be 24 hours a day with another adult, who has access to a phone and preferably a car. They have to be able to tolerate gory descriptions of blood running down the legs and risk of hysterectomy and so on. This is probably the majority of progressive obstetric opinion.

Robson: Two votes were taken at the recent British Maternal and Fetal Medicine Society meeting in Oxford concerning the management of placenta praevia. The first related to the question, 'How would you manage a major placenta praevia who has not bled?', which is the sort of patient that you are talking about. Of the 300 or so delegates, only a handful indicated they would electively admit the woman to hospital. In other words, the majority of practising obstetricians in the audience would manage a major placenta praevia that had not bled as an outpatient. Where there was 'equipoise' was the management when there had been bleeding. Interestingly, there was still a substantial body of opinion in favour of outpatient management.

Neilson: Dr Hall, you mentioned your disbelief that there was an association between abruption and ruptured membranes. When I reviewed this a little while ago, the association seemed to be not with ruptured membranes *per se*, but with chorioamnionitis, which may of course be related to ruptured membranes.

I have been aware of one local difficulty that has stemmed from the chapter in the Confidential Enquiry for which you were responsible, which advocated that planned delivery for women at high risk of haemorrhage of one sort or another should take place in a maternity unit with on-site bloodbank. There are clearly many maternity units in the UK and elsewhere that do not have on-site bloodbanks. Could you develop that a little further? If a maternity unit is very close to a major hospital, for example, with bloodbank facilities, is that acceptable? Is there a certain distance that makes you anxious?

Hall: Distance is not really the issue. There are some hospital sites where it could take a long time for something to get from one end of the site to the other. It is certainly true that there were cases – and I pronounced on management on the basis of anecdotes within the report – where the bloodbank that was available was 60 miles away, or a similar unacceptable distance. It is an ideal to which one would aspire, but the key point is how the system works in practice. If you can have an arrangement whereby the bloodbank that is closely adjacent can provide huge amounts of blood quickly, then if it works there is no problem.

Neilson: Let us move on to postpartum haemorrhage (PPH). Are there any comments about that?

Hall: The results of the WHO Multicentre Randomised Trial of Misoprostol in the Management of the Third Stage of Labour[2] were disappointing in a way, because the misoprostol came out just on the other side of the arbitrary level that you had set as being acceptable. The choice of the level of effect that would be acceptable was arbitrary. I wonder whether its major advantages, in terms of being storable without refrigeration, do not outweigh the disadvantages.

Gülmezoglu: That is true, and the level was arbitrary, although we felt that an increase of 35% or over was a fairly large difference. We should also consider that difference in relation to the level of adverse effects, which is fairly high. I did not show these data, but the relative risks of severe shivering and temperature rise are fairly high. There is definitely an advantage in terms of oral administration but, when we look at other essential interventions that we are promoting, we are looking at intravenous or intramuscular antibiotics, or at magnesium sulphate. If oxytocin injectable 10 iu is the gold standard, we should recommend it.

MacLean: You made a comment about infusion of syntocinon saline, presumably maternal intravenous infusion. However, there was a recommendation about 20 years ago about injection into the cord, to manage retained placenta, into cord vessels, where you did not have easy access either to theatre or to anaesthetists. I just want to clarify that you mean maternal administration. Do you have any thoughts on ways of managing retained placenta without having to get to theatre?

Gülmezoglu: Perhaps that was not very clear. I meant umbilical vein infusion, not maternal.

Neilson: Is there any information on misoprostol injection into the umbilical vein? Obviously, you need to dissolve it.

Robson: Do you have any feel for the proportion of women in developing countries who have access to routine oxytocin at delivery? I am just interested to know what proportion of the delivering obstetric population in developing countries does not have access to third-stage oxytocics.

Gülmezoglu: Dr Graham may know this better than me. In some places, such as India, oxytocin is less expensive than misoprostol. Sometimes we get carried away with the oral administration and so on but my gut feeling would be that, in institutions and healthcare centres, oxytocin should be available. Unlike ergometrine, it is fairly stable. Ergometrine is much less stable and it degenerates but I do not have the data to support that.

Graham: The easiest way to consider that is to look at it in terms of the proportion of deliveries that take place with a health professional. Most of those health professionals practise in health facilities. You will not have oxytocin outside of a health facility in most settings. The global figure now is 45% of deliveries occurring with a health professional but in places like Bangladesh it is only 8%. In other words, 92% take place outside of facilities and without health professionals, so they will have no oxytocin. That percentage varies enormously, as I said earlier, but certainly fewer than half the world's deliveries have obvious access to oxytocics.

De Bernis: I support that. I would like to make one point, because technology could help with some issues. For that, we have Uniject™ (Path, Seattle, WA), which is a dose of 10 ml already prepared in a syringe, for unique use. A factory in Mexico is trying to produce this and we are establishing the system in Mexico. We hope to be able to propose this technology for many countries. It could help not only at facility level but also in countries where a number of births occur at home, and the health worker can supply Uniject without risk of misuse and danger. This is something new that we are seeing in this area. It is also a reason to promote more and more systematic use of it.

Gülmezoglu: The WHO trial should not be taken out of context. That was within the context of active management and in hospitals. Beyond that, we need more research, which is being done. A trial is being conducted in the Gambia comparing oral ergometrine with misoprostol used by traditional birth attendants at home deliveries.

We are working on a protocol in South Africa where we will test misoprostol, at a higher dose, for the treatment of PPH. Those are separate questions.

Yentis: Could I reveal my ignorance here and ask the obstetricians a question? I have never heard of saline being given down an umbilical vessel: if this reduces the need for theatre by 20%, why is everyone not doing it?

Gülmezoglu: The first publication about umbilical vein injection goes back to the beginning of the 20th century, or even to the 19th century.

Yentis: That would explain it!

Robson: I can offer another possible explanation: some cases of retained placenta in hospital are the result of overexuberant pulling on the cord by doctors leading to the cord snapping, in which case you cannot then give an oxytocic.

References

1. Logue M. Management of the third stage of labour. A midwife's point of view. *J Obstet Gynaecol* 1990;10 Suppl 2:5510–12.
2. Gülmezoglu AM, Villar J, Ngoc NN, Piaggio G, Carroli G, Adetoro L, *et al.* WHO multicentre double-blind randomized controlled trial to evaluate the use of misoprostol in the management of the third stage of labour. *Lancet* 2001;358:689–95.

SECTION 6

SPECIFIC PROBLEMS OF MORTALITY AND MORBIDITY II

Chapter 22

Cardiac disease

Michael de Swiet

Introduction

Heart disease is the most common indirect cause of maternal mortality in the UK and was responsible for 35 maternal deaths in the report for the triennium 1997–99 (Confidential Enquiries into Maternal Deaths 1997–99).[1] Indeed, because of the more rapid decline in direct than in indirect deaths, heart disease now causes as many deaths as thromboembolism, which is the leading direct cause of maternal mortality.

Although sporadic fatalities occur in all forms of heart disease in pregnancy, maternal mortality is most likely in myocardial infarction, dissecting aneurysm and in conditions where pulmonary blood flow cannot be increased. Table 22.1 lists the deaths from the various forms of heart disease given in the CEMD report for 1997–99. But when cardiomyopathy (12 cases) and pulmonary hypertension (seven cases) are listed with dissecting aneurysm (five cases) and myocardial infarction (five cases), these dominate the series, with other causes only contributing one or two cases each (Table 22.2).[1] This pattern also applies to the whole period from 1991 to 1999 (dissecting aneurysm was only included within cardiac mortality from the 1991–1993 triennium.) Between 1991 and 1993, a total of 105 cardiac deaths was noted: 26 from cardiomyopathy and myocarditis, 21 from dissecting aneurysm and 18 each from pulmonary hypertension and myocardial infarction. All other causes only accounted for 22 deaths, approximately 20% of the total (Table 22.3).[1–3]

Cardiomyopathy and myocarditis

Traditionally, cardiomyopathy is divided into dilated and restrictive cardiomyopathy. In pregnancy, dilated cardiomyopathy is responsible for more cardiac deaths than is restrictive cardiomyopathy. There is one form of dilated cardiomyopathy, puerperal cardiomyopathy, that is specific to pregnancy and has a particularly high mortality. Some forms of dilated cardiomyopathy show clinical or pathological features that suggest infection and the condition is then labelled 'myocarditis'. By far the most

Table 22.1. Maternal deaths due to cardiac disease, UK 1997–99[1]

Cause	Deaths (*n*)
Congenital	
Primary pulmonary hypertension	3
Pulmonary hypertension cause unknown	1
ASD, Eisenmenger syndrome	2
ASD closed, residual pulmonary hypertension	1
Total PHT	7
Bicuspid aortic valve, endocarditis	1
Coarctation repair, endocarditis	1
Previous ASD surgery, ? dysrhythmia	1
Total congenital	10
Acquired	
Puerperal cardiomyopathy	7
Cardiomyopathy and myocarditis	5
Total cardiomyopathy	12
Aneurysm of thoracic aorta and its branches	5
Myocardial infarction	5
Endocarditis, normal mitral valve	1
Heart failure cause unknown	2
Total acquired	25
Total cardiac deaths	35

ASD = atrial septal defect; PHT = pulmonary hypertension

common form of restrictive cardiomyopathy is hypertrophic obstructive cardiomyopathy (HOCM). Both restrictive and dilated cardiomyopathy may be inherited.

Hypertrophic obstructive cardiomyopathy

The precise cause of HOCM is unknown, although rapid advances are being made in the molecular genetics of the condition.[4] The pathological features are hypertrophy and

Table 22.2. Maternal deaths due to cardiomyopathy, pulmonary hypertension, aneurysm of the thoracic aorta, myocardial infarction and other cardiac causes, UK 1997–99[1]

Cause	Deaths (*n*)
Cardiomyopathy	12
Pulmonary hypertension	7
Aneurysm of thoracic aorta and its branches	5
Myocardial infarction	5
Heart failure cause unknown	2
Bicuspid aortic valve; endocarditis	1
Coarctation repair; endocarditis	1
Previous ASD surgery, dysrhythmia	1
Endocarditis, normal mitral valve	1
Total cardiac deaths	35

ASD = atrial septal defect

Table 22.3. Maternal deaths due to cardiomyopathy, pulmonary hypertension, aneurysm of the thoracic aorta, myocardial infarction and other cardiac causes UK 1991–99;[1-3] Crown copyright material reproduced with permission of the Controller of HMSO and the Queen's Printer for Scotland

Cause	1997–99	1994–96	1991–93	Totals
Cardiomyopathy and myocarditis	12	9	5	26
Aneurysm of thoracic aorta and its branches	5	7	9	21
Myocardial infarction	5	6	8	19
Pulmonary hypertension	7	7	4	18
All other heart disease				22
Aortic valve disease	1	2		3
Mitral valve disease		1	2	3
Atrial septal defect (ASD)			2	2
Ventricular septal defect			2	2
Heart failure cause unknown	2			2
Aneurysm of coronary vein			1	1
Anomalous coronary arteries		1		1
Chromosome 3 abnormality			1	1
Previous ASD surgery; ? dysrhythmia	1			1
Coarctation repair; endocarditis	1			1
Endocarditis, normal mitral valve	1			1
Non-bacterial endocarditis			1	1
Left ventricular hypertrophy		1		1
Myocardial fibrosis			1	1
Pericarditis		1		1
Total cardiac deaths	35	34	36	105

disorganisation of cardiac muscle, particularly of the left ventricular outflow tract. The patient presents with chest pain, syncope, dysrhythmias or symptoms of heart failure; death is thought to be caused by left ventricular outflow tract obstruction and/or dysrhythmia. The diagnosis can usually be made by echocardiography, which shows abnormally thickened and disorganised cardiac muscle.

Oakley *et al.*[5] have reported extensive experience of the management of this condition in pregnancy from the Hammersmith Hospital, London. These authors originally advocated beta-adrenergic blockade in all cases to reduce the risk of syncope resulting from obstruction of the left ventricular outflow tract; this is now reserved for symptomatic patients. Patients should not be allowed to become hypovolaemic because this also increases the risk of obstruction of the left ventricular outflow tract. They should not lie supine because of the risk of caval obstruction and subsequent decrease in venous return. Particular care should be taken to give adequate fluid replacement if there is antepartum haemorrhage and also to avoid postpartum haemorrhage. During labour, patients with HOCM should be given epidural anaesthesia with caution, as this causes relative hypovolaemia by increasing venous capacitance in the lower limbs.

Puerperal cardiomyopathy

The incidence of puerperal cardiomyopathy (also known as peripartum cardiomyopathy and pregnancy cardiomyopathy) in the UK is probably less than one in 5000. The condition usually arises in the puerperium. The pathogenesis of this condition is unknown; therefore, some authors have denied that puerperal cardiomyopathy is a specific entity and considered the condition to be another form of congestive cardiomyopathy caused by hypertension. Rand *et al.*[6] postulated an immunological cause on the basis of antibodies to heart muscle present in cord blood and serum from the mother in a case of pregnancy cardiomyopathy. Alternatively, the combination of multiparity and low social class has suggested that the condition is due to an undefined nutritional defect. Melvin *et al.*[7] described three cases of puerperal cardiomyopathy due to myocarditis, proven by endomyocardial biopsy at cardiac catheterisation, and these authors propose that infection may be an important cause. Cunningham *et al.*[8] reviewed 28 cases of obscure cardiomyopathy occurring in 106 000 pregnancies in Texas. In only seven cases was the condition truly idiopathic, which indicates the rarity of the condition, but these patients fared badly. Four were dead within eight years.

At presentation, there is no other predisposing cause for the heart failure and the heart is grossly dilated. The patients are not necessarily multiparous, black, relatively elderly, nor of poor social class, in the sporadic cases seen in the UK. Pregnancy has often been complicated by hypertension. Multiple pregnancy is another risk factor. Pulmonary, peripheral and particularly cerebral embolisation is a major cause of morbidity and mortality, and this occurs at a rate of 25–50%.[9] The majority of deaths occur around the time of presentation, but some women have protracted illnesses and die up to eight years later. However, if the patient recovers fully from the initial episode, the long-term prognosis is good. There is always concern about the risk of recurrence in future pregnancies. For this reason, any patient who develops pulmonary oedema peripartum should be investigated thoroughly in case the diagnosis of peripartum cardiomyopathy is made unjustifiably. The prognosis in future pregnancies has been defined by Elakyam[10] and much depends upon whether the patient has recovered from the previous episode, as judged by echocardiography. Table 22.4 clearly shows that the prognosis is much worse if the patient still had evidence of previous cardiomyopathy. Most would consider pregnancy to be contraindicated in this group: three of 12 such patients died (25%), by comparison with no mortalities in 23 patients where the echocardiograph was normal at the onset of pregnancy. Nevertheless, pregnancy, even if not fatal, was associated with deterioration in 10–20% of the latter group. Thus, a cautious attitude should be adopted towards all women who have had previous puerperal cardiomyopathy.

Table 22.4. Pregnancy excluding abortion following puerperal cardiomyopathy;[10] copyright © 2001 Massachusetts Medical Society; all rights reserved

	Patients (*n*)	Symptoms of failure (%)	> 20% decrease in LVEF (%)	Decrease in LVEF at follow-up (%)	Death
Dysfunction at onset	12	50	33	42	3
Normal at onset	23	26	17	9	0

LVEF = left ventricular ejection fraction

Dissecting aneurysm

In the last ten years, dissecting aneurysm has been the second most common cause of cardiac mortality (Table 22.3). Coarctation of the aorta, Marfan's syndrome and Ehlers–Danlos disease (see below) are the conditions traditionally associated with dissection but, in practice, none of these conditions is at all common in women dying in pregnancy from dissection and the cause of the dissection is usually uncertain. The patients described in the CEMD report have often been seriously ill for some time, even days, before they die. This is in contrast to the deaths from myocardial infarction, which are usually sudden. Therefore there is the potential to save some of these women. Obstetricians and others caring for pregnant women need to be aware of the risks of dissection. The definitive diagnosis is usually made by echocardiography. However, even a chest X-ray may be helpful in showing widening of the mediastinum. As with pulmonary embolism, the unjustified reluctance of doctors to order chest X-rays in pregnancy costs lives.

Pulmonary vascular disease

In normal pregnancy, the pulmonary blood flow has to increase *pari passu* with systemic flow and the pulmonary vascular resistance also falls. The failure to increase pulmonary blood flow occurs because of obstruction, either within the pulmonary blood vessels or at the mitral valve.

The situation is documented clearly in Eisenmenger syndrome, where until now there has been no effective treatment and where the maternal mortality is 30–50%.[11,12] Maternal mortality (40%) had not improved in a UK survey of 15 pregnancies.[12] Elevations in pulmonary vascular resistance are also found in vasculitis, such as due to systemic lupus erythematosus, in cor pulmonale, patients with single ventricle, pulmonary veno-occlusive disease and in primary pulmonary hypertension.[13] In the latter condition, the maternal mortality is around 50%.[11]

In contrast, in Fallot's tetralogy where the pulmonary vascular resistance is normal, the reported maternal mortality varies from 4–20%.[11,14] Furthermore, the figure of 20% is based on only one maternal death in five pregnancies in Jacoby's study.[14]

As indicated above, Eisenmenger syndrome has a high maternal mortality rate. Only over the last 10–15 years has there been any form of surgical treatment and the opportunities for this – heart and lung transplantation – rarely arise. Most patients with Eisenmenger syndrome who die in pregnancy do so in the puerperium. Although deaths are occasionally sudden, due to thromboembolism, this is not usually so. More frequently, these patients die from a slowly falling systemic $P\text{O}_2$ with an associated decrease in cardiac output. This is because the pulmonary vascular resistance is high and fixed. Any fall in the shunt ratio or in the cardiac output will cause a fall in pulmonary blood flow. For example, in pre-eclampsia, the pulmonary vascular resistance increases and the cardiac output falls.[15] These factors would therefore decrease pulmonary blood flow, which could account for the observed deterioration in Eisenmenger syndrome associated with hypertensive pregnancy.[11]

What can be offered to the pregnant patient with Eisenmenger syndrome? Unfortunately, abortion would appear to be the answer. The maternal mortality associated with abortion is only 7%, in comparison with 30% for continuing pregnancy.[16] However, if the patient decides to continue with the pregnancy, prophylactic anticoagulation, probably with subcutaneous heparin, should be offered, because of the risk of thromboembolism, both systemic and pulmonary. Labour should not be induced unless there are good obstetric reasons. Induced labour carries a higher risk of caesarean section, which is associated with a particularly high maternal mortality in Eisenmenger syndrome.

There is controversy concerning the place of epidural anaesthesia for the management of labour. Although epidural anaesthesia should decrease pulmonary blood flow by decreasing the systemic vascular resistance, this may not occur; at least, it did not in the case studied by Midwall *et al.*[17] On balance, a carefully administered elective epidural anaesthetic at the beginning of labour is probably preferable to emergency epidural or general anaesthesia if it is suddenly decided that instrumental delivery is necessary.

If the patient does become hypotensive, with increasing cyanosis and decreasing cardiac output, it has been shown that high inspired oxygen concentrations can decrease pulmonary vascular resistance and increase pulmonary blood flow and peripheral oxygen saturation.[17] In addition, beta-sympathomimetic agents, such as phenylephrine, methoxamine and noradrenaline (norepinephrine), will increase systemic resistance and thus increase pulmonary blood flow.[18] However, drugs such as tolazline, phentolamine, nitroprusside and isoprenaline, which have been used to decrease pulmonary vascular resistance in other clinical situations, probably should not be given, because they will also decrease the systemic vascular resistance.[18] If systemic resistance decreases more than pulmonary resistance, pulmonary blood flow will decrease rather than increase. The same problem occurs with dopamine and β-sympathomimetic drugs, which have been given to increase cardiac output. They too will decrease systemic resistance and, if systemic resistance decreases more than the cardiac output increases, pulmonary blood flow will fall.

Two other pulmonary vasodilators deserve mention. There is evidence of thromboxane/epoprostenol imbalance in primary pulmonary hypertension, with too much thromboxane production and too little epoprostenol production.[13] In these circumstances, epoprostenol infusion may act as a relatively selective pulmonary vasodilator.[19] The drug has to be given by intravenous infusion, but it might just tip the balance in the deteriorating patient with Eisenmenger syndrome to allow improved pulmonary blood flow and better myocardial oxygenation. Also, nitric oxide has now been identified as the endothelium-derived relaxing factor, which in turn is a powerful vasodilator. When inhaled, it can be a relatively selective pulmonary vasodilator and it has been shown to be effective both in the neonate and in adults with pulmonary hypertension. Unfortunately, anecdotal experience with inhaled nitric oxide has not been favourable for patients with Eisenmenger syndrome and fixed pulmonary resistance.

A report has suggested that the endothelin antagonist bosentan (Tracleer™, Actelion, Switzerland) may be helpful.[20] It can be taken orally. Although there is little or no experience of bosentan use in pregnancy, the prognosis for pulmonary vascular disease is so poor that any treatment that could be effective should be considered, whatever the fetal risk. Bosentan could certainly be used after delivery, which is when most pregnant women with pulmonary vascular disease die.

Cor pulmonale, pulmonary veno-occlusive disease and primary pulmonary hypertension

Where there is pulmonary hypertension and vascular disease in small blood vessels in cor pulmonale, pulmonary veno-occlusive disease and primary pulmonary hypertension, the maternal mortality is still high and termination of pregnancy is still the management of choice.[21]

Primary pulmonary hypertension is particularly worrying because, although it is a rare condition, it commonly presents in young women. It may be familial. The genetics and cell biology of pulmonary vascular disease are currently the subjects of intense research.[13] Primary pulmonary hypertension has also been associated with taking appetite-suppressant drugs.[22] There has also been concern about the association between the development of primary pulmonary hypertension and combined oral contraceptive use.

Because of the risk of thrombotic microangiopathy, anticoagulation should be continued in pregnancy or instigated if the patient is not already on such therapy. The options are similar to those in patients with artificial heart valves; either warfarin to maintain international normalised ratio at approximately 2 or high-dose low molecular weight heparin aiming for anti-Xa level about 0.8 units/ml.

The problem in these conditions still appears to be one of maintaining adequate pulmonary blood flow for adequate oxygenation. Although blood cannot be shunted directly from the pulmonary to the systemic circuit as in Eisenmenger syndrome, excessive vasodilatation in the systemic circulation during epidural anaesthesia could still decrease preload to the right ventricle and therefore further decrease pulmonary blood flow.

Unfortunately, as in Eisenmenger syndrome, selective pulmonary vasodilators are not available. The options include nifedipine, nitroprusside and oxygen and the effects of epoprostenol infusion and nitric oxide inhalation are being investigated. Oral epoprostenol analogues are becoming available but have not yet been used in pregnancy.[23] Nifedipine may of course be taken on a long-term basis, although the doses needed can be high, of the order of 240 mg per day. Although nifedipine is used to control systemic blood pressure in pregnancy, the effects of such high doses on the fetus are uncertain.

Manoeuvres that suddenly increase venous return (ergometrine injection, movement from supine to left lateral position) should be avoided, as should those that increase vagal tone (e.g. bladder catheterisation). Several patients with primary pulmonary hypertension have died in association with bradycardia and atrioventricular block, which suggest vagally mediated mechanisms.

These patients should be delivered in an intensive care environment with elective insertion of a Swan–Ganz catheter (notwithstanding the risk in patients with pulmonary hypertension) and facilities for pacing. If circumstances permit, there are arguments for elective testing of various potential pulmonary vasodilators on the day before delivery to see which (if any) will work in the event that the patient deteriorates. To maintain haemodynamic stability, Abboud *et al.*[24] used intrathecal morphine as an analgesic in labour in a patient with primary pulmonary hypertension. Intrathecal morphine gives highly effective analgesia, with little change in maternal haemodynamics and little transfer to the fetus. The most common adverse effects are pruritus and late respiratory depression. The immediate results in this case were excellent as judged clinically and by Swan–Ganz monitoring. Unfortunately, the patient died seven days later from acute right ventricular strain. The theoretical advantage of epidural morphine over epidural block with local anaesthesia is the lack of haemodynamic effects. Yet conventional epidural anaesthesia when skilfully applied can be beneficial in primary pulmonary hypertension,[25] and fentanyl (an opiate) and bupivacaine have been combined with success for delivery in primary pulmonary hypertension. Even if epidural block in any of its forms gives a superior haemodynamic profile, it is also tempting to recommend caesarean section and general anaesthesia, which offers a controlled process with less physical stress for the mother in the short term.[26] The anaesthetist's experience is likely to dictate the more suitable form of anaesthesia in these difficult and rare situations.

Myocardial infarction

Myocardial infarction is rare in pregnancy and in young women in general. Only 1% of admissions for myocardial infarction occur in women younger than 45 years.[27] In 1996, Badui and Enciso[28] cited only 109 cases of myocardial infarction in pregnancy in the literature since 1922. Most of these cases were in women aged 30–40 years (mean age 32 years). However, the increasing incidence of myocardial infarction in women and the increasing age at which women become pregnant may result in an increased incidence of myocardial infarction in pregnancy.

The immediate mortality from myocardial infarction in pregnancy is 19%;[28] some women die up to four years after the original event, making the overall mortality 32%. The overall mortality from myocardial infarction rises during pregnancy from nil in the first trimester to 50% in the puerperium: surprisingly, younger patients are more likely to have myocardial infarction in the puerperium and therefore have a higher mortality.[29] Pregnancies in these younger patients have frequently been complicated by pre-eclampsia.

The precise mechanism of myocardial infarction is open to speculation. Women have a high incidence of coronary spasm and atypical mechanisms seem to be common in pregnancy. Beary *et al.*[30] suggest that the group of patients with myocardial infarction occurring in the puerperium includes those most likely to have spasm or coronary artery thrombosis not associated with atherosclerotic narrowing. The syndrome of myocardial infarction with normal coronary arteries occurring in young women is well documented. In the non-pregnant state, the prognosis is good if they survive the initial episode. Primary dissection of the coronary arteries is another cause of myocardial infarction, particularly peripartum,[31] when some cases have been associated with beta-sympathomimetic tocolysis. Coronary artery dissection in general is rare but more than 70% of cases occur in women and 25% of these have occurred at the end of pregnancy or immediately afterwards.[32] This is presumably another example of the tendency for pregnancy-induced changes in vessel walls to cause any fault in arteries such as coronary, splenic, adrenal or even the aorta to rupture in pregnancy.

Because arteries do seem particularly 'fragile' in pregnancy (see dissecting aneurysm above), caution is necessary concerning angioplasty immediately following myocardial infarction in pregnancy or even concerning coronary arteriography, which itself may precipitate dissection. Anomalous origin of the coronary arteries and arteritis due to systemic lupus erythematosus or Kawasaki's disease are other rare causes of myocardial infarction in pregnancy.

Other causes of cardiac mortality

Rheumatic heart disease is still a major cause of mortality in developing countries. Mitral stenosis is the usual killer and, again, the problem lies in maintaining pulmonary blood flow, although in this case the obstruction is between the left atrium and left ventricle rather than in the pulmonary blood vessels themselves.

Nevertheless, in rheumatic heart disease maternal mortality can be very low. Szekely *et al.*[33] reported 26 mortalities in 2856 pregnancies (about 1%) complicated by rheumatic heart disease between 1942 and 1969. Half of the deaths were due to pulmonary oedema, which became less common once mitral valvotomy was freely available. These authors reported no maternal deaths in about 1000 pregnancies occurring in 1960. Rush *et al.*[34] also reported a maternal mortality of 0.7% in 450 mothers with rheumatic heart disease in South Africa. In Ehlers–Danlos syndrome, the arterial and classic forms have also been associated with high mortality, due to arterial dissection and bleeding.[35] The Ehlers–Danlos syndrome is characterised on the basis of the specific collagen defect and in Ehlers–Danlos syndrome type IV, the maternal mortality is said to be as high as 25% in North America.[36] Further review of the literature based on 50 pregnancies in women with Ehlers–Danlos type IV has estimated the maternal mortality to be 20% per pregnancy.[37] This high mortality, which is largely due to haemorrhage from major blood vessels, has been disputed by Pope and Nicholls[38] in a different series from the UK, implying a different referral population or genetic heterogeneity. There is also a high fetal loss rate attributable to premature rupture of the membrane if either father or mother has Ehlers–Danlos syndrome.[39] This is presumably due to a collagen defect in the fetal membranes.

Morbidity

With regard to morbidity, the best recent study comes from Canada, where 562 pregnant women with structural heart disease or significant arrhythmias from 13 cardiac centres and obstetric teaching hospitals were followed prospectively during 617 pregnancies between 1994 and 1999.[40] The majority of the patients had congenital heart disease. There were 81 pregnancies in patients with valvular heart disease and 32 pregnancies in patients with cardiomyopathy. Only three patients had pulmonary hypertension; presumably more patients with pulmonary hypertension had their pregnancies terminated, which was a specific reason for exclusion from the study.

The aim of the study was to define risk factors for adverse maternal and fetal outcomes. Only adverse maternal outcomes will be considered here. Primary cardiac events occurred in 80 pregnancies and were defined as pulmonary oedema, significant dysrhythmia requiring treatment, stroke, cardiac arrest or cardiac death. Predictors of cardiac events were prior cardiac event, left heart obstruction (mitral valve area <2 cm^2, aortic valve area <1.5 cm^2 or left ventricular outflow tract gradient > 30 mmHg) and reduced systemic ventricular contractility with ejection fraction of less than 40% (Table 22.5). Each predictor was given a score of 1. Half the pregnancies were assessed and it was found that the risk of a cardiac event with a score 0 was 5%, with score 1 was 27% and with score greater than 1 was 75%. These scores were then tested with the other half of the study population and similar results were obtained. The value of

Table 22.5. Predictors of cardiac events in 617 pregnancies of women with heart disease;[40] reproduced with permission from Lippincott, Williams and Wilkins

Predictor	Odds ratio[a]	95% CI	*P*
Prior cardiac event	6	3–14	< 0.001
NYHA class >II or cyanosis	6	2–22	0.009
Left heart obstruction	6	3–14	< 0.001
Systemic ventricular dysfunction	11	4–34	< 0.001

NYHA = New York Heart Association Gradings of Heart Disease severity (Grades I to IV)

this study lies in its simplicity. Only four predictors are significant. If none is present (and the patient does not have pulmonary hypertension or a lesion-specific risk factor such as dissection in Marfans syndrome), the risks of cardiac event are small and the authors suggest that the woman may deliver in a community hospital. If more than one predictor is present, the risk of a serious cardiac event is extremely high. Interestingly, the authors found that method of delivery and continuing or initiation of drug therapy were not independent risk factors predicting cardiac events. Therefore, much agonising about the route of delivery in cardiac patients on the grounds of their health is probably unnecessary.

Many clinicians still believe that 'every pregnancy was so many nails of a coffin of a woman with heart disease'.[41] Chesley[42] has reported a group of 38 patients with 51 pregnancies occurring after they were diagnosed as having severe rheumatic heart disease. These were compared with a group of 96 women with equally severe rheumatic heart disease who did not have any pregnancies after diagnosis. The mean survival time (14 years) was no less and, in fact, was greater in the group who did have further pregnancies compared with the group that did not (12 years). I would agree with Chesley[42] that pregnancy does not affect the long-term survival of a woman with rheumatic heart disease, providing that she survives pregnancy itself.

References

1. Drife J, Lewis G, editors. *Why Mothers Die 1997–99. The Confidential Enquiries into Maternal Deaths in the United Kingdom.* London: RCOG Press; 2001.
2. Department of Health, Welsh Office, Scottish Home and Health Department, Department of Health and Social Services, Northern Ireland. *Report on Confidential Enquiries into Maternal Death in the United Kingdom, 1994–96*. London: The Stationery Office; 1998.
3. Department of Health, Welsh Office, Scottish Home and Health Department, Department of Health and Social Services, Northern Ireland. *Report on Confidential Enquiries into Maternal Death in the United Kingdom, 1991–93*. London: HMSO; 1996.
4. Spirito P, Seidman CE, McKenna WJ, Maron BJ. The management of hypertrophic cardiomyopathy. *N Engl J Med* 1997;336:775–85.
5. Oakley GDG, McGarry K, Limb DG, Oakley CM. Management of pregnancy in patients with hypertrophic cardiomyopathy. *BMJ* 1979;1:1749–50.
6. Rand RH, Jenkins BM, Scott DG. Maternal cardiomyopathy of pregnancy causing stillbirth. *Br J*

Obstet Gynaecol 1975;82:172–5.
7. Melvin KR, Richardson PJ, Olsen EGJ, Daly K, Jackson G. Peripartum cardiomyopathy due to myocarditis. *N Engl J Med* 1982;307:731–4.
8. Cunningham FG, Pritchard JA, Hankins GDV, Anderson PL, Lucas MJ, Armstrong KF. Peripartum heart failure: idiopathic cardiomyopathy of compounding cardiovascular events. *Obstet Gynecol* 1986;67:157–68.
9. Homans DC. Peripartum cardiomyopathy. *N Engl J Med* 1985;312:1432–7.
10. Elakyam U, Tummala PP, Rao K, Akhter MW, Karaalp IS, Wani OR, *et al.* Maternal and fetal outcomes of subsequent pregnancies in women with peripartum cardiomyopathy. *N Engl J Med* 2001;344:1567–71.
11. Morgan Jones A, Howitt G. Eisenmenger syndrome in pregnancy. *BMJ* 1965;1:1627–31.
12. Yentis SM, Steer PJ, Plaat F. Eisenmenger's syndrome in pregnancy: maternal and fetal mortality in the 1990s. *Br J Obstet Gynaecol* 1998;105:921–2.
13. Strange JW, Wharton J, Phillips PG, Wilkins MR. Recent insights into the pathogenesis and therapeutics of pulmonary hypertension. *Clin Sci (Colch)* 2002;102:253–68.
14. Jacoby WJ. Pregnancy with tetralogy and pentalogy of Fallot. *Am J Cardiol* 1964;14:866–73.
15. Littler WA, Redman CW, Bonnar J, Beilin LJ, Lee Gde J. Reduced pulmonary arterial compliance in hypertensive pregnancy. *Lancet* 1973;1:1274–8.
16. Gleicher N, Midwall J, Hockberger D, Jaffin H. Eisenmenger's syndrome and pregnancy. *Obstet Gynecol Surv* 1979;34:721–41.
17. Millwall J, Jaffin H, Herman MV, Kuper Smith J. Shunt flow and pulmonary haemodynamics during labour and delivery in the Eisenmenger syndrome. *Am J Cardiol* 1978;42:299–303.
18. Devitt JH, Noble WH. Eisenmenger's syndrome and pregnancy. *N Engl J Med* 1980;302:751.
19. Jones K, Higenbottam T, Wallwork J. Pulmonary vasodilation with prostacyclin in primary and secondary hypertension. *Chest* 1989;96:748–89.
20. Rubin LJ, Badesch DB, Barst RY, Galie N, Black CM, Keogh A, *et al.* Bosentan therapy for pulmonary arterial hypertension. *N Engl J Med* 2002;346:896–903.
21. Bowers C, Devine PA, Chervenak FA. Dilation and evacuation during the second trimester of pregnancy in a woman with primary pulmonary hypertension. A case report. *J Reprod Med* 1988;33:787–8.
22. Abenheim F, Moride Y, Brenot F, Rich S, Benichou J, Kurz X, *et al.* Appetite suppressant drugs and risk of primary pulmonary hypertension. *N Engl J Med* 1992;335:609–16.
23. Okano Y, Yoshioka T, Shimouchi A, Satoh T, Kunieda T. Orally active prostacyclin analogue in primary pulmonary hypertension. *Lancet* 1997;349:1365.
24. Abboud TK, Raya J, Noueihed R, Daniel J. Intrathecal morphine for relief of labour pain in a parturient with severe pulmonary hypertension. *Anesthesiology* 1983;59:477–9.
25. Slomka F, Salmeron S, Zetlaoui P, Cohen H, Simonneau G, Samii K. Primary pulmonary hypertension and pregnancy: anesthetic management of delivery. *Anesthesiology* 1988;69:959–61.
26. Oakley C, editor. *Heart Disease in Pregnancy*. London: BMJ Publishing Group; 1997.
27. Peterson DR, Thompson DJ, Chinn N. Ischemic heart disease prognosis. A community-wide assessment. *JAMA* 1972;219:1423–7.
28. Badui E, Enciso R. Acute myocardial infarction during pregnancy and puerperium: a review. *Angiology* 1996;47:739–56.
29. Ginz B. Myocardial infarction in pregnancy. *J Obstet Gynaecol Br Cwlth* 1970;77:610–15.
30. Beary JF, Summer WR, Bulkley BH. Postpartum acute myocardial infarction: a rare occurrence of uncertain etiology. *Am J Cardiol* 1979;43:158–61.
31. Jewett JF. Two dissecting coronary artery aneurysms postpartum. *N Engl J Med* 1978;278:1255–6.
32. Vicari R, Eybel C, Monson D. Survival following spontaneous coronary artery dissection: surgical repair by extrusion of intramural haematoma. *Am Heart J* 1986;111:593–4.
33. Szekely P, Turner R, Snaith L. Pregnancy and the changing pattern of rheumatic heart disease. *Br Heart J* 1973;35:1293–303.
34. Rush RW, Verjans M, Spracklen FHN. Incidence of heart disease in pregnancy. A study done at Peninsular Maternity Services Hospital. *S Afr Med J* 1979;55:808–10.
35. Peaceman AM, Cruikshank DP. Ehlers–Danlos syndrome and pregnancy: association of type IV disease with maternal death. *Obstet Gynecol* 1987;69:428–31.
36. Rudd NL, Nimrod C, Holbrook KA, Byers PH. Pregnancy complications in type IV Ehlers–Danlos Syndrome. *Lancet* 1983;i:50–3.
37. Lurie S, Manor M, Hagay ZJ. The threat of type IV Ehlers–Danlos syndrome on maternal well-being during pregnancy: early delivery may make the difference. *J Obstet Gynecol* 1998;18:245–8.
38. Pope FM, Nicholls AC. Pregnancy and Ehlers–Danlos syndrome type IV. *Lancet* 1983;i:249–50.

39. Levick K. Pregnancy loss and fathers with Ehlers–Danlos syndrome. *Lancet* 1989;ii:1151.
40. Siu SC, Sermer M, Colman JM, Alvarez N, Mercier L, Morton BC, *et al.* Prospective multicenter study of pregnancy outcomes in women with heart disease. *Circulation* 2001;104:515–21.
41. Webster JC. The conduct of pregnancy and labour in acute and chronic affections of the heart. *Transactions of the American Gynecological Society* 1913;38:223.
42. Chesley LC. Severe rheumatic cardiac disease and pregnancy: the ultimate prognosis. *Am J Obstet Gynecol* 1980;136:552–8.

Chapter 23

Cancer during pregnancy

Allan B MacLean

The statistics

Between 1991 and 1999, and among 370 indirect, 111 fortuitous or coincidental and 225 late maternal deaths recorded from the Confidential Enquiries, there were 96 cancer deaths.[1–3] This represents 14% of indirect, coincidental and late deaths or, if direct deaths are included in the denominator, 9% of all maternal deaths recorded in these publications. During this time, there were almost 6 700 000 births, representing one cancer death in 69 781. As Drife[4] explains, these figures include late deaths, whereas maternal deaths, by the World Health Organization definition, include only direct and indirect deaths.

Table 23.1 shows data adapted from Drife[4] covering 1985 to 1999, with one death from neoplasia in every 83 000 deliveries. Before this, from the beginning of the Confidential Enquiries in 1952 to 1984 there were 386 deaths caused by neoplasia, representing almost 5% of all maternal deaths and one cancer death in 62 361 births. The variation in cancer deaths may relate more to careful and thorough enquiry than biological factors and a reduction in death from other causes.

These 96 deaths between 1991 and 1999, approximately ten per year, represent only a small fraction of the 75 000 women (73 666 with malignant neoplasms or 74 949 with any neoplasm) who died of cancer in 1999. There are no comparisons for pregnant and non-pregnant women but in 1999 there were 641 cancer deaths in women between 15 and 34 years of age. Cancer mortality rates for women aged 15–34 years and 35–49 years have fallen steadily between 1960 and 1997. Cancer is the cause of 24% of all deaths in the UK and is the cause of death of 46% of women who die before the age of 65 years. Deaths from breast, lung and large bowel cancer account for 47% of all female cancer deaths.[5]

The anatomical sites of the cancers recorded in the Confidential Enquiries are listed in Table 23.2. Lymphomas and leukaemias are a heterogenous group and include acute leukaemia and non-Hodgkin lymphomas. Brain and nervous system tumours include astrocytoma, glioma, meningioma, pituitary and spinal tumours, as well as cerebral tumours, not otherwise specified according to autopsy findings. Gastrointestinal tract cancers include carcinoma of the colon, rectum and stomach.

Table 23.1. Deaths from neoplasia reported in the Confidential Enquiries into Maternal Deaths 1985–1999[4]

	Births (n)	Deaths from neoplasia (n)	Indirect deaths (n)	Fortuitous deaths (n)	Late deaths	
					Indirect (n)	Fortuitous (n)
1985–87	2 293 700	16	4	9	–	2
1988–90	2 374 800	25	4	10	2	9
1991–93	2 346 800	17	1	10	4	1
1994–96	2 228 600	27	2	8	5	12
1997–99	2 123 600	52	12	6	16	18
Totals	11 367 500	137	23	43	27	42

There are no data for the UK relating to cancer incidence or registration during pregnancy to allow comparison between women who are diagnosed during or soon after pregnancy, or those who have previously undergone cancer treatment and embark on a pregnancy, and those who die. It is estimated that cancer is diagnosed in association with pregnancy in about one in 1000.[6,7] Cervical and breast cancer together account for approximately 50% of cancer diagnoses.

Lambe and Ekbom[8] used the Swedish Cancer Registry to link with a nationwide fertility registry that included information on the number and dates of live births. Between 1960 and 1990, there were 32 848 cancers registered for ages 15–44 years: 428 of these (1.3%) were diagnosed during pregnancy and 1425 (4.3%) during 'the lactation period' (the 12 months after birth). The overall incidences during pregnancy and lactation were 15.6 and 51.6 respectively per 100 000 live births. The most frequent sites were skin (malignant melanoma 3.6/100 000 live births), cervix (2.4/100 000) and breast (2.0/100 000). Table 23.3 has been adapted from the table in their article: expected numbers during pregnancy and lactation were estimated from female age-specific and period-specific population rates, and 'observed to expected'

Table 23.2. Cancer deaths by site;[1–3] Crown copyright material reproduced with permission of the Controller of HMSO and the Queen's Printer for Scotland

Cancer site/type	Deaths (n)
Lymphomas and leukaemias	15
Brain and nervous system	13
Gastrointestinal tract	10
Pancreas	8
Malignant melanoma	7
Sarcoma (bone and striated muscle)	7
Carcinoma, unknown primary	6
Cervix	5
Lung	5
Breast	5
Ovary	5
Bladder	2
Other	8

Table 23.3. Ten most common sites of cancers coinciding with childbearing: observed and expected ratios of these sites during pregnancy and lactation;[8] reproduced with permission from the BMJ Publishing Group

	During pregnancy			During lactation		
	Observed	Expected	Ratio	Observed	Expected	Ratio
Melanoma	100	90.3	1.11	171	120.5	1.42
Cervix[a]	102	158.0	0.65	213	210.7	1.01
Breast[a]	114	156.6	0.73	248	208.6	1.19
Nervous system	32	71.7	0.45	129	95.6	1.35
Ovary[a]	54	62.6	0.86	70	83.4	0.84
Colon	24	31.9	0.75	57	42.3	1.35
Endocrine	20	33.2	0.60	46	44.2	1.04
Hodgkin's[a]	24	31.2	0.77	58	41.7	1.40
Thyroid	17	50.0	0.34	118	66.7	1.77
Leukaemia[a]	24	29.1	0.82	39	38.7	1.01
All sites	428	880.7	0.49	1425	1174.0	1.21

[a] adjusted for under-reporting in the first and second trimester

ratios were calculated for the ten most common sites. Observed cases for cervix, breast, ovary, Hodgkin's disease and leukaemia were adjusted based in observed numbers for the third trimester, to counter the under-reporting of cases in earlier pregnancy when termination followed diagnosis of cancer. During pregnancy, the observed to expected ratio was only above unity for melanoma (1.11; 95% CI 0.88–1.32) and for all sites was 0.49 (95% CI 0.44–0.59). During lactation, the observed to expected ratio for all sites was 1.21 (1.15–1.28). The reduced ratio during pregnancy and higher ratio in the subsequent 12 months may reflect pregnancy-associated delay in diagnosis.

Does pregnancy increase the risk of death for those patients with cancer?

In the past, cancer deaths in pregnancy have been either indirect deaths, i.e. resulting from previous existing disease or deaths from diseases that developed during pregnancy and were not due to direct obstetric causes but were aggravated by the physiological effects of pregnancy, and fortuitous and now coincidental deaths, i.e. from unrelated causes that happen to occur in pregnancy or the puerperium. Until more information is available about tumour behaviour, it is inappropriate to designate some cancers as being aggravated by pregnancy and others as not. The most recent Confidential Enquiry[3] has grouped together all the cancer deaths to facilitate pattern recognition and identify key messages.

Cancers and their growth, recognition, dissemination and management, may be influenced by pregnancy in one of several ways:

- alterations in blood flow
- alterations from increased sex hormone levels
- alterations from increased unbound corticosteroid levels

- alterations from reduced cellular immunity
- alterations due to the effect of placental and other growth factors.

It was once believed that cervical cancer was influenced by mechanical effects of vaginal delivery, breast cancer by oestrogens and melanoma by melanocyte-stimulating hormone or whatever the hormone is that causes the pigment changes in the nipples and linea nigra. The scientific details no longer fit these explanations and will be discussed in greater detail below. However, it is fair to say that we have little idea what most of these factors do *in vitro*, for example in cell culture or laboratory situations, and even less what they do *in vivo*.

What is apparent from cancer mortality associated with pregnancy is that, although there appears to be no difference in survival stage-for-stage, prognosis is compromised by later presentation or sometimes by delay in starting treatment. These points are expanded below. The Confidential Enquiries continue to contain cautionary tales of missed or delayed diagnosis. Patients who complain of vaginal bleeding, breast changes, vomiting and bowel upset, abdominal pain, headache and backache are frequently found in antenatal clinics but these symptoms will sometimes reflect an underlying cancer. The omission of any form of examination to assess for pathology must be challenged.

Cervical carcinoma in pregnancy

There are no UK data on the frequency of cervical cancer during pregnancy. Johnstone[9] in Edinburgh stated that 'the condition mitigates strongly against the occurrence of pregnancy, and is therefore a rare complication', while Munro Kerr in Glasgow reported an incidence of one in 2000 pregnancies.[10] This figure is identical to that quoted by Williams[11] in the USA and similar to the one in 2205 calculated by Hacker *et al.*[12] from 11 papers published between 1960 and 1977. It is acknowledged that the incidence of invasive carcinoma of the cervix associated with pregnancy in the USA has declined in the last 20 years[6,13] and this is probably also true for Europe and the UK.

Behaviour of cervical carcinoma during pregnancy

Older textbooks[11,14] reported that pregnancy produced rapid growth and extension of tumour and 'worsens the prognosis'. Pregnancy and other hormonal changes are regarded as co-factors acting with human papillomavirus; various events including eversion of the squamocolumnar junction and trauma at delivery may increase the risk for cervical neoplasia.[15] However, there is no evidence that when early-stage disease is found during pregnancy the prognosis is worse than that for non-pregnant women of similar age. For example, Hacker *et al.*[12] reported a review of 1657 cases of invasive carcinoma of the cervix seen during or in the first 12 months postpartum and found that there was no difference in survival for stages IB or II compared with data from the International Federation of Gynecology and Obstetrics (FIGO) Annual Report.

Prognosis for cervical cancer (and probably many other cancers) is presumably dependent on a short interval between diagnosis and treatment.[16] If treatment is delayed as long as the doubling-time, theoretically the tumour will double in size. It has been calculated previously that the potential doubling-time of cervical tumours, using bromodeoxyuridine and cell kinetics, was 4.4 days, although there was considerable heterogeneity and no pregnant patients were included in the study.[17] It therefore comes as a surprise that reports of treatment delay in pregnancy do not appear to compromise outcome. Prem *et al.*[18] described their experience in treating 100 cervical cancer patients during or within 18 months of pregnancy with radium and external beam radiotherapy. Five women whose diagnosis of stage I cancer was made between 20 and 34 weeks had opted to delay their treatment for between 11 and 17 weeks before being delivered by caesarean section. None of the five mothers was compromised by this delay, leading the authors to comment that deliberate delay of treatment in the third trimester to reduce the fetal hazards of preterm delivery did not appear to adversely affect the prognosis. Subsequent reports have provided similar reassurance. Duggan *et al.*[13] reported on 19 pregnant patients who accepted the advice for immediate treatment with a mean diagnosis to treatment interval of 17 days (range 2–42 days); there were nine fetal and two neonatal deaths. Eight patients with stage Ia or Ib disease between 11 and 31 weeks requested postponement of treatment with a mean diagnosis–treatment interval of 144 days (53–212 days); neonatal outcome was normal and all mothers remained free of disease after treatment with a median follow-up of 23 months. Sorosky *et al.*[19] also described eight women with stage Ib lesions who requested that treatment be delayed for between three and 40 weeks – this latter patient had conceived in the cycle after diagnosis and refused therapy until a viable fetus could be delivered. All eight patients were managed by caesarean section and radical hysterectomy and were alive and disease-free after mean follow-up of three years. Van Vliet *et al.*[20] reported on 12 pregnant women, six of whom were more than 20 weeks and stage Ib or IIa and had treatment delayed for two to ten weeks. Six patients were less than 20 weeks and stage Ib or IIb and had immediate treatment. One patient in each group died after a relapse but the remaining five patients in the delayed-treatment group were disease-free after a median follow-up of 82 months. All these authors suggest that delayed treatment to achieve greater fetal maturity is a reasonable option.

The problem with generalisations about behaviour is that there are always exceptions. It is believed that pregnancy does not accelerate progression of cervical intraepithelial neoplasia towards invasion. However, Dudan *et al.*[21] reported on 48 patients who underwent cone biopsy during pregnancy for carcinoma *in situ*; one patient advanced to stage Ia two months later and three advanced to stage Ib, two, five and 12 months later. It is recognised that cone biopsy during pregnancy may not remove the whole lesion,[12] and it is possible that these reported examples of progression may have been lesions missed during the cone biopsy.

Second, Hacker *et al.*[12] reported that pregnant women who were seen with stage III or IV disease had a five-year survival of only 16% compared with 28% for the FIGO data.[22] It was suggested that the difference might be related to problems with radiation dosimetry during or soon after pregnancy.

Third, behaviour is influenced by histological type. Certain tumours such as villoglandular papillary adenocarcinoma are usually indolent,[23] while neuroendocrine small cell carcinoma are aggressive and fortunately are rarely complicated by pregnancy.[24,25] Therefore, management of these lesions must be individualised.

Diagnosis and management of cervical cancer during pregnancy

The diagnosis of cervical cancer usually follows the assessment of an abnormal smear – colposcopy during pregnancy is outside the remit of this chapter but occasionally invasive cancer will be found. Additionally, the diagnosis can follow the investigation of the patient with threatened abortion or antepartum haemorrhage. The rarity of cervical cancer makes the junior obstetric trainee's interpretation of the appearances of the cervix uncertain. Contact bleeding will occur for various reasons but, if there is any uncertainty, the patient should undergo colposcopy and directed biopsy.

Staging of the lesion is more difficult when the uterus is enlarged with a pregnancy. Intravenous urography must be omitted to prevent X-ray exposure to the fetus but magnetic resonance imaging (MRI) would be appropriate.

Treatment should be individualised according to histological type, stage and treatment options. In the past, it was a major success to avoid serious haemorrhage and keep the mother alive: Sarwey[26] in 1899 (quoted by Williams, 1930) reported on 603 collected cases where the mortality at the time of labour or early puerperium was 43.3% and 8.0% of the patients died undelivered. Johnstone[9] stated that it was better to perform a caesarean section, followed by supravaginal hysterectomy, to remove the uterus from the neighbourhood of the septic cervix: subsequent treatment was radium if there was some hope of cure. Treatment during pregnancy was also by radium, which often induced abortion but, if not, the pregnancy was allowed to continue or the uterus was evacuated later. If the mother's condition was hopeless, all due consideration was given to the interests of the child.

Modern treatment is described by Crawford and Shepherd.[27] In the first and second trimesters, radical hysterectomy and lymphadenectomy can be performed with the fetus *in utero*.[28] In the late mid-trimester (gestation not defined, but presumably after 24 weeks), the mother is given corticosteroids to accelerate fetal lung maturation and, once maturity is confirmed, caesarean section is performed, with radical hysterectomy and pelvic lymphadenectomy. A classical section has advantages over a lower-segment incision for avoiding the encroaching tumour and associated increased vascularity. It is suggested that, if the patient presents in labour, an emergency section is necessary to avoid vaginal delivery and tumour dissemination. However, Hacker *et al.*[12] reported that the five-year survivals for stages Ib and II were 30% after abdominal delivery and 56% after vaginal delivery: for all stages the five-year survival after abdominal delivery was 33%, after vaginal delivery 46% and after pretreatment spontaneous or therapeutic abortion 63%. They stated that classical caesarean section remains the recommended method of delivery, but if patients delivered vaginally there was no evidence to suggest the prognosis was jeopardised. The data for Sood *et al.*[29] contradict those of Hacker *et al.*[12] They include 56 women who had cervical cancer diagnosed during pregnancy and 27 whose cancer was diagnosed up to six months after delivery. Of the postpartum group, one of the seven patients who had been delivered by caesarean section developed a recurrence, but ten of the 17 who had been delivered vaginally developed recurrences. The authors concluded that women who had their cancer diagnosed postpartum had worse survival than those diagnosed during pregnancy and were at significant risk of recurrent disease, especially if delivered vaginally.

Comments have been made above about the possibility of delaying management without sacrificing the fetus. An alternative approach is to use chemotherapy. Marana *et al.*[30] describe the management of a patient who was diagnosed with a stage IIb squamous cell carcinoma measuring 5 cm in width, using cisplatin and bleomycin. The cervical tumour 'shrank' to 3 cm in width, until the patient was delivered at 38 weeks. The patient then refused further treatment and returned one year later with recurrence; however, the child, three years of age at time of publication, was growing normally with no evidence of sequelae after exposure to the chemotherapy.

A final thought in this section concerns a small but growing group of women who have undergone radical trachelectomy for fertility-sparing management of their early-stage cervical cancer. The number of subsequent pregnancies is small but will increase.[31] Inevitably there will be some who have residual but occult disease after trachelectomy, which will become apparent in the subsequent pregnancy. The information described above about management of cervical cancer during pregnancy and planned delay while awaiting fetal maturity may not apply to the behaviour of recurrent cancer.

Breast cancer and pregnancy

There is much evidence to link breast cancer with hormonal events, including the use of the combined oral contraceptive pill and hormone replacement therapy. Similarly, pregnancy seems to cause a short-term increase in breast cancer. In a Swedish study, women within three years of their last childbirth had an estimated risk of 1.21 (95% CI 1.02–1.44) compared with women whose last birth was ten or more years earlier, after adjusting for parity and age at first birth.[32] Similarly, a Norwegian study observed a short-term increase in the risk of breast cancer after a full-term pregnancy, with a maximum risk of three to four years after delivery followed by a subsequent decrease in risk.[33] A pregnancy that ends with preterm labour has less transient increased risk, but less long-term protection.[34,35] There is controversy as to whether termination of pregnancy increases the risk of breast cancer, but two case–controlled studies where the study design prevented differential reporting of a history of abortion did not support this link.[36,37] Bartholomew and Grimes[38] reviewed other studies reported via Medline and emphasised the results from large cohort studies that refute the association.

Pregnancy also increases the risk of breast cancer developing in carriers of *BRCA1* and *BRCA2* mutations.[39] Carriers of these mutations who have children are significantly more likely to develop breast cancer by the age of 40 years than carriers who are nulliparous, and each pregnancy is associated with an increased risk of cancer. An early age at first pregnancy does not protect these carriers against breast cancer.[40]

Only about 3% of women diagnosed with breast cancer will be pregnant or lactating[41] and one breast cancer will be found during every 3000–10 000 pregnancies.[42] Unfortunately, when the diagnosis is made during or soon after pregnancy the prognosis is worse, particularly if the woman is aged less than 30 years.[43–45] Stage for stage, it is believed that the prognosis is similar[46–48] and some of the differences are due to more advanced stage at (delayed) diagnosis, or delays with treatment.[49]

A study at Imperial College, London,[50] compared the histopathology and immunohistochemistry of 14 breast cancers found shortly after pregnancy or lactation, with 13 tumours in age-matched but non-pregnant patients. The incidence of axillary lymph node metastases was high in both groups (78% in pregnant and 90% in non-pregnant), but tumours in the pregnancy/lactation group had a significantly higher incidence of cancerisation of lobules (79% versus 15%) and of grade III invasive ductal carcinomas (80% versus 33%). Tumours occurring during pregnancy but not lactation were mostly oestrogen and progesterone receptor negative. All tumours occurring during pregnancy and lactation that were tested for c-erbB2 overexpression were negative, whereas the four tumours that occurred shortly after delivery were positive for c-erbB2 overexpression. The reasons for these more aggressive changes are not clear. A comparison of hormone levels (oestradiol, oestriol, prolactin and progesterone) at 16 and 27 weeks between pregnant women in Shanghai and Boston found higher levels among the Chinese women, who have paradoxically a lower incidence of breast cancer than American women.[51] A high level of α-fetoprotein in maternal serum during any pregnancy is associated with a low overall incidence of breast cancer and a low incidence of advanced cancer at diagnosis, particularly for a pregnancy at a young age.[52,53] On the other hand, women who have elevated levels of human chorionic gonadotrophin due to trophoblast disease have an increased risk (standardised incidence ratio of 1.3; 95% CI 1.0–1.7) of breast cancer.[54] Smoking during a first pregnancy may increase the risk of early-onset breast cancer, while a small placenta or pre-eclampsia reduce the risk of breast cancer.[55,56]

Treatment of breast cancer during pregnancy

Treatment during pregnancy will require discussion between patient, oncologist and obstetrician regarding possible complications, for example with preterm delivery versus the risk of remaining pregnant and starting therapy. Generally, the data for immediate treatment are reassuring, and patient delay or refusal to undergo therapy has serious consequences.[41,49]

Surgery is usually the first-line treatment, with mastectomy and axillary clearance being the preferred option, deferring reconstruction until post delivery. Alternatively, if the cancer is early-stage and detected in the second trimester or later, lumpectomy followed by chemotherapy is possible and radiotherapy is not started until after the birth of the child.[57]

If chemotherapy is used in the first trimester, it is likely to be followed by spontaneous abortion.[58] Subsequently, it appears to be relatively safe to use, without serious fetal or neonatal effects. In a series of 22 women managed at the MD Anderson Cancer Center in Texas, 18 underwent modified radical mastectomy followed by combination chemotherapy with 5-fluorouracil, doxorubicin and cyclophosphamide.[59]

The use of radiotherapy to treat breast cancer in pregnancy is not absolutely contraindicated, but an appropriate thickness of lead shielding should be used to reduce fetal dose.[60,61]

There are cautions about the use of tamoxifen during pregnancy.[62] There have been a small number of reports of spontaneous abortion, birth defects and fetal deaths after the use of tamoxifen. Isaacs *et al.*[63] describe a case report where tamoxifen was used to control widely disseminated metastatic breast cancer.

Pregnancy after treatment of breast cancer

Effects of treatment on fertility

It has been suggested that up to 7% of women who are fertile after treatment for breast cancer will subsequently have children.[64] Most young women will no longer undergo surgical or radiation ovarian ablation,[65] but it is recognised that chemotherapy may cause premature ovarian failure depending on the patient's age and the treatment regimen. Cyclophosphamide, which is an alkylating agent, can damage resting cells, while methotrexate and fluorouracil (as combination cyclophosphamide, methotrexate and fluorouracil [CMF]) are cell cycle-specific; that is, they affect dividing cells. Bonadonna and Valgussam[66] reported that 96% of women over 40 years of age and receiving six or 12 cycles of CMF for breast cancer developed amenorrhoea after treatment, whereas 54% of women under 40 years experienced amenorrhoea that was reversible in 23%. Resumption of menstruation did not confirm restoration of fertility but was more likely in younger than older women.

The information about the effect of doxorubicin on fertility is limited, but 9% of women less than 35 years old and receiving fluorouracil, doxorubicin and cyclophosphamide developed permanent amenorrhoea.[67] The taxanes (paclitaxel and docetaxel) are used in treating breast cancer, but are too new for their impact on fertility to be understood yet.[68]

To date, there is no evidence that any of these cytotoxic drugs used before a pregnancy has adverse effects on fetal development or on the neonate.[69]

Risk of recurrence

Generally the prognosis is good for a subsequent pregnancy after early stage cancer,[70–72] with evidence of a 'healthy-mother effect'.[73] Among 41 patients collected over 30 years at Memorial Sloan-Kettering Cancer Centre, there was a five-year survival rate of 80%.[74] In a nationwide French study,[75] the ten-year survival rate of 68 patients who had subsequent pregnancies was 71%. The survival of the node-negative patients was 90% at ten years, and there was no difference between those who had subsequent pregnancies and those who did not. In another study,[76] the ten-year survival rate was 56% among 16 patients with node-positive disease and 55% for patients who did not become pregnant. It appears that carcinoma antigen 15–3 may be a useful marker for monitoring pregnant breast cancer patients.[77]

Interval before attempting conception

Several authors have recommended that pregnancy should be delayed for at least two years after breast cancer treatment.[78,79] It is likely that this timescale helps to differentiate those with a better prognosis for long-term survival from those with more aggressive disease. A five-year survival rate of 54% has been reported with an interval of less than six months, compared with 78% from six months to two years and 100% for those patients who waited for more than five years.[80] As younger patients have significantly lower survival rates and higher local and distant relapse rates than older patients, those under 33 years of age might be better advised to delay pregnancy for at least three years, to reduce the risk of relapse.[81]

Averette *et al.*[82] have recommended that decisions about future conception should be based on the prognosis for the individual patient. They advise that patients with stage IV disease (with a five-year survival rate of less than 15%) should not consider a pregnancy, and that patients with stage III disease should consider deferring pregnancy for at least five years after treatment. Patients with recurrent stage I or II tumours should not contemplate conception because of the intensity of the required treatment, and the poor prognosis.

Finally, it seems that in pregnancy after treatment of breast cancer there is an increased chance of spontaneous pregnancy loss.[71]

Leukaemia and lymphoma

There are probably good reasons for not grouping these malignancies, but the latest Confidential Enquiry has done this; collectively, they are the greatest contributor to maternal deaths. It might be presumed that they are coincidental because they occur in women of reproductive age but many have been classified as 'indirect' or 'late indirect'. Some deaths have occurred in women who had previously undergone treatment and were thought to be in remission while they planned their pregnancy.

Acute leukaemias may be diagnosed on the results from full blood counts performed during pregnancy. Treatment cannot be delayed and requires effective cytotoxic drugs. It is not always possible to avoid fetal exposure in the first trimester: Brell and Kalaycio[83] quote a 17% risk of congenital malformations in such circumstances.

Hodgkin's lymphoma has a peak age of incidence around 20 years and occurs once every 1–6000 pregnancies.[84] There is no convincing evidence that pregnancy alters the lymphoma or that the lymphoma affects pregnancy outcome.[6] Non-Hodgkin's lymphomas are more aggressive and are often at an advanced stage, or with extra-nodal disease (cervical, uterine, ovarian or breast) at presentation.[84,85] Pregnancy may complicate staging (X-ray) assessment and again combination chemotherapy is necessary, whatever the gestation.

Cerebral and nervous system tumours

Some of these tumours are of low-grade behaviour but are influenced by pregnancy and alterations in blood volume, fluid retention and altered vascularity, such as meningiomas, acoustic neuromas and pituitary adenomas. Other tumours, such as astrocytoma and glioblastoma multiforme, are highly malignant and aggressive in behaviour. The distribution of histological types shows no difference between pregnancy and non-pregnancy women.[6] However, the growth of some cerebral tumours including meningiomas may be influenced because they contain progesterone or other hormone or growth receptors.[86]

Sometimes these patients will have had symptoms of headaches or back pain plus ataxia, motor dysfunction or sensory changes. Others present with dramatic onset of drowsiness, confusion and disorientation and deteriorate rapidly.

Colorectal tumours

Fox[86] has summarised the role of reproductive factors in colonic carcinoma, in that although these tumours are more frequently seen in men, carcinomas of the descending and sigmoid colon are more common in women under the age of 55 years. Although they contain oestrogen and progesterone receptors, there is no evidence that these hormones influence the risk or behaviour of colon cancer.

During pregnancy the cancers are more likely to be rectal. The prognosis is worse than for non-pregnant women, probably because of delays in diagnosis.[6] Although haemorrhoids and rectal bleeding are common in pregnancy, persistent or continual symptoms must be investigated. The flexible sigmoidoscope has obvious advantages over a rigid instrument, but bowel preparation should be less vigorous than in the non-pregnant patient.

Ovarian tumours

The frequency with which ovarian or adnexal cysts or tumours are identified during pregnancy is quoted as between one in 81 and one in 2489.[87] The majority of these will be functional cysts, or benign cystadenomas or dermoids. Only 3–6% of these tumours that require surgery are malignant.

The majority of ovarian cysts are asymptomatic and discovered during scanning: 25% will be more than 10 cm. Some will be present with pain from torsion or leakage. Rarely, tumours will be identified because of elevated α-fetoprotein levels.

If a cyst is identified in the first trimester, the scan should be repeated at 14 weeks: corpus luteal cysts involute by 12 weeks and, if the cyst persists and is more than 10 cm in size, surgery should be planned. If the cyst is less than 5 cm, intervention is usually unnecessary. If it is between 5 cm and 10 cm, the patient should be kept under observation, and surgery should be planned if there is an increase in size or symptoms to suggest torsion.[88]

If the ovarian tumour is neoplastic, more than one-third will be of germ cell origin, that is, dysgerminoma, teratoma or endodermal sinus tumour. Surgery can be limited to unilateral oophorectomy but staging must be thorough. Only one-third will be epithelial in type, and these will often be of borderline histology and low malignant potential. The remainder will be stromal cell or miscellaneous. Again, surgery during pregnancy can be limited usually to removal of the tumour but, as before, thorough assessment for evidence of spread beyond the ovary must be sought. The findings at laparotomy and adverse histological features may determine the need for chemotherapy. There is limited evidence, for example the administration of bleomycin, etoposide and cisplatin for germ cell tumours, that these agents can be given after surgery and before delivery. Once again, delays in investigation to make a diagnosis or give appropriate treatment have proved fatal.

Melanoma

Obstetricians know that pregnancy is associated with changes in skin pigmentation such as chloasma, and have suspected that pregnancy and melanoma do not go well together. Although melanoma is a significant contributor to cancer deaths in pregnancy, the information on melanoma is not as sinister as might be supposed. The report from the World Health Organization Melanoma Programme[89] referred to 388 women with primary stage I melanoma, 92 who were pregnant at the time of diagnosis, 85 who had never been pregnant, 68 who were between pregnancies and 143 who had completed their families. Those who were pregnant had a thicker tumour (2.38 mm) than the other groups (1.49 mm, 1.48 mm and 1.96 mm respectively; $P = 0.002$) and had a worse prognosis, but not when adjusted for thickness.

It is not known why the melanoma is thicker in pregnancy, but there has often been clinical delay before the diagnosis is made. Johnston[90] and Fox[86] have reviewed evidence linking oestrogens and oestrogen receptors with melanoma behaviour. Earlier studies that suggested the presence of oestrogen receptors may have been misleading because of non-specific binding to tyrosine: more recent studies using immunohistocytochemical techniques have failed to demonstrate their presence.[90] The reasons for the increased melanoma thickness remain unexplained.

The management of melanoma in pregnancy is by surgical excision; more advanced or recurrent disease is more difficult. The use of the cytotoxic dacabazine has an uncertain effect in the fetus,[6] but its use in the second and third trimesters has been described.[90] If the tumour metastasises, there is a 25% chance of placental and fetal involvement.[91]

Mackie *et al.*[89] describe the prognosis after melanoma treatment as 90% disease-free five-year survival if the tumour thickness is less than 1.5 mm, less than 50% survival if thickness is more than 3.5 mm and 70% if 1.5–3.5 mm. Therefore, women who have had a melanoma can be advised about the safety of pregnancy on the basis of tumour thickness, site, evidence of spread and not on the basis of hormonal status. As the majority of stage II patients who return with recurrence do so within two years of treating the primary, they recommend a delay of two years between surgery and starting a family: Borden[91] advises waiting three years.

Other tumours and general considerations

The information about the other tumours listed in Table 23.2 is sparse. Some of the tumours, such as sarcomas, are more likely to be seen in younger women and some, such as lung tumours, are going to be seen for the same reasons that they are increasing among all women.

The one tumour that is unique to pregnancy is choriocarcinoma. Its contribution to maternal mortality in this country is minimal. Newlands[92] has reported the results of treatment from the Charing Cross Hospital, London, where patients with choriocarcinoma in the low-risk group have a disease-specific survival of 100% and those in the high-risk group, treated with etoposide, methotrexate and actinomycin D, alternating weekly with vincristine and cyclophosphamide (EMA/CO), have an overall survival of 86%. Berkowitz *et al.*[93] remind us that 1% of pregnancies that follow gestational trophoblastic disease will be another pregnancy with gestational trophoblastic disease, but the outcome for pregnancies after chemotherapy for persistent gestational trophoblastic disease is good, although it is associated with a 2.5% major and minor congenital abnormality rate.

Woolas *et al.*[94] reported a 1.7% abnormality rate among the Charing Cross Hospital patients, but also noted a higher than expected stillbirth rate.

Generally, the information about the outcome of pregnancy when chemotherapy is given before or during pregnancy is reassuring. Certain regimens, as discussed for breast cancer but also relevant to lymphoma, are associated with ovarian failure. Partridge and Garber[95] balance this optimism by stating that patients or parents must be advised that long-term outcome is restricted by small numbers, different tumours and the variety of drugs used, the absence of comprehensive assessments during follow-up examinations and the fact that methotrexate at least is known to be toxic in early pregnancy.

The use of radiotherapy is not an absolute contraindication in pregnancy and Fenig *et al.*[60] describe its use for breast carcinoma and supradiaphragmatic lymphoma, provided that special attention is paid to the treatment technique and appropriate shielding of the fetus.

A further fetal consideration is the risk of metastatic tumour. This has been described for melanoma but is not thought to occur for other tumours. However, placental metastases have been recorded, for example for breast cancer.[96]

Just as radiotherapy can be used judiciously during pregnancy, X-ray imaging may be appropriate and necessary in certain or suspected tumours. Nicklas and Baker[97] give some reassurance that a standard chest X-ray does not expose the fetus to significant radiation. MRI does not appear to cause fetal effects and is probably the imaging procedure of choice.

Finally, the diagnosis and treatment of cancer during pregnancy raise important psychosocial issues. Schover[98] describes the continuing anxieties, which include the child's health, future fertility and possible pregnancies in the future – some of these issues have been mentioned above. However, although there are increasing numbers of counselling services provided through oncology or cancer centres, they may be less aware of the factors involving the pregnancy. This emphasises the desirability of communications between those caring for the patient, as well as with the patient herself.

References

1. Department of Health, Welsh Office, Scottish Home and Health Department, Department of Health and Social Services, Northern Ireland. *Report on Confidential Enquiries into Maternal Death in the United Kingdom, 1991–93*. London: HMSO; 1996.
2. Department of Health, Welsh Office, Scottish Home and Health Department, Department of Health and Social Services, Northern Ireland. *Why Mothers Die. Report on Confidential Enquiries into Maternal Death in the United Kingdom, 1994–96*. London: The Stationery Office; 1998.
3. Lewis G, Drife J, editors. *Why Mothers Die 1997–1999. The Confidential Enquiries into Maternal Deaths in the United Kingdom*. London: RCOG Press; 2001.
4. Drife J. The contribution of cancer to maternal mortality. In: O'Brien PMS, MacLean AB, editors. *Hormones and Cancer*. London: RCOG Press; 1999. p. 299–310.
5. Cancer Research UK. CRC cancer stats. CRUK; 2000 [http:www.cancerresearch.uk.org].
6. Antonelli NM, Dotters DJ, Katz VL, Kuller JA. Cancer in pregnancy: a review of the literature. Part I & II. *Obstet Gynecol Surv* 1996;51:125–42.
7. Kaiser HE, Nawab E, Nasir A, Chmielarczyk W, Krenn M. Neoplasms during the progression of pregnancy. *In Vivo* 2000;14:277–85.
8. Lambe M, Ekbom A. Cancers coinciding with childbearing: delayed diagnosis during pregnancy? *BMJ* 1995;311;1607–8.
9. Johnstone RW. *A Textbook of Midwifery*. 8th ed. London: A & C Black; 1936.
10. Munro Kerr, cited by Donald I. *Practical Obstetric Problems*. 4th ed. London: Lloyd-Luke; 1972. p 224.
11. Williams JW. *Obstetrics*. 6th ed. New York: Appleton; 1930.
12. Hacker NF, Berek JS, Lagasse LD, Charles EH, Savage EW, Moore J. Carcinoma of the cervix associated with pregnancy. *Obstet Gynecol* 1982;59:735–46.

13. Duggan B, Muderspach LI, Rowan LD, Curtin JP, d'Ablaing G III, Morrow CP. Cervical cancer in pregnancy: reporting on planned delay in therapy. *Obstet Gynecol* 1993;82:598–602.
14. Donald I. *Practical Obstetric Problems*. 4th ed. London: Lloyd-Luke; 1972.
15. MacLean AB. Hormones and cancer of the cervix, vulva, vagina and ovary. In: Sturdee D, Oláh K, Keane D, editors. *The Yearbook of Obstetrics and Gynaecology*. Vol. 9. London: RCOG Press; 2001. p.137–43.
16. Menczer J. Diagnosis and treatment delay in gynaecological malignancies. Does it affect outcome? *Int J Gynecol Cancer* 2000;10:89–94.
17. Bolger BS, Cooke TG, Symonds RP, MacLean AB, Stanton PD. Measurement of cell kinetics in cervical tumours using bromodeoxyuridine. *Br J Cancer* 1993;68:166–71.
18. Prem KA, Makowski EL, McKelvey JL. Carcinoma of the cervix associated with pregnancy. *Am J Obstet Gynecol* 1966;95:99–108.
19. Sorosky JI, Squatrito R, Ndubisi BU, Anderson B, Podczaski ES, Mayr N, *et al.* Stage I squamous cell cervical carcinoma in pregnancy: planned delay in therapy awaiting fetal maturity. *Gynecol Oncol* 1995;59:207–10.
20. van Vliet W, van Loon AJ, ten Hoor KA, Boonstra H. Cervical carcinoma during pregnancy: outcome of planned delay in treatment. *Eur J Obstet Gynecol Reprod Biol* 1998;79:153–7.
21. Dudan RC, Yon JL, Ford JH, Averette HE. Carcinoma of the cervix and pregnancy. *Gynecol Oncol* 1973;1:283–9.
22. Kottmeier HL, editor. *FIGO Annual Report on the Results of Treatment in Carcinomas of the Uterus, Vagina and Ovary*. No. 15. Stockholm: Pogo Prints; 1973. p. 370.
23. Hoffman JS, Bazzurini L, Laird L, Murphy JC, Magriples U, Lewis J. Term delivery following conservative treatment for villoglandular papillary adenocarcinoma of the uterine cervix: report of a case and analysis of the literature. *Gynecol Oncol* 2001;81:310–3.
24. Balderston KD, Tewari K, Gregory WT, Berman ML, Kucera PR. Neuroendocrine small cell uterine cervix cancer in pregnancy: long-term survival following combined therapy. *Gynecol Oncol* 1998;71:128–32.
25. Ohwada M, Suzuki M, Hironaka M, Irie T, Sato I. Neuroendocrine small cell carcinoma of the uterine cervix showing polypoid growth and complicated by pregnancy. *Gynecol Oncol* 2001;81:117–19.
26. Sarwey 1899. Carcinom u. Schwangerschaft. *Veit's Handbuch Gyn* 1899. Bd. 1: iii, 2te Hälfte, 1ste Abth. ff.489–532. Cited by Williams JW. *Obstetrics*. 6th ed. New York: Appleton; 1930. p. 688.
27. Crawford R, Shepherd JH. Radical hysterectomy. In: Luesley DM, Barrasso R, editors. *Cancer and Pre-cancer of the Cervix*. London: Chapman and Hall; 1998. p. 319–33.
28. Monk BJ, Montz FJ. Invasive cervical cancer complicating intrauterine pregnancy: treatment with radical hysterectomy. *Obstet Gynecol* 1992;80:199–203.
29. Sood AK, Sorosky JI, Mayr N, Anderson B, Buller RE, Niebyl J. Cervical cancer diagnosed shortly after pregnancy: prognostic variables and delivery routes. *Obstet Gynecol* 2000;95:832–8.
30. Marana HR, de Andrade JM, da Silva Mathes AC, Duarte G, da Cunha SP, Bighetti S. Chemotherapy in the treatment of locally advanced cervical cancer and pregnancy. *Gynecol Oncol* 2001;80:272–4.
31. Shepherd JH, Crawford RA, Oram DH. Radical trachelectomy: a way to preserve fertility in the treatment of early cervical cancer. *Br J Obstet Gynaecol* 1998;105:912–6.
32. Leon DA, Carpenter LM, Broeders MJ, Gunnarskog J, Murphy MF. Breast cancer in Swedish woman before age 50: evidence of a dual effect of completed pregnancy. *Cancer Causes Control* 1995;6:283–91.
33. Albrektsen G, Heuch I, Kvale G. The short term and long term effect of a pregnancy on breast cancer risk: A prospective study of 802,457 parous Norwegian women. *Br J Cancer* 1995;72:480–4.
34. Hsieh CC, Wuu J, Lambe M, Trichopoulos D, Adami HO, Ekbom A. Delivery of premature newborns and maternal breast-cancer risk. *Lancet* 1999;353:1239.
35. Melbye M, Wohlfahrt J, Andersen AM, Westergaard T, Andersen PK. Preterm delivery and risk of breast cancer. *Br J Cancer* 1999;80:609–13.
36. Tang MT, Weiss NS, Malone KE. Induced abortion in relation to breast cancer among parous women: a birth certificate registry study. *Epidemiology* 2000;11:177–80.
37. Newcomb PA, Mandelson MT. A record-based evaluation of induced abortion and breast cancer risk (United States). *Cancer Causes Control* 2000;11:777–81.
38. Bartholomew LL, Grimes DA. The alleged association between induced abortion and risk of breast cancer: biology or bias? *Obstet Gynecol Surv* 1998;53:708–14.
39. Johannsson O, Loman N, Borg A, Olsson H. Pregnancy-associated breast cancer in BRCA1 and BRCA2 germline mutation carriers. *Lancet* 1998;352:1359–60.
40. Jernstrom H, Lerman C, Ghadirian P, Lynch HT, Weber B, Garber J, *et al.* Pregnancy and risk of early breast cancer in carriers of BRCA1 and BRCA2. *Lancet* 1999;354:1846–50.

41. Saunders CM. Breast cancer in and after pregnancy. In: O'Brien PMS, MacLean AB, editors. *Hormones and Cancer*. London: RCOG Press; 1999. p. 311–21.
42. Sivanesaratnam V. Management of the pregnant mother with malignant conditions. *Curr Opin Obstet Gynecol* 2001;13:121–15.
43. Guinee VF, Olsson H, Moller T, Hess KR, Taylor SH, Fahey T, *et al*. Effect of pregnancy on prognosis for young women with breast cancer. *Lancet* 1994;343:1587–9.
44. Kroman N, Wohlfahrt J, Andersen KW, Mouridsen HT, Westergaard T, Melbye M. Parity, age at first childbirth and the prognosis of primary breast cancer. *Br J Cancer* 1998;78:1529–33.
45. Olson SH, Zauber AG, Tang J, Harlap S. Relation of time since last birth and parity to survival of young women with breast cancer. *Epidemiology* 1998;9:669–71.
46. Petrek JA. Pregnancy safety after breast cancer. *Cancer* 1994, 74: 528–31.
47. Gemignani ML, Petrek JA, Borgen PI. Breast cancer and pregnancy. *Surg Clin North Am* 1999;79:1157-69.
48. Ibrahim EM, Ezzat AA, Baloush A, Hussain ZH, Mohammed GH. Pregnancy-associated breast cancer: a case–control study in a young population with a high-fertility rate. *Med Oncol* 2000;17:293–300.
49. Yip CH, Taib NA, Abdullah MM, Wahid I. Breast cancer in pregnancy – our experience with six patients in the University Hospital, Kuala Lumpur. *Med J Malaysia* 2000;55:308–10.
50. Shousha S. Breast carcinoma presenting during or shortly after pregnancy and lactation. *Arch Pathol Lab Med* 2000;124:1053–60.
51. Lipworth L, Hsieh CC, Wide L, Ekbom A, Yu SZ, Yu GP, *et al*. Maternal pregnancy hormone levels in an area with a high incidence (Boston, USA) and in an area with a low incidence (Shanghai, China) of breast cancer. *Br J Cancer* 1999;79:7–12.
52. Richardson BE, Hulka BS, Peck JL, Hughes CL, van den Berg BJ, Christianson RE, *et al*. Levels of maternal serum alpha-fetoprotein (AFP) in pregnant women and subsequent breast cancer risk. *Am J Epidemiol* 1998;148:719–27.
53. Melbye M, Wohlfahrt J, Lei U, Norgaard-Pedersen B, Mouridsen HT, Lambe M, *et al*. Alpha-fetoprotein levels in maternal serum during pregnancy and maternal breast cancer incidence. *J Natl Cancer Inst* 2000;92:1001–5.
54. Erlandsson G, Weiderpass E, Lambe M, Ekbom A. Hydatidiform moles and the long-term risk of breast cancer (Sweden). *Cancer Causes Control* 2000;11:117–20.
55. Innes KE, Byers TE. Preeclampsia and breast cancer risk. *Epidemiology* 1999;10:722–32.
56. Troisi R, Weiss HA, Hoover RN, Potischman N, Swanson CA, Brogan DR, *et al*. Pregnancy characteristics and maternal risk of breast cancer. *Epidemiology* 1998;9:641–7.
57. Bernik SF, Bernik TR, Whooley BP, Wallack MK. Carcinoma of the breast during pregnancy: a review and update on treatment options. *Surg Oncol* 1998;7:45–9.
58. Giacalone PL, Laffargue F, Benos P. Chemotherapy for breast carcinoma during pregnancy: a French national survey. *Cancer* 1999;86:2266–72.
59. Berry DL, Theriault RL, Holmes FA, Parisi VM, Booser DJ, Singletary SE, *et al*. Management of breast cancer during pregnancy using a standardized protocol. *J Clin Oncol* 1999;17:855–61.
60. Fenig E, Mishaeli M, Kalish Y, Lishner M. Pregnancy and radiation. *Cancer Treat Rev* 2001;27:1–7.
61. Antolak JA, Strom EA. Fetal dose estimates for electron-beam treatment to the chest wall of a pregnant patient. *Med Phys* 1998;25:2388–91.
62. *Association of the British Pharmaceutical Industry Compendium of Data Sheets*. London: Datapharm Ltd; 1999. p. 1799.
63. Isaacs RJ, Hunter W, Clark K. Tamoxifen as systemic treatment of advanced breast cancer during pregnancy – case report and literature review. *Gynecol Oncol* 2001;80:405–8.
64. Saunders CM, Baum M. Breast cancer and pregnancy: A review. *J R Soc Med* 1993;86:162–5.
65. Scottish Cancer Trials Breast Group ICRF Breast Unit. Adjuvant ovarian ablation versus CMF chemotherapy in premenopausal women with pathological stage II breast carcinoma: the Scottish trial. *Lancet* 1993;341:1293–8.
66. Bonadonna G, Valgussa P. Adjuvant systemic therapy for resectable breast cancer. *J Clin Oncol* 1985;3:259–75.
67. Sutton R, Buzdar A, Hortobagyi GN. Pregnancy and offspring after adjuvant chemotherapy in breast cancer patients. *Cancer* 1990;65:847–850.
68. Hensley ML, Reichman BS. Fertility and pregnancy after adjuvant chemotherapy for breast cancer. *Crit Rev Oncol Hematol* 1998;28:121–8.
69. Falconer AD, Ferns P. Pregnancy outcomes following treatment of cancer. *J Obstet Gynecol* 2002;22:43–4.
70. von Schoultz E, Johansson H, Wilking N, Rutqvist LE. Influence of prior and subsequent pregnancy on breast cancer prognosis. *J Clin Oncol* 1995;13:430–34.

71. Velentgas P, Daling JR, Malone KE, Weiss NS, Williams MA, Self SG, *et al.* Pregnancy after breast carcinoma: outcomes and influence on mortality. *Cancer* 1999;85:2424–32.
72. Gelber S, Coates AS, Goldhirsch A, Castiglione-Gertsch M, Marini G, Lindtner J, *et al.* Effect of pregnancy on overall survival after the diagnosis of early-stage breast cancer. *J Clin Oncol* 2001;19:1671–5.
73. Sankila R, Heinavaara S, Hakulinen T. Survival of breast cancer patients after subsequent term pregnancy: 'healthy-mother effect'. *Am J Obstet Gynecol* 1994;170:818–23.
74. Harvey JC, Rosen PP, Ashikara R, Robbins GF, Kinne DW. The effect of pregnancy on the prognosis of carcinoma of the breast following radical mastectomy. *Surg Gynecol Obstet* 1981;153:723–5.
75. Mignot L, Morvon F, Berdah J, Querleu D, Laurent JC, Verhaeghe M, *et al.* Pregnancy after breast cancer. Results of a case-control study. *Presse Med* 1986;15:1961–4.
76. Ariel I, Kempner R. The prognosis of patients who become pregnant after mastectomy for breast cancer. *Int Surg* 1989;74:185–7.
77. Botsis D, Sarandakou A, Kassanos D, Kontoravdis A, Rizos D, Protonotariou E, *et al.* Breast cancer markers during normal pregnancy. *Anticancer Res* 1999;19:3539–41.
78. Isaacs JH. Cancer of the breast in pregnancy. *Surg Clin North Am* 1995;75:47–51.
79. Di Fronzo LA, O'Connell TX. Breast cancer in pregnancy and lactation. *Surg Clin North Am* 1996;76:267–78.
80. Clark RM, Chua T. Breast cancer and pregnancy: the ultimate challenge. *Clin Oncol* 1989;1:11–18.
81. de la Rochefordiere A, Asselain B, Campana F, Scholl SM, Fenton J, Vilcoq JR, *et al.* Age as prognostic factor in premenopausal breast carcinoma. *Lancet* 1993;341:1039–43.
82. Averette HE, Mirhashemi R, Moffat FL. Pregnancy after breast carcinoma: the ultimate medical challenge. *Cancer* 1999;85:2301–4.
83. Brell J, Kalayeio M. Leukaemia in pregnancy. *Semin Oncol* 2000;27:667–77.
84. Pohlman B, Macklis RM. Lymphoma and pregnancy. *Semin Oncol* 2000;27:657–6.
85. Wang PH, Chao KC, Lin G, Chao HT, Yuan CC, Ng HT. Primary malignant lymphoma of the cervix in pregnancy. A case report. *J Reprod Med* 1999;44:630–2.
86. Fox H. Pathology of hormone-dependent cancers. In: O'Brien PMS, MacLean AB, editors. *Hormones and Cancer*. London: RCOG Press; 1999. p. 3–19.
87. Zanotti KM, Belinson JL, Kennedy AW. Treatment of gynecologic cancers in pregnancy. *Semin Oncol* 2000;27:686–98.
88. Overton TG, Vatish M, Thornton S. Abdominal pain in pregnancy. In: MacLean AB, Stones RW, Thornton S, editors. *Pain in Obstetrics and Gynaecology*. London: RCOG Press. p. 308–24.
89. MacKie RM, Bufalino R, Morabito A, Sutherland C, Cascinelli N. For the World Health Organization Melanoma Programme. Lack of effect of pregnancy on outcome of melanoma. *Lancet* 1991;337:653–5.
90. Johnston SRD. Effects on melanoma of hormone replacement therapy, hormonal contraception and pregnancy. In: O'Brien PMS, MacLean AB, editors. *Hormones and Cancer*. London: RCOG Press, 1999. p. 328–39.
91. Borden EC. Melanoma and pregnancy. *Semin Oncol* 2000;27:654–6.
92. Newlands ES. Human chorionic gonadotrophins monitoring, hormonal contraception and pregnancy in patients with trophoblastic disease. In: O'Brien PMS, MacLean AB, editors. *Hormones and Cancer*. London: RCOG Press; 1999. p. 136–44.
93. Berkowitz RS, Tuncer ZS, Bernstein MR, Goldstein DP. Management of gestational trophoblastic diseases: subsequent pregnancy experience. *Semin Oncol* 2000;27:678–85.
94. Woolas RP, Bower M, Newlands ES, Seckl M, Short D, Holden L. Influence of chemotherapy for gestational trophoblastic disease on subsequent pregnancy outcome. *Br J Obstet Gynaecol* 1998;105:1032–5.
95. Partridge AH, Garber JE. Long-term outcomes of children exposed to antineoplastic agents *in utero*. *Semin Oncol* 2000;27:712–26.
96. Dunn JS Jr, Anderson CD, Brost BC. Breast carcinoma metastatic to the placenta. *Obstet Gynecol* 1999;94:846.
97. Nicklas AH, Baker ME. Imaging strategies in the pregnant cancer patient. *Semin Oncol* 2000;27:623–32.
98. Schover LR. Psychosocial issues associated with cancer in pregnancy. *Semin Oncol* 2000;27:699–703.

Chapter 24

Epilepsy in pregnancy

Catherine Nelson-Piercy

Introduction

Epilepsy is the most common chronic neurological disorder to complicate pregnancy, affecting approximately 0.5–0.6% of pregnancies in the UK.[1,2] Epilepsy is classified according to clinical type of seizure. These may be broadly divided into primary generalised epilepsy (including tonic–clonic seizures, absences and myoclonic jerks) and partial (focal) seizures, with or without secondary generalisation.[3] Temporal lobe seizures (complex [meaning loss of consciousness] partial seizure) are a form of partial seizure. They are often associated with an aura, a duration of one minute or more and confusion after the event.[3] Absences (*petit mal*), in contrast, are normally of a few seconds' duration, have a rapid onset, rapid recovery and are precipitated by hyperventilation. Absences are associated with 3 Hz spike-and-wave discharge on the electroencephalogram (EEG).[3] The clinical features of tonic–clonic seizures resulting from primary generalised epilepsy and secondarily generalised partial seizures are similar. There may be no aura associated with the latter. Pointers to a diagnosis of primary generalised epilepsy are myoclonic jerks and photosensitivity.[3]

Most cases of epilepsy are idiopathic and no underlying cause is found. Secondary epilepsy may be encountered in pregnancy with patients who have previously undergone surgery to the cerebral hemispheres or who have intracranial mass lesions. This should always be considered if the first seizure occurs in pregnancy. Epilepsy may be a feature of the antiphospholipid syndrome. Most women with epilepsy enter pregnancy with the diagnosis already established. Other causes of seizures in pregnancy include eclampsia, cerebral vein thrombosis, thrombotic thrombocytopenic purpura, cerebral infarction, drug and alcohol withdrawal, hypoglycaemia (complicating insulin therapy) and, rarely, seizures related to post-dural puncture headaches.[4] If a first fit occurs in pregnancy and eclampsia is excluded, imaging with computed tomography or magnetic resonance imaging of the brain is appropriate.[5]

Table 24.1. Maternal deaths due to epilepsy from the Confidential Enquiries into Maternal Deaths; Crown copyright material reproduced with permission of the Controller of HMSO and the Queen's Printer for Scotland[6–9] (full data not available for all deaths)

	Total	Trimester 1	Trimester 2	Trimester 3 antepartum	Total	Postpartum
1988–90	9	2		4	8	1
1991–93	6			3	4	2
1994–96	19			10	14	5
1997–99	9	2	1	1	4	2

Epilepsy as a cause of maternal death

Maternal deaths due to epilepsy as ascertained by the Confidential Enquiries into Maternal Deaths in the UK (CEMD) 1988–99 are summarised in Table 24.1.[6–9] There have been 43 deaths in a total of 11 years; approximately four per year. In the 1994–96 CEMD report,[6] there were 19 deaths due to epilepsy. Most deaths were antenatal; ten were in the third trimester. In ten women, the cause of death was aspiration, but epileptic seizures may be fatal in themselves. Only five women had poorly controlled epilepsy, but two women died despite not having had a seizure for the previous two years. Associated risk factors for death in mothers with epilepsy as identified from the CEMD report[6–9] include obesity (eight of 19 deaths, 1994–6), comorbidity (asthma, diabetes, alcoholism), coexistent pseudo-seizures, non-adherence to prescribed medications, socially disadvantage and bathing (three of nine deaths, 1997–99).

In a prospective study of 400 pregnancies in women with epilepsy from the Northern region, there were two maternal deaths (0.5%) related to seizures.[2] The problem with data of maternal deaths in epilepsy is that even outside pregnancy there is a risk of sudden unexpected death in epilepsy (SUDEP).[10] This risk has been estimated at one in 1000 per year in the epileptic population but reaches one in 200–300 in high-risk populations such as those with severe epilepsy and learning difficulties.[11] An American prospective cohort study[12] found an incidence of SUDEP of 1.21/1000 patient-years, although the incidence was higher in women (1.45/1000). SUDEP accounted for 18% of all deaths. One and possibly two of the nine cases of maternal death in the 1997–1999 CEMD report[9] fulfilled the criteria for SUDEP, where a person with epilepsy dies suddenly and no other cause of death is found. Few deaths are witnessed but evidence suggests that cases of SUDEP represent ictal or immediate post-ictal deaths in people with a history of generalised tonic–clonic seizures in both primary generalised and localisation-related epilepsy.[13] Death may be related to cardiac arrhythmia. Risk factors for SUDEP include high seizure frequency, increasing numbers of antiepileptic drugs (AEDs), low IQ and early-onset epilepsy.[10,12] SUDEP is uncommon in those with good seizure control.

Fertility in epilepsy

A large study[14] has demonstrated decreased fertility rates in women with epilepsy. The proportion of anovulatory cycles is increased in women with temporal lobe epilepsy.[15]

Controversy exists regarding a possible association between sodium valproate and polycystic ovary syndrome (PCOS).[16] In one study, PCOS was more common in women beginning valproate therapy before the age of 20 years. Valproate may cause weight gain, leading to insulin resistance, polycystic ovaries and menstrual irregularities. Obesity rather than valproate therapy may therefore be the link. Certainly, valproate therapy should be avoided in adolescents, in those with obesity or menstrual irregularities, and should be discontinued if these develop during therapy. Recently, the association between sodium valproate therapy and PCOS has been challenged.[17]

The failure rate of the combined oral contraceptive pill is increased in women with epilepsy. In one study, 24% of unplanned pregnancies in women with epilepsy were due to failure of the oral contraceptive pill[2] (see below under 'Contraception').

Effect of pregnancy on epilepsy

In general, pregnancy does not affect the frequency of seizures. About 25% of women report improvement and 10–30% of women experience an increased seizure frequency in pregnancy. In one study,[18] seizure frequency remained unchanged in 54%, increased in 22% and decreased in 24%. Women with poorly controlled epilepsy, especially those who fit more than once a month, are more likely to deteriorate in pregnancy.[15] There is no relation to the seizure type or the course of epilepsy during previous pregnancies. Reasons for deterioration in seizure control during pregnancy include: pregnancy itself; stress; poor compliance with anticonvulsant medication (due to fears regarding teratogenicity); decreased drug levels related to nausea and vomiting in early pregnancy or to increased volume of distribution and increased drug clearance; lack of sleep towards term and during labour; lack of absorption of anticonvulsant drugs from the gastrointestinal tract during labour and hyperventilation during labour.

By far the most common cause of an increase in seizure frequency in pregnancy is decreased compliance. Many women intentionally decrease or discontinue their AEDs before conception or once pregnancy is confirmed. In one prospective study, nearly two-thirds of women were incompletely compliant with their AED regimens in pregnancy.[2] There is no difference in the change of seizure frequency between trimesters,[17] although the risk of seizures is greatest peripartum (see below).

Effect of epilepsy on pregnancy

The majority of women with epilepsy have uncomplicated pregnancies with normal deliveries and healthy children. The fetus is relatively resistant to short episodes of hypoxia and there is no evidence of adverse effects of single seizures on the fetus. Some workers have documented fetal bradycardia during and after maternal convulsions but there are no data relating to any long-term effects on the offspring. Status epilepticus is dangerous for both mother and fetus and should be vigorously treated. Fortunately, it has been estimated to affect from less than 1.0%[15] to 2.5%[19] of pregnancies in women with epilepsy.

Although some workers have suggested an increased risk of obstetric complications such as miscarriage, pre-eclampsia, premature labour, antepartum haemorrhage and caesarean section,[20] most recent prospective studies have not indicated any increase in adverse pregnancy outcome[15] and a large population-based study from Iceland found no increase in adverse events during pregnancy, although the caesarean rate was doubled.[21]

The risk of a child itself developing epilepsy is also increased (4–5%) if either parent has epilepsy. Maternal epilepsy carries a higher risk than paternal epilepsy. If there is a previously affected sibling, the risk is 10%. If both parents have epilepsy, the risk is 15–20%.[22] Genetic factors are important in the generalised epilepsies but also play a role in partial epilepsies.[23] The high frequency of concordant monozygotic pairs with the same major epilepsy syndrome in twin studies suggests that there are syndrome-specific genetic determinants rather than a broad genetic predisposition to seizures.[23] The risk of a woman with idiopathic epilepsy having a child who develops epilepsy is increased if she herself had onset of epilepsy before the age of ten years.[22] A recent study suggests that a history of miscarriage in women with epilepsy is associated with an increased risk of epilepsy in liveborn children (12.8%) compared with children of women with epilepsy without a history of miscarriage (4.7%).[24]

Adverse effects of antiepileptic drugs

The main concern of epilepsy in pregnancy stems from the two- to three-fold increased risk of congenital abnormalities in the fetus due to AEDs taken by the mother (Table 24.2).[25–28] Until recently, it was thought that even women with epilepsy not receiving AEDs had a slightly increased risk (4%) compared with the general population (3%).[29] This has been challenged in a large study from Boston,[28] in which 98 infants of mothers with a history of epilepsy but not taking AEDs in pregnancy did not have a higher frequency of malformations than 508 control infants.

Phenytoin, primidone, phenobarbitone, carbamazepine and sodium valproate all cross the placenta and are teratogenic. The major malformations caused by anticonvulsants are neural tube defects (ten times background incidence; particularly valproate [1.0–3.8%][25] and carbamazepine [0.5–1.0%][25,30,31] but also phenytoin and phenobarbitone [0.3–0.4%]), orofacial clefts (particularly carbamazepine, phenytoin and phenobarbitone),[25] congenital heart defects (particularly phenytoin, phenobarbitone and valproate)[25] and hypospadias (carbamazepine).[25] There is little difference in the overall level of risk for major malformations between individual drugs,[13,25] although the risk of neural tube defects is much higher with valproate. The risk of major malformations for any one drug is about 6–7%[13,21,25–28] (i.e. twice to three times the background level) (Table 24.2). The risk increases with the number of drugs, so for those taking two or more anticonvulsants the risk is 10–15%[32] and, for those taking the combination of valproate, carbamazepine and phenytoin or phenobarbitone, the risk is extremely high. A study in 1994 suggested a magnitude of over 50%,[33] and a more recent study in 1997 found an incidence of major congenital malformations of 43%[25] and a relative risk of 11 (95% CI 2.1–57.6) for the combination of all four drugs compared with phenytoin monotherapy.[25] This Dutch study used pooled data from five European prospective studies. When compared with control children not exposed to AEDs, a significant increase in the risk of major congenital malformations was found for children exposed to carbamazepine monotherapy (RR 4.9; 95% CI 1.3–18) and

Table 24.2. Recent studies demonstrating an increased risk of congenital malformations in offspring of mothers receiving antiepileptic drugs (AEDs) – definition of congenital malformations differs between studies

Study	Women receiving AEDs (*n*)	Control women (*n*)	Congenital malformation rate in group receiving AEDs (%)	Odds ratio for congenital malformations OR (95% CI)
Sabers[26]	151	38 983	5.3	3.53(2.3–10.3)
Fonager[27]	235	17 259	6.4	2.2 (1.3–3.8)
Fairgrieve[2]	400	not known	5.0 (3.1–7.6%)	2.15(1.3–3.37)
Samren[25]	192	158	16.0	2.3 (1.2–4.7)
Holmes[28]	223	508	20.6 (major and minor)	2.8 (1.1–9.7)

valproate monotherapy (RR 4.9; 95% CI 1.6–15]). When comparing different AED regimens in 1221 pregnancies from the five studies and after adjustment for study centre, the increased risk of malformations for monotherapy with phenobarbitone was RR 4.2 (95% CI 1.0–18.6), with carbamazepine was RR 2.8 (95% CI 1.1–7.3) and with valproate was RR 3.7 (95% CI 1.0–18.6). There was no association between different types of epilepsy and the risk of major congenital malformations.[25]

Minor malformations (fetal hydantoin syndrome) occur in 5–30% of infants exposed to phenytoin in pregnancy, and fetal valproate and carbamazepine syndromes have also been described. Although specific syndromes have been ascribed to phenytoin, carbamazepine[34] and valproate, there is considerable overlap and many have craniofacial abnormalities. Features of these AED syndromes include dysmorphic features (V-shaped eyebrows, low-set ears, broad flat nasal bridge, irregular teeth), hypertelorism and hypoplastic nails and distal digits. Hypoplasia of the midface could be a marker for cognitive dysfunction.[28]

A large study examining the frequency of major malformations, hypoplasia of the midface and fingers and growth restriction[28] has confirmed a higher risk (OR 4.2; 95% CI 1.1–5.1) for infants exposed to two or more drugs compared with those exposed to only one drug (OR 2.8; 95% CI 1.1–9.7]). For sodium valproate, there appears to be a dose–response relationship for the risk of major congenital malformations, particularly neural tube defects. Offspring of mothers receiving more than 1000 mg/day of sodium valproate were at significantly increased risk (RR 6.8; 95% CI 1.4–32.7) compared with children of mothers receiving 600 mg or less per day. Furthermore, there were no neural tube defects in 54 of those receiving less than 1 g per day of valproate, two in 30 women receiving 1.0–1.5 g per day and three in eight women receiving more than 1.5 g a day.[25] This study also demonstrated the absence of a dose–response relationship for phenytoin and carbamazepine and a non-significant dose–response relationship for phenobarbitone.[25]

These data provide the rationale for using daily doses of valproate of less than 1000 mg/day if possible without jeopardising seizure control. As well as the total daily dose affecting malformation rates, peaks in maternal serum levels may increase the fetal risk. Thus it is preferable to prescribe a slow-release formulation more often (see below under 'management').

Trigonocephaly, a form of craniosynostosis resulting from premature fusion of the metopic suture and associated with reduction in IQ, has been described in the babies of

17 mothers receiving valproate monotherapy and may be part of the fetal valproate syndrome.[35]

Further anxiety has been raised concerning valproate therapy in pregnancy because of the reported association of maternal valproate use and impaired psychomotor development in the children.[36,37] One case–control study from Canada[36] of 116 children born to women with epilepsy demonstrated an odds ratio for developmental disorders of 4.82 (95% CI 1.27–18.37) with polytherapy and 9.38 (95% CI 1.75–50.22) with valproate monotherapy. Another study by Adab *et al.*[37] found an incidence of additional educational needs of 30% (OR 3.4; 95% CI 1.63–7.10) in children of mothers receiving valproate monotherapy, compared with only 3.2% (OR 0.26; 95% CI 0.06–1.15) for carbamazepine monotherapy and 24% (OR 2.51; 95% CI 1.04–6.07) for polytherapy with valproate. These are worrying data but derive from a retrospective questionnaire study with a 57% response rate. Clinical geneticists, to whom such patients are often referred, believe that neurodevelopmental delay may be a highly significant, yet poorly recognised, aspect of fetal exposure to sodium valproate.[38] Further prospective studies are needed.

Various theories exist to explain the mechanism for teratogenesis of AEDs, including a genetic deficiency of the detoxifying enzyme epoxide hydrolase, leading to the accumulation of toxic metabolites, cytotoxic free radicals and folic acid deficiency.[15,28] Phenytoin and phenobarbitone particularly, but also carbamazepine and valproate, interfere with folate metabolism. The risk of neural tube defects in the general population can be decreased by the use of preconceptual and first-trimester folic acid.[39] Disappointingly, in one study, although the risks of cardiac, urinary tract and oral cleft defects were decreased with maternal multivitamin supplementation containing folic acid in women receiving folate antagonists such as sulfasalazine and trimethoprim, this beneficial effect of multivitamins was not seen in women receiving AEDs.[40] One explanation for these findings is that drugs such as valproate may cause congenital malformations and neural tube defects by some other, non-folic acid-dependent mechanism.

There is not much information as to the teratogenic effects of the newer anticonvulsant drugs – vigabatrin, lamotrigine, levetiracetam, topiramate and gabapentin. They may be prescribed in combination with other anticonvulsants and it is therefore difficult to ascertain the teratogenic risk of these drugs in isolation. There are few data as to their use in human pregnancy but in animal studies vigabatrin and topiramate demonstrate teratogenicity. Lamotrigine, levetiracetam and gabapentin are not teratogenic in animals. Lamotrigine carries a theoretical risk because it is a weak inhibitor of dihydrofolate reductase and may interfere with folate metabolism; in practice it seems to carry a similar risk of teratogenesis to other AEDs in monotherapy. Published data from the worldwide prospective (1992–98) pregnancy registry for prospective first-trimester exposures of monotherapy and polytherapy with lamotrigine quote a malformation rate of 8/123 (6.5%; 95% CI 3.1%–12.8%).[41] More recent data from the GlaxoSmithKline lamotrigine pregnancy registry for prospective first trimester exposures show risks of major defects of three in 168 live births (1.8%; 95% CI 0.5%–5.5%) for monotherapy, five in 50 (10%; 95% CI 3.7%–22.6%) for polytherapy including valproate and five in 116 (4.3%; 95% CI 1.6%–10.3%]) for polytherapy excluding valproate.[42] Data from the UK prospective register of epilepsy and pregnancy with outcome data available for 1060 cases yield relative rates of major structural malformations of 2.2% (95% CI 0.4–11.6%) for no AED, 2.2% (95% CI 1.1–4.6%) for carbamazepine monotherapy, 8.4% (95% CI 5.4–12.8%) for valproate monotherapy and 3.9% (95% CI 1.7–8.8%) for lamotrigine monotherapy.[43] Whether the risk of lamotrigine monotherapy is low enough to justify replacement of an older AED such as valproate for lamotrigine pre-pregnancy is not yet known. The benzodiazepines (e.g. clobazam, clonazepam) normally used as add-on therapy are not teratogenic in monotherapy.

Management of epilepsy in pregnancy

Pre-pregnancy counselling

It should be assumed that all women of childbearing age may become pregnant, and therefore any opportunity to counsel such women should not be missed. Only 44% of pregnancies in 400 women with epilepsy were planned.[2] Control of epilepsy should be maximised before pregnancy. For women still having seizures, the lowest dose of the most effective treatment giving best control of seizures is appropriate; 80% of patients with epileptic seizures are well controlled by one or two AEDs. Polytherapy should be avoided if possible. Most women with epilepsy are on monotherapy, and of these the most common are carbamazepine and valproate. Although carbamazepine may have a slightly lower overall risk of teratogenesis than sodium valproate, phenytoin or phenobarbitone, sodium valproate is currently the treatment of choice for primary generalised epilepsy. It may be that levetiracetam will prove to be an acceptable and effective alternative to valproate.

If a woman has been free of seizures for two years or more, withdrawal of the AED may be considered. The risk of recurrent seizures is about 25% (80% of which will occur within four months after tapering of the dose begins and 90% of which will occur within the first year).[3] The risk of recurrence is about 40% by two years after drug withdrawal.[44] Recurrence risk is increased to over 50% in women with a known structural lesion, an abnormal EEG, onset of seizures in adolescence and those with a history of frequent seizures requiring more than one AED.[3] Factors associated with a low risk of recurrent seizures following discontinuation of AED are a normal EEG, onset in childhood and seizures that have been easily controlled with one drug.[3] Patients with juvenile myoclonic epilepsy require lifelong treatment with AEDs. If a decision is taken to stop treatment, AEDs should be withdrawn slowly in order to reduce the risk of withdrawal-associated seizures. This is particularly important for benzodiazepines and phenobarbitone. Decisions regarding cessation of AEDs should be fully informed after counselling, particularly concerning the risk of losing a driving licence in the event of a seizure. The current recommendations are to stop driving from the start of the period of drug withdrawal and for a period of six months after cessation of treatment even if there is no recurrence of seizures.[15]

All women (with or without epilepsy) should be advised to take 0.4 mg daily of folic acid for at least 12 weeks before conception. Worryingly, in one study[45] only 45% of women took preconceptional folic acid despite national guidance based on clear evidence for a benefit in reducing neural tube defects.[39] Since babies of women receiving AEDs are at high risk of neural tube defects, the higher dose of preconceptual folic acid (5 mg rather than 400 μg per day) is recommended.[15] In one prospective study,[2] only 11% of women with epilepsy took appropriate folic acid. In the UK prospective pregnancy registry, only 33% of women had been prescribed folic acid preconceptually.[43] Of concern, however, is the study demonstrating that maternal multivitamin supplements, including folic acid, did not reduce the increased incidence of cardiovascular, urinary tract abnormalities or oral clefts in the infants of mothers receiving AEDs.[40] Although there is no definite evidence that folic acid in any dose reduces the risk of neural tube defects in women with epilepsy, the recommendation that women taking AEDs should receive 5 mg daily of folic acid before conception and throughout pregnancy is logical.

The dose of sodium valproate should be lowered if possible to below 1 g per day, and therapy should be changed to a thrice-daily regimen and modified-release preparation in order to lower peak concentrations and reduce the risk of malformations. This is because of evidence of a dose-dependent teratogenic effect.[25] It is preferable to prescribe sodium valproate 300 mg three times daily, rather than 500 mg twice daily. It is important to achieve these changes before pregnancy because the neural tube closes by day 26, often before the woman realises she is pregnant.[46] Baseline anticonvulsant concentrations should be checked before conception.[46]

Antenatal management

As women with epilepsy may be from socially deprived populations, every effort should be made to ensure that they receive and understand the need for regular multidisciplinary antenatal care. Folic acid should be continued throughout pregnancy, as with AEDs there is a small risk of folate deficiency anaemia.[5] There is no need to change the anticonvulsant used in pregnancy if the woman is well controlled. Doses of sodium valproate should be reduced to below 1 g per day if possible and a slow-release formulation used in three divided doses if this has not been established pre-pregnancy. No evidence exists for a dose-dependent teratogenic effect of carbamazepine. However, carbamazepine may also be given as a slow-release formulation if seizure control deteriorates during pregnancy. Prenatal screening for congenital abnormalities with nuchal translucency scanning and detailed ultrasound at 18–20 weeks should be offered. A repeat scan at about 22 weeks is advisable if cardiac defects are suspected.

The altered pharmocokinetics in pregnancy mean that drug levels are likely to change and, for most drugs, concentration of the free drug falls. This is because of the increased plasma volume and the enhanced renal and hepatic drug clearance. These effects are partly offset by changes in protein binding. Protein levels fall in pregnancy and protein binding of drugs decreases, resulting in increased free drug levels. For drugs that are largely protein-bound such as phenytoin, this effect partly counteracts the above factors, leading to reduced free drug levels, so changes in dosage are rarely needed in pregnancy. However, for drugs with little protein binding, such as carbamazepine and lamotrigine, this effect of reduced protein binding is not significant and the predominant result of pharmacokinetic changes of pregnancy is marked reductions in free drug levels and thereby a need in many patients to increase the dosage during pregnancy. In practice, it is useful to have a baseline drug level early in pregnancy to ensure compliance and to guide any increases that may be necessary. If a woman is seizure-free, there is no need to measure serial drug levels or adjust the dose. In women who have regular seizures and who are dependent upon critical drug levels, it is worth monitoring drug levels (preferably of the free drug), since they are likely to fall and increasing doses of anticonvulsants should be guided by serum concentrations. In women with regular seizures, it is frequently necessary to increase the dose of sodium valproate, carbamazepine and especially lamotrigine[47] in pregnancy. Doses of lamotrigine may need to be increased two- to three-fold during pregnancy. Problems may arise with therapeutic drug monitoring because most plasma assays measure the total of bound and free AED concentrations and these ratios change in pregnancy. Anticonvulsant dosage should be altered on clinical grounds.

Vitamin K (10–20 mg orally) should be prescribed in the last four weeks of pregnancy.[48] This is because vitamin K-dependent clotting factors may be reduced in the babies of women taking hepatic enzyme-inducing drugs, increasing the risk of haemorrhagic disease in the newborn.

In the latest CEMD report,[9] there was one death in a woman with epilepsy from status epilepticus that had a clear temporal association with the administration of dexamethasone to induce fetal lung maturity. There is certainly not enough evidence to justify withholding systemic corticosteroids in prematurity in women with epilepsy. Indeed, some authorities recommend an increased dose of corticosteroids (to compensate for increased metabolism) to induce fetal lung maturation in women receiving hepatic microsomal enzyme-inducing AEDs.[15] This recommendation has not been widely adopted.

Intrapartum management

The risk of seizures increases around the time of delivery: 1–2% of women with epilepsy will have a seizure during labour and a further 1–2% will fit in the first 24 hours postpartum.[15,49] Therefore, women with epilepsy should be advised to deliver in hospital and should not be left unattended in labour.[15,46]

Most women with epilepsy have vaginal deliveries and caesarean section is only required for obstetric indications or if there are recurrent generalised seizures in labour.[15,46] If seizures that are not rapidly self-limiting occur in labour, intravenous lorazepam (4 mg over two minutes) or diazemuls (10 mg) may be appropriate. For women who have had seizures during previous deliveries, an option is to use rectal carbamazepine or intravenous sodium valproate or phenytoin to replace the usual oral therapy and ensure adequate absorption during labour.

Postnatal management

The neonate should receive 1 mg intramuscular vitamin K. In the prospective study of Fairgrieve,[2] only 36% infants received appropriate vitamin K. Women with epilepsy require particular care in the immediate puerperium because of the increased risk of seizures. They should not be left unattended and should be supervised in the bath.

All women with epilepsy should be strongly encouraged to breastfeed.[15] Sadly, in some countries mothers receiving AEDs tend to choose formula-feeding.[50] Babies whose mothers received phenobarbitone in pregnancy may experience withdrawal if they are not breastfed and, although this is rare with the newer anticonvulsants, it provides a logical reason to encourage breastfeeding in all epileptic mothers. Although most anticonvulsants are secreted into breast milk, the dose of phenytoin, carbamazepine or sodium valproate that the baby receives is only a fraction (3–5%) of the therapeutic dose for neonates and, in any case, is likely to be less than that received *in utero*. The ratio between breast milk and serum concentration is 0.36 for phenobarbitone, and doses received by the neonate may reach over 50% of therapeutic levels. Similarly, the median ratio for lamotrigine in one study of ten infants of nine women was 0.61 (range 0.47–0.77).[47] In addition, phenobarbitone, primidone and lamotrigine[47] may accumulate in breastfed babies because of slow elimination by the neonate. Lamotrigine is metabolised mainly by glucuronidation and the capacity to glucuronidate is not fully developed in newborns.[47] Lamotrigine should not be initiated in breastfeeding mothers.

If the mother's dose of anticonvulsant was increased during pregnancy, it should be slowly decreased two to three weeks after delivery. Maternal plasma concentrations of lamotrigine increase significantly during the first two weeks after delivery, with a median increase in the plasma concentration/dose ratio of 170%.[47] This is likely to reflect a normalisation of induced metabolism of lamotrigine in pregnancy and may indicate that doses of lamotrigine should be decreased sooner after delivery. If a baby of a mother taking AEDs is unusually sleepy or has to be woken for feeds, the mother should be encouraged to feed before rather than after taking her anticonvulsants. This should avoid peak serum and therefore breast milk levels.

General advice in pregnancy and the puerperium

Various patient information leaflets are available for women with epilepsy, some dealing with the specific issues concerning pregnancy. Practical advice concerning their safety and that of their baby or child in the event of a generalised seizure should be given. This includes bathing infants with somebody else around, changing nappies on the floor, placing hot drinks at a distance while feeding or holding the baby, using a pram or buggy with a 'dead man's handle', use of safety harnesses and gates and domestic safety.[15]

The following recommendations appear in successive CEMD reports: 'Epilepsy is a potentially fatal disease whether the patient is pregnant or not. General practitioners and midwives should check with relatives that they know what to do in case of a fit and should provide instruction, particularly on the need to place the patient in the recovery position once the fit is over. Pregnant women who are at risk of fits should be advised not to bathe alone, or should use a shower instead.'[6]

'Women with epilepsy need specific specialist advice in pregnancy. The ideal treatment for pregnant epileptic women, which has already been instigated in some centres, is a dedicated clinic to encompass pre-pregnancy counselling and attended by obstetrician, neurologist/obstetric physician and a specialist midwife or neurological nurse.'

'Women with epilepsy should also be made aware of the dangers of bathing in pregnancy. They should be advised to bathe only in shallow water with someone else in the house, or alternatively to shower.'[9]

Contraception

Women taking hepatic enzyme-inducing drugs (phenytoin, primidone, carbamazepine, phenobarbitone, topiramate and oxcarbazepine) require higher doses of oestrogen to achieve adequate contraception. They should be given a combined oral contraceptive pill containing at least 50 μg oestrogen, be instructed to take two pills containing 30μg[1] or be advised to use a different form of contraception. More effective contraception can be achieved by tricycling followed by a four-day pill-free interval. Higher doses of the progesterone-only pill are also required. Women should be advised to take two rather than one daily pill of norethisterone (350 μg) or levonorgestrel (30 μg). An alternative is medroxyprogesterone acetate. This is entirely metabolised by 'first-pass effect' in the liver and therefore a higher dose is not required. A double dose is also required of the 'morning-after pill'. Particular caution is needed when first introducing hepatic enzyme inducing drugs. A detailed drug history, including oral contraceptive use, should be taken. Valproate, clonazepam, vigabatrin, lamotrigine, gabapentin and tiagabine do not induce hepatic enzymes.

Conclusions

Most pregnancies in women with epilepsy are associated with a successful outcome. However, timely and appropriate counselling concerning the teratogenic risks of AEDs and how to minimise them is not yet available to the majority. GPs, neurologists, general physicians, obstetricians and midwives should be encouraged to volunteer such advice and counselling at any appropriate opportunity to any woman with epilepsy within or approaching childbearing years. Such advice is particularly important when starting or changing AEDs. Pregnant women with epilepsy require specialist management.

Acknowledgements

The author wishes to thank Dr Michael D O'Brien, Consultant Neurologist, Guy's Hospital, London, for his help and advice in the preparation of this manuscript.

References

1. O'Brien MD, Gilmour-White S. Epilepsy and pregnancy. *BMJ* 1993;307:492–5.
2. Fairgrieve SD, Jackson M, Jonas P, Walshaw D, White K, Montgomery TL, *et al.* Population based, prospective study of the care of women with epilepsy in pregnancy. *BMJ* 2000;321:674–5.
3. Browne TR, Holmes GL. Epilepsy. *N Engl J Med* 2001;344:1145–51.
4. Shearer VE, Jhaveri HS, Cunningham FG. Puerperal seizures after post-dural puncture headache. *Obstet Gynecol* 1995;85:255–60.
5. Nelson-Piercy C. Neurological disorders. In: Nelson-Piercy C. *Handbook of Obstetric Medicine*. 2nd ed. London: Martin Dunitz; 2002. p. 156–79.
6. Department of Health, Welsh Office, Scottish Home and Health Department, Department of Health and Social Services, Northern Ireland. *Why Mothers Die. Report on Confidential Enquiries into Maternal Death in the United Kingdom, 1994–96*. London: The Stationery Office; 1998.
7. Department of Health, Welsh Office, Scottish Home and Health Department, Department of Health and Social Services, Northern Ireland. *Report on Confidential Enquiries into Maternal Death in the United Kingdom, 1991–93*. London: HMSO; 1996.
8. Department of Health, Welsh Office, Scottish Home and Health Department, Department of Health and Social Services, Northern Ireland. *Report on Confidential Enquiries into Maternal Death in the United Kingdom, 1988–90*. London: HMSO; 1994.

9. Lewis G, Drife J, editors. *Why Mothers Die 1997–1999. The Confidential Enquiries into Maternal Deaths in the United Kingdom*. London: RCOG Press; 2001.
10. Nilsson L, Farahmand BY, Perssson PG, Thiblin I, Thaman T. Risk factors for sudden unexpected death in epilepsy: a case–control study. *Lancet* 1999;353:888–93.
11. Nashef L, Fish DR, Garner S, Sander JW, Shorvon SD. Sudden death in epilepsy: a study of incidence in a young cohort with epilepsy and learning difficulty. *Epilepsia* 1995;36:1187–94.
12. Walczak TS, Leppik IE, D'Amelio M, Rarick J, So E, Ahman P, *et al.* Incidence and risk factors in sudden unexpected death in epilepsy: a prospective cohort study. *Neurology* 2001;56:519–25.
13. Nashef L, Garner S, Sander JW, Fish DR, Shorvon SD. Circumstances of death in sudden death in epilepsy: interviews of bereaved relatives. *J Neurol Neurosurg Psychiatry* 1998;64:349–52.
14. Wallace H, Shorvon S, Tallis R. Age-specific incidence and prevalence rates of treated epilepsy in an unselected population of 2,052,922 and age-specific fertility rates of women with epilepsy. *Lancet* 1998;352:1970–3.
15. Crawford P, Appleton R, Betts T, Duncan J, Guthrie E, Morrow J, *et al.* Best practice guidelines for the management of women with epilepsy. *Seizure* 1999;8:201–17.
16. Isojarvi JIT, Laatikainen TJ, Knip M, Pakarinen AJ, Juntunen KT, Myllyla VV. Obesity and endocrine disorders in women taking valproate for epilepsy. *Ann Neurol* 1996;39;579–84.
17. Genton P, Bauer J, Duncan S, Taylor AE, Balen AH, Eberle A, *et al.* On the association between valproate and polycystic ovary syndrome. *Epilepsia* 2001;42:295–304.
18. Vidovic MI, Della Marina BM. Trimestral changes of seizure frequency in pregnant epileptic women. *Acta Med Croatica* 1994;48:85–7.
19. Sawhney H, Vasishta K, Suri V, Khunnu B, Goel P, Sawhney IMS. Pregnancy with epilepsy – a retrospective analysis. *Int J Gynaecol Obstet* 1996;54:17–22.
20. Yerby MS. Pregnancy, teratogenesis, and epilepsy. *Neurol Clin* 1994;12:749–71.
21. Olafsson E, Hallgrimsson JT, Hauser WA, Ludvigsson P, Gudmundsson G. Pregnancies of women with epilepsy: a population-based study in Iceland. *Epilepsia* 1998;39:887–92.
22. Ottman R, Lee JH, Risch N, Hauser WA, Susser M. Clinical indicators of genetic susceptibility to epilepsy. *Epilepsia* 1996;37:353–61.
23. Berkovic SF, Howell RA, Hay DA, Hopper JL. Epilepsies in twins: genetics of the major epilepsy syndromes. *Ann Neurol* 1998;43:435–45.
24. Schupf N, Ottman R. Risk of epilepsy in offspring of affected women: association with maternal spontaneous abortion. *Neurology* 2001;57:1642–9.
25. Samren EB, van Duijn CM, Koch S, Hiilesmaa VK, Klepel H, Bardy AH, *et al.* Maternal use of antiepileptic drugs and the risk of major congenital malformations: a joint European prospective study of human teratogenesis associated with maternal epilepsy. *Epilepsia* 1997;38:981–90.
26. Sabers A, Arogvihansen B, Dam M, Fischerrasmussen W, Gram L, Hansen M *et al.* Pregnancy and epilepsy: a retrospective study of 151 pregnancies. *Acta Neurol Scand* 1998;97:164–70.
27. Fonager K , Larsen H, Pedersen L, Sorensen HT. Birth outcomes in women exposed to anticonvulsant drugs. *Acta Neurol Scand* 2000;101:289–94.
28. Holmes LB, Harvey EA, Coull BA, Huntington KB, Khoshbin S, Hayes AM, *et al.* The teratogenicity of anticonvulsant drugs. *N Engl J Med* 2001;344:1132–8.
29. Friis ML, Holm NV, Sindrup EH, Fogh-Andersen P, Hauge M. Facial clefts in sibs and children of epileptic patients. *Neurology* 1986;36:346–50.
30. Rosa FW. Spina bifida in infants of women treated with carbamazepine during pregnancy. *N Engl J Med* 1991;324:674–7.
31. Jones KL, Lacro RV, Johnson KA, Adams J. Pattern of malformations in the children of women treated with carbamazepine during pregnancy. *N Engl J Med* 1989;320:1661–6.
32. Nakane Y, Okuma T, Takahashi R, Sato Y, Wada T, Sato T, *et al.* Multi-institutional study on the teratogenicity and fetal toxicity of antiepileptic drugs: a report of a collaborative study group in Japan. *Epilepsia* 1980;21:663–80.
33. Lindhout D, Hoppener RJEA, Meinardi H. Teratogenicity of antiepileptic drug combinations with special emphasis on epoxidation (of carbamazepine). *Epilepsia* 1984;25:77–83.
34. Ornoy A, Cohen E. Outcome of children born to epileptic mothers treated with carbamazepine during pregnancy. *Arch Dis Child* 1996;75:517–20.
35. Lajeunie E, Barcik U, Thorne JA, Ghouzzi VE, Bourgeois M, Renier D. Craniosynostosis and fetal exposure to sodium valproate. *J Neurosurg* 2001;95:778–82.
36. Ohtsuka Y, Silver K, Lopes-Cendes I, Andermann E, Tsuda T. Effect of antiepileptic drugs on psychomotor development in offspring of epileptic mothers. *Epilepsia* 1999;40 Suppl 2:296.
37. Adab N, Jacoby A, Smith D, Chadwick D. Additional educational needs in children born to mothers with epilepsy. *J Neurol Neurosurg Psychiatry* 2001;70:15–21.

38. Turnpenny P. Epilepsy and anticonvulsants in pregnancy. *Seizure* 2000;9:6–7.
39. Medical Research Council (MRC) Vitamin Study Research Group. Prevention of neural tube defects: results of the MRC vitamin study. *Lancet* 1991;338:131–7.
40. Hernandez-Diaz S, Werler MM, Walker AM, Mitchell AA. Folic acid antagonists during pregnancy and the risk of birth defects. *N Engl J Med* 2000;343:1608–14.
41. Reiff-Eldridge R, Heffner CR, Ephross SA, Tennis PS, White AD, Andrews EB. Monitoring pregnancy outcomes after prenatal exposure through prospective pregnancy registries: a pharmaceutical company commitment. *Am J Obstet Gynecol* 2000;182:159–63.
42. GlaxoSmithKline International. Lamotrigine pregnancy registry. Interim report 1 September 1992 through 30 September 2001.
43. Morrow JI, Craig JJ, Russell AJC, Morrison P, Parsons L, Guthrie E, *et al.* Epilepsy and pregnancy: A prospective register in the United Kingdom. *J Neurol Sci* 2001;187 Suppl 1:s299.
44. Medical Research Council Antiepileptic Drug Withdrawal Study Group. Randomised study of antiepileptic drug withdrawal in patients in remission. *Lancet* 1991;337:1175–80.
45. Huttly WJ, Wald NJ, Walters JC. Folic acid supplementation before pregnancy remains inadequate. *BMJ* 1999;319:1499.
46. Cleland PG. Management of pre-existing disorders in pregnancy: epilepsy. *Prescriber's Journal* 1996;36:102–9.
47. Ohman I, Vitols S, Tomson T. Lamotrigine in pregnancy: pharmacokinetics during delivery, in the neonate, and during lactation. *Epilepsia* 2000;41:709–13.
48. Deblay MF, Vert P, Andre M, Marchal F. Transplacental vitamin K prevents haemorrhagic disease of infant of epileptic mother. *Lancet* 1982;1:1247.
49. Bardy A. Epilepsy and pregnancy. A prospective study of 154 pregnancies in epileptic women [dissertation]. Helsinki: University of Helsinki, Finland; 1982.
50. Ito S, Moretti M, Liau M, Koren G. Initiation and duration of breast-feeding in women receiving antiepileptics. *Am J Obstet Gynecol* 1995;172:881–6.

Chapter 25

Specific problems of mortality and morbidity II

Discussion

Discussion following Professor de Swiet's paper

Drife: I have been troubled, as I am sure you have, by the report of the death of a young woman who appears not to have been informed that she is in effect playing Russian roulette with a six-shooter, with three of the chambers loaded. I do not personally believe that people have the right, because of our sensitivities, not to be given that information. The idea of people having the right to refuse to hear that quite important information seems bizarre to me. The human right of the patient is to know exactly what is happening.

Because of the ethnic concerns that we all have about not trampling insensitively into a difficult area, we are standing back a little too far from it. If we are really keen to ensure that the lives of these young women are saved, and if the only logical method at this point in our knowledge is to say that they should avoid going through a full-term pregnancy – I am thinking of pulmonary vascular disease cases – it would be a strategy to involve the whole community if we perceive that this risk is particularly high in certain ethnic groups. Rather than trying to educate the patient when she is already pregnant, and through an interpreter who may or may not transfer the information in the way that we would like, we should speak to community leaders and people who have a position of influence in communities. We should tell them that this is a risk we are concerned about, as a group, and ask what they suggest would be the best way of putting that information across, when we perceive – rightly or wrongly – that there is a strong social pressure on these girls to become pregnant, even if they kill themselves in so doing.

Neilson: Can you encapsulate that into a recommendation?

Drife: I was listening for a hiss of disapproval to what I was saying, around the room. Since we have not had that, perhaps we could crystallise it a little more, into awareness of the risk among (1) healthcare professionals, (2) individual patients and (3) communities in which the risks appear to be increased, so that it is a community awareness, rather than an individual awareness.

Neilson: Together with an individual awareness?

Drife: Yes, it is not either/or.

Marteau: Professor De Swiet, you seem to have this unrealistic optimism that there are data that might guide these consultations but, sadly, there are no data to devise the most effective and sensitive way of giving this kind of information.

Probably, the best way forward will be to use the very good practice – which is obviously not an evidence base – that has evolved for communicating bad news. One does not decide to hold back on information until someone has asked for it, but one goes gently and is able to assess how much detail people want. People need to be given the information.

I wonder whether part of this recommendation could be about general training in communication skills. I will come back to that in my presentation. It is rather like motherhood and apple pie – who will be against it? We need evidence-based training in effective and sensitive communication.

De Swiet: I would have taken exactly the same attitude as Professor Drife, until I took part in a debate a couple of days ago about this question of imparting a 50% risk of maternal mortality to the patient. It was implied that imparting this entailed a degree of paternalism and that it took away the patient's autonomy. Whatever this group says, I think I will change my practices. I think I will say the same as you are saying, which is that I will try to ensure that the woman really does want to know what the risks are before I tell her.

Marteau: But in order for her to know what the risks are, she needs to know that there is some kind of risk. I am suggesting, based on common sense rather than anything else, that rather than jumping in and saying, 'Do you realise that you have a one in two chance of dying', we should start by saying that there is a fairly high risk and that death is a possible outcome. There is a whole debate about numbers, presenting absolute and relative risk, and how one frames the information, but unless the woman knows that this is even on the cards, how can she know whether she wants more information?

De Swiet: I accept that. From a practical point of view, one is obviously going to say that this could be a risky business.

Bewley: I just despair about all this rights-based talk in medical encounters! I would point out that death, in that situation, represents a 100% removal of your autonomy, and it is just not an irrelevant thing. You must not be stung by being called paternalistic. It is not the paternalism that is bad – there is good paternalism and bad paternalism. I would much prefer to phrase this in terms of your duty to the patient, which is to look after her, care for her and talk to her. It is not a question of whether to break bad news, because withholding bad news is taking everything away from her, and that would be bad paternalism. It is a question of how, not whether, to break bad news. I would echo everything that Professor Marteau is saying. Do not be stung by people saying you are paternalistic – that is the last thing you are, Professor De Swiet!

Robinson: There are things that people need to know and that is what professional care is about. However, what we have a continual problem with – and I must deal with at least three women a week – are those who are grossly dissatisfied with the way in which risk has been conveyed. What they have is an authoritarian picture: 'Thou shalt, or shalt not.'

The other component is that a great deal of risk seems to us to be conveyed, particularly by midwives opposed to doing home births, in a dishonest and exaggerated way. I will give you the example of one area where every single woman who tried to book a home birth was told that she had placenta praevia. After we had had the fifth woman with placenta praevia, who went in and had a perfectly normal vaginal delivery, we said that the next one we had would be funded by the Maternity Defence Fund to sue. Of course we could not and would not have done that, but it stopped it!

It worries us that people come to us with stories of what they have been told about risk. They have simply been told, 'You are at risk', or 'You are at high risk', but they either have not been told, or they have not understood, what the components of that risk are. When we try to tease this out, we find that some of them – from our lay knowledge – have high and genuine risk factors, which they have not taken on board because they rejected the authoritarian approach. In others, the genuine risk or the statistical risk was in fact very low. We have to have honesty. Risk should not be used so that professionals get you to do what they want you to do and adopt their preferred method of operating. It should enable you to make choices for yourself. That is one side of the story.

There are also strong cultural elements in this, dealing with other communities. The translation issue worries us enormously. I sat on the Turkish kidney case that lasted from November until April 2002 at the GMC. The President of the GMC was trying to explain to a poor Turkish woman, the mother of two young children, who had donated one of her healthy kidneys to her much richer sister-in-law, what risk she might have run. He asked whether she had understood and whether she had agreed to it. Was it informed consent? This went backwards and forwards and he was being very patient and very sweet. Eventually, she said, with some asperity, 'Yes, I understand what you are saying, but we are all in the hands of Allah.' She was content to leave this to Allah, whether she lived or died, and whether her children were motherless or not. This was a vignette of the conceptual difficulties. We are not sufficiently well educated in this, but we are more than happy to work with anybody, to share anything that we have. Like Professor Marteau, I agree that we need better hard information on the way to do it.

Cooper: I would like to share an amusing anecdote from *Anaesthesia* in February this year, which addressed the subject of risk. This compared risks of clinical problems with those of everyday life. Your risk of dying from anaesthesia is substantially lower than your risk of dying by being struck by lightning but you are about ten times less likely to achieve six balls on the National Lottery. I doubt that many of the population understand that.

Neilson: We should probably move on. The group feels that the assessment of risk needs to be communicated in a sensitive manner and in understandable terms. This includes cultural sensitivity.

Marteau: I would like to push very strongly for putting this within the context of training. It is like apple pie and motherhood. One of the issues is that most of us have an unrealistic view of our skills – particularly in the area of communication. Most people will read the recommendations and say, 'Yes, I agree with that. Yes, I'm pretty good at that!' However, on closer inspection, it will not necessarily be there.

We need to grasp this firmly. It is one of the issues that is bubbling up under a good deal of what we are looking at. There needs to be evidence-based training that involves giving people feedback on what they are doing and having some evidence that the training is making a difference.

De Swiet: So the educational component would be two-fold. One would be so that people really know what the risks are and, second, they would need training in how to communicate them. That second part, if there is a place for it, might be a more general recommendation from the group with regard to everything we have been saying, rather than just with regard to heart disease.

Drife: I agree with Ms Robinson that one of the ways in which we have shot ourselves in the foot as doctors has been by overplaying risks that in absolute terms are low, so that when we have a real risk, people do not believe us. However, am I right in my understanding that many of these conditions pre-date pregnancy by quite a long way? Or are they often discovered at the booking clinic or at 18 weeks? My understanding about some of the conditions is that the woman has lived with risk for some length of time. Therefore, perhaps we should make a recommendation about the timing of informing the woman as to the increased risks of pregnancies.

De Swiet: My impression is that, in two-thirds of the patients with pulmonary vascular disease, this risk would have been known, or could have been inferred, beforehand. In at least one-third, however, it appears *de novo* in pregnancy.

Neilson: We need to discuss whether assessment of risk in women with cardiac disease should be taking place in the community or in secondary or tertiary centres.

Yentis: Having spent a long time at the Chelsea and Westminster Hospital, London, building a multidisciplinary cardiac clinic so that we can assess the risk properly, I would be uneasy about suggesting that anyone can assess the risk in any location – even with a protocol.

The problem with the Toronto study is that their overall severity of illness was very mild – much less than in the cases we have had reported to the Obstetric Anaesthetists Association registry of cardiac disease. I am not sure how useful a tool it will be, applied to the UK population. Even if it were a good tool, I would be worried about other people applying it who did not have specialist insight into the problems that these women have.

De Swiet: The alternative is to get people who, five years ago, had a diagnosis of mitral valve prolapse on the basis of a systolic murmur, to go to a tertiary centre to have that risk assessed. I understand exactly what you are saying and so perhaps the truth is somewhere between these viewpoints.

Yentis: I suspect you are right. We see quite a few people with mitral valve prolapse and reassure them, with the confidence that they are being reassured by people who can reassure them!

Neilson: Are you saying that that expertise does not exist in some district hospitals?

Yentis: The fear is that you have someone who on the face of it is quite well, and perhaps had an atrial septal defect repaired as a child, but who has residual primary hypertension that will not be picked up. Or that they could have some connective tissue disease and no one appreciates that what they have is cardiomegaly, while in fact they have primary hypertension. It is a matter of babies and bathwater, or tuna and dolphin – if you make the net too wide, you lose some of the tuna, or vice versa.

Nelson-Piercy: This is a related point. It is not where the assessment happens but who does it that is the issue. As with epilepsy, we have to think outside this room. These women with heart disease – the sorts of heart disease that one is concerned about – are often under follow-up by cardiologists. One should not remove them from the equation, and the same is true for almost any medical disorder you care to mention.

Part of this education must be of the physicians caring for these women. Some of them will say that they are not under follow-up, and they present a problem, but this is where the general practitioner comes in. We cannot envisage some kind of superstructure whereby, within obstetrics and midwifery, we can cover it all – because we cannot. We need the help of the primary-care doctors, and of the other specialist physicians. I would suggest it should be done by a clinician who has working knowledge of the risks and a working knowledge to undertake that assessment.

Oates: Before it expired, I attended the Specialist Services Commissioning Group. The favoured model of service delivery – which almost exactly mimics what the Royal College of Psychiatrists suggests for serious psychiatric disorders following delivery – is the 'hub and spoke' method. For every tertiary centre of excellence, there are identified clinicians with a special interest at health authority level (secondary level), backed up by specialist multidisciplinary teams. They have this 'hub and spoke' relationship with the centre of excellence, which allows dissemination of knowledge. I think there is a technical term for groups of professionals who can meet up locally and share things. It is a halfway house between having the tertiary centre and the jobbing people with a specialist interest in secondary care.

When the various Royal Colleges work out the competencies for specialist registrars to become, say, cardiologists, one of the things they will have to do will be to provide evidence that they are up-to-date with obstetric cardiology. We should avoid making recommendations that are just aspirational and utopian fantasies – they have to have some way of being translated into action. The hub and spoke method is a practical and sensible way of translating the knowledge of people like us, who are specialists, into the realities of everyday life.

De Swiet: This goes much further than recommendations about heart disease, which is a relatively uncommon condition – even though it is a high cause of maternal mortality. This really relates to all of the plans that Dr Nelson-Piercy and others have had about a model for obstetric medicine.

Robson: Cardiac disease is the one branch of obstetric medicine where you are on shaky ground. The vast majority of even obstetric physicians are not capable of dealing with the sort of cardiac disease that you are talking about. I would regard the most important phrase in your presentation as 'the identification of the one and only cardiac physician with knowledge of obstetrics in any one region', because there would be only one. By and large, if the infrastructure was there that clearly identified that person, this would make the management of these patients substantially more co-ordinated.

De Swiet: But, in general, there is not even one cardiologist who does know anything about pregnancy.

Robson: But that may be important to recognise.

De Swiet: For the time being, we need an obstetric physician working together with a cardiologist.

Robson: I do not dispute that, but the point I am trying to make is that it is vital that there is a cardiologist identified, who either currently has, or should aspire to obtain, knowledge of obstetrics.

Yentis: Perhaps it would be better to issue a recommendation that each maternity unit has its own scheme for ensuring that at-risk patients with this sort of condition are picked up, assessed and referred as appropriate, and leave individual units to do that? We should perhaps even say that we recommend that this is audited – or is that going too far?

Lewis: I will go against that. The new concept that I would like to see supported is a 'managed clinical network', not hub and spoke. A managed clinical network is the way we are going. Under this scheme, given that we now have a new system of commissioning, we would envisage that, in every region, everyone would have a pathway and know where to send people with particular conditions. If you propose a 'managed clinical network', people will begin to understand what you are talking about and we can then discuss it and refine it.

Neilson: That is not incompatible with what Dr Yentis was saying – it is just that the initiative is not necessarily at hospital level but at a regional level.

Bewley: I would like to add something about research. In a way, I know that if you have good clinicians, you achieve a better outcome, but we have to prove that. There is evidence that if you use guidelines and if you have a high volume of work then, for example in cancer, you achieve better outcomes. We hope that this new profession of obstetric physicians will produce better outcomes, but we need to research that because we have some bad examples from the tertiary centres in fetal medicine that have shown that, if you send pregnancies with certain fetal anomalies into tertiary centres, the outcome is no better in spite of more intervention with the women. We cannot say we know that this team working will produce better outcomes in diseases that are often very difficult to treat.

Discussion following Dr Nelson-Piercy's and Professor MacLean's papers

Tuffnell: I may have misunderstood the Confidential Enquiry recommendation about cervical smears in pregnancy, but the way it seems to have been interpreted locally within our region is that all women with bleeding in early pregnancy should have cervical smears. That has raised a degree of consternation from practising jobbing gynaecologists and also from oncologists, because they feel that this is not necessarily the right way to go. Could you comment on that?

MacLean: If a patient has a convincing history of previous negative cytology, then it is probably unnecessary to reassess her. If a patient presents with a poorly documented or inconsistent story of previous cervical cytology, then you should perhaps use the opportunity. However, you must be aware that about 20–25% of cervical carcinomas will give you falsely negative smears, so that you cannot rely solely on cytology. In fact, in my chapter, I have suggested that patients who continue to bleed should be assessed in the colposcopy clinic. Colposcopists will groan with dismay but it is just that you have the advantage of having a patient in an appropriate position with an adequate light, so that you can have a better view than is ever possible in the labour ward. If you feel that the patient needs a smear, then you can take a smear. If you feel that the patient has something abnormal, you can at least consider whether to proceed to biopsy.

You cannot rely on smears. If the patient has a good smear history, then it is probably unnecessary.

De Swiet: Dr Nelson-Piercy, would you agree that magnesium is not an anticonvulsant and that the sort of brain stem reflex that some obstetricians have, that fits = magnesium, is inappropriate? Perhaps the most appropriate approach might be magnesium *plus* an anticonvulsant, in some circumstances.

Nelson-Piercy: Yes, I would agree. I culled the slide with the relative incidence of fitting due to epilepsy and fitting due to eclampsia on a labour ward, and the former is much more common. However, in practical terms, I do not think that giving magnesium to a woman who is having an epileptic tonic-clonic seizure is likely to do any harm. I would prefer it if people would think and review the notes. If a woman has never had a tonic-clonic seizure before, the diagnosis of eclampsia needs to be seriously considered.

De Swiet: I guess we get into problems, not so much with chronic epilepsy but with *de novo* epilepsy in pregnancy, because of such things as cerebral vein thrombosis. It is then that you might need to use both magnesium and anticonvulsants.

Nelson-Piercy: Yes. I also culled the slide that said that anyone who fits in pregnancy for the first time requires cerebral imaging, a blood count and film (to exclude TTP), and all those things to exclude everything else, because I did not want to insult this audience since I knew they knew that.

While I have the floor, can I raise a serious issue? As a country, we need more neurologists, especially ones with a special interest in epilepsy. I would go further and say that we need clinicians with a special interest in epilepsy in pregnancy. It is rather like the cardiology argument. With all due respect, the classification of epilepsy is not understood by most general physicians. I would not expect most obstetricians to understand it and therefore you need someone else to help with these very difficult decisions about which drugs to use and whether to stop the drug.

Greer: Dr Nelson-Piercy's presentation was highly informative. I wondered how many of the deaths that are seen in epilepsy could be attributed to subclinical status. Also, I wondered whether we should discriminate between those women who have tonic-clonic seizures and those who do not. I appreciate that the nomenclature in the classification of epilepsy is complex and beyond the reach of most general physicians and obstetricians.

However, I wonder whether patients who do not have generalised seizures could have different advice. Perhaps they could stop their therapy if they are not going to be exposed to tonic-clonic seizures.

You recommend monitoring levels, and I do the same, but that goes against the vast majority of neurologists in the country, who do not monitor levels. They push the drug up if the patient fits and they lower it if they have adverse effects. I take the view that it is helpful to know if they are compliant and also that antenatal care is about preventive rather than reactive medicine, and so I do monitor levels – although I probably do not change the dosage as much as I did in the past.

The folic acid issue is certainly a problem and I wonder whether we should lobby to get pharmacists to make this information available. Very few women with epilepsy on anticonvulsants know about folic acid, which is amazing. We have pharmacists dispensing anticonvulsant therapy and I wondered whether we could have an insert in the pack for women of childbearing age to make them aware of the need for folic acid in pregnancy. This is a very simple measure that could happen at pharmacy level or at drug company level. Finally, I was not sure about the American study that you cited[1] –

my recollection is that they were on low doses of folic acid, and not on 5 mg, which might be confusing. Lastly, you mentioned the issue about the steroid hormones and the pill but, for obstetricians in general, you should also be aware that you have to double the dose of steroids for fetal lung maturation from 12 mg to 24 mg, for the same reason.

Nelson-Piercy: I will try to answer those points in the order in which they were raised. The issue of differentiating major convulsive seizures from partial seizures is difficult. I, too, have gone to neurologists say, 'Surely, she could stop?' When you speak to women who have 20 absences a day, it is actually almost as debilitating as having one tonic-clonic seizure. Neurologists will argue that there is always the risk of secondary generalisation and, in my experience, they are not very keen to stop the drugs, even if women have never had a major convulsive seizure. I hear what you are saying, but we, as non-neurologists, do not understand enough about the risk of secondary generalisation, or that we should undermine the morbidity associated with non-major seizures, which can be very distressing for the woman.

Greer: I was not advocating that – I just wanted to know what you thought.

Nelson-Piercy: I bow to my neurological colleagues and, on the whole, they will not, and I do not either.

Yes, subclinical status could be a feature and Professor De Swiet may be able to enlighten me. However, many of these women died in circumstances where it was not possible to tell whether they had been fitting or not and, if they had been fitting, how long they had been fitting for, because the deaths are not witnessed. So yes, it is entirely possible that they could have died of status epilepticus. The problem is that you can only differentiate status from sudden unexpected death in epilepsy (SUDEP) if it is witnessed. The best practice guidelines do not recommend doubling the dose of steroids for fetal lung maturation. Rather worryingly, in the last Confidential Enquiry, one woman died where there was a very definite temporal association with the dexamethasone or betamethasone and her death, so much so that the assessors worried whether there was causality here.

I questioned several neurologists about antenatal steroids. They asked what was the minimum dose required to achieve fetal lung maturation. As that question was not answerable, they thought the doses were so massive anyway that doubling them was not an evidence-based thing to do. We do not actually do that.

Millward-Sadler: I would like to come back to this whole question of SUDEP. When I have been reviewing the autopsies, I have been very concerned that it has been a diagnosis of presumption and that very often other causes of sudden death, such as a fulminating case of pre-eclampsia, have not been adequately excluded. Also, it is very rare to have drug levels established at autopsy, to confirm whether or not there has been compliance, to add feedback to the general audit.

On an anecdotal basis, with regard to the comments about bathing, in the last year I personally have carried out two autopsies in epileptics who drowned. One was on a cruise, having a good time, and perhaps became a little too excited in the jacuzzi. The other was a gardener who happened to fall into a garden pool. This is a mode of death that is not specific to pregnancy, but we have the opportunity to target a particular group with specific advice about the risk.

Robinson: I would like to raise a question about a subgroup that may be at higher risk. When I was running a women's refuge, there were many women with epilepsy. When I was reviewing the literature, particularly looking at domestic violence in pregnancy, there were several stories of women in this group who had epilepsy and who had had previous head injuries from their violent partners. Therefore, among this non-compliant epileptic group, who do not come to appointments and do not comply with medication, there may be a small subgroup in which domestic violence is very much part of the picture.

Domestic violence is of course a chronic problem in women's lives, and not an acute problem. They are in and out of the refuge, going back to the same blokes and then coming back in again. They come from all social classes, as I am sure you are aware. It might be useful to bear that in mind. The original cause of the epilepsy may have been head injuries from domestic violence.

Nelson-Piercy: I would just highlight the *BMJ* editorial once again, which pointed out that you can fit after a single event of concussion and you can fit after a head injury. This does not mean to say that you have idiopathic epilepsy, so Ms Robinson is absolutely right. It may be that they do not have epilepsy at all – they may have had one isolated concussion and myoclonus, and been labelled as epileptic because that is a more socially acceptable term than 'a bang on the head'.

Hall: Did you look at perinatal mortality at all?

Nelson-Piercy: I think one study did,[2] but I did not use those data for this presentation. I do not think the perinatal mortality rate was any different – it was just the malformations. There were some terminations because of identifiable malformations and, if you take those out, the overall perinatal mortality rate is no different, in that one study in the UK. I am not 100% sure about that.

Oates: There is quite a large number of women in psychiatry who are receiving anticonvulsants as mood stabilisers. Many of these will become pregnant and they have a very high risk of recurrence following delivery. This is an issue that I do not think my colleagues in psychiatry are aware of. This is not just an issue of epilepsy.

The other point is that the risk of epilepsy – its rate and prevalence – among the psychiatric and learning disabled population is three or four times higher than in the general population, so psychiatric comorbidity is not an unusual occurrence with epilepsy. Do you find that you have to handle these problems on your own, or is this an area for specialists? We will have so many specialists coming out of this meeting that there will be no generalists left in the world, will there?

Nelson-Piercy: In my experience, we commonly encounter women on anti-epileptic drugs in the psychiatric population. Their management is very much by the psychiatrist in combination with the obstetrician at the moment. I do not become involved, other than to make some comments about congenital malformations. This is a group in whom it is particularly difficult to work out what, if anything, they wish to know about their risks, especially, as you rightly say, because they are not in a position where you would ever recommend stopping the drugs. If they were, the psychiatrist has usually thought of that beforehand. The alternative is lithium, which, as you say, probably has just as high a teratogenic risk as valproate and carbamazepine.

Marteau: I wonder if the pendulum is swinging too far now against giving risk information in a brutal way that increases anxiety, so that some people feel that it is better to say nothing. We should be very careful about the adverse effects of false reassurance. Are you aware of any evidence of the harm that women experience from being informed of the risks associated with epilepsy or indeed any of these conditions?

There is only a small amount of evidence that I am aware of, of the harm of people being falsely reassured – going through pregnancy, being told that everything is fine, and subsequently giving birth to a child with a fetal abnormality.

Nelson-Piercy: Do not misunderstand me – I am a complete advocate of pre-pregnancy counselling and, as Professor De Swiet mentioned, I am very directive. I give the information, even if it is not requested, because I feel that it is our duty as healthcare professionals to enable women to make an informed choice. I have previously been criticised for relaying this information at 14 or 15 weeks, because people say that is unfair, and that all I am doing is inducing anxiety.

I have anecdotal evidence of the results of my counselling, which is that when they go to Dr Bewley for their fetal medicine scan, they are halfway up the wall – according to her – because of what I have told them. I do not for one minute imagine that we do not induce a huge amount of anxiety. I have always been very wary of how I express things. Sometimes, you try your hardest, but you still upset the patient – but that does not mean that it was wrong to tell them.

The important issue for epilepsy is that, even if you have missed the boat for that pregnancy, that is the time when you give the pre-pregnancy counselling for the next pregnancy. That is the only time, often, that I have the chance to meet the patient, so I am often giving advice that is designed to help her to decide what to do in her next pregnancy – not this pregnancy. That is why I have included 'pregnancy' in my list of opportunities for pre-pregnancy counselling.

References

1. Hernandez-Diaz S, Werler MM, Walker AM, Mitchell AA. Folic acid antagonists during pregnancy and the risk of birth defects. *N Engl J Med* 2000;343:1608–14.
2. Fairgrieve SD, Jackson M, Jonas P, Walshaw D, White K, Montgomery TL, *et al*. Population based, prospective study of the care of women with epilepsy in pregnancy. *BMJ* 2000;321:674–5.

SECTION 7

PSYCHOLOGICAL MORBIDITY

Chapter 26

Post-traumatic stress disorder – a consumer view

Jean Robinson

One of the difficulties that lay groups have in communicating with professional audiences is that we use another language – one that has a different hinterland – so our meanings may be misunderstood. Our value to professionals, we hope, is that we bring raw data, unfiltered by researchers, which provides examples of the impact both of clinical care and of policies not only on individuals but on family and community life. As a pressure group with forty years' experience of watching maternity care, the Association for Improvements in the Maternity Services (AIMS) may have something to offer.

First I would like to take this opportunity on behalf of consumers to express our thanks to Dr Gwyneth Lewis and all who work on the Confidential Enquiries into Maternal Deaths (CEMD) and to let you know how grateful we are. Although AIMS members know of your reports from our quarterly journal, many women and their families are unaware of the work you do and how valuable it is. We have been particularly pleased to see the faster production of the reports in recent years and the increased effort put into disseminating the findings. We make criticisms, of course, because that is our job and naturally we want the Enquiries to be even better, but that does not detract from our recognition of their importance and value to us all.

There is still room for improvement. We have continually said that the missing factor is the parents' voice in infant deaths and that of the surviving family in cases of maternal death. This means that some essential threads of causality are missed. At present, the Enquiries work from records and statements of staff alone. We know, from contact with hundreds of families, especially since the Access to Health Records Act and the Data Protection Act, how inadequate the records alone are in putting together the full story of what contributes to both good and bad care.

We would stress that we are not trying to create a culture of blame. Our primary aim is to help families to achieve emotional resolution and, like them, we want identification of underlying causes. Our clients are more interested in truth and understanding than anything else and we find that this is what helps their recovery most. Indeed, they become distressed if they feel that individual staff members are being scapegoated. When we have occasionally suggested to bereaved families that they should send their story to one of the Confidential Enquiries – although there is no official niche for it – they have been enormously relieved. It is only excessive delay, dishonesty and cover-up that set up a cycle of bitterness and anger.

Post-traumatic stress reactions

To come to the nub of our concerns, AIMS is delighted that suicide is now identified as the leading cause of maternal death. We have been urging for many years that the CEMD should take more interest in this problem. Even so, the incidence is still underestimated because the Enquiries cover deaths only up to one year after delivery. We know that there are suicides related to childbirth beyond that time, and we are dealing with clients two or three years after a birth whom we believe to be at risk.

When women tell us about their preferences for place of birth and type of care, reducing their risk of psychiatric morbidity is often mentioned. This can be a primary reason for women choosing a home birth. While they are often criticised for such choices, which are sometimes seen by obstetricians as irresponsible and self-indulgent, in fact they have usually made their decisions with care. We provide information but also try to be as supportive as we can, since we know that stress in pregnancy may be linked to restricted fetal growth.[1]

Both AIMS and the National Childbirth Trust were alarmed by the recommendation by the latest CEMD that midwives should be prepared to decline responsibility for high-risk cases where the involvement of a consultant obstetrician is essential.[2] We are afraid that this recommendation could actually increase the risk of maternal death. We are seeing an increasing number of cases of women choosing to give birth alone if the local maternity unit refuses to provide a midwife. Such cases are increasing since NHS trusts have realised that, although they are required to provide maternity services, they are not legally compelled to do so in the home. Women, however, have the right to give birth anywhere they choose. When high-risk women tell AIMS that they would rather die than give birth in hospital again, lay supporters are left out on a limb. We now understand that the recommendation was inserted to give midwives confidence to challenge obstetricians' decisions when women had been referred back for community care inappropriately. That is understandable, but nothing was said about the woman's view.

The biggest disappointment for us is that, although depression and psychosis are mentioned in the latest CEMD report,[2] there is not a single reference in the chapter on deaths from psychiatric causes to post-traumatic stress disorder (PTSD). Yet, as a consumer group running a busy helpline, post-traumatic stress reactions and PTSD are the most common serious postnatal problem we encounter and we receive at least one new report a week.

We find that it is common for women to ruminate extensively about their experience of childbirth. They have been shown to retain vivid memories of such events for at least 20 years.[3] After listening to many women, we have found that good experiences, as well as bad, can set up echoes that reverberate down the years, increasing confidence and self-esteem, and that 'good' births can also be therapeutic. Damaging experiences, therefore, may not only be harmful in themselves, but may also mean the loss of the long-lasting benefits of these empowering birth experiences to families and society.

We first drew attention to birth trauma damage 17 years ago.[4] Our clients with these problems include doctors, health visitors, nurses and professional women from all walks of life, as well as the poorest and least articulate. The overwhelming majority of women who come to us in a suicidal state do not have postnatal depression alone, but have either severe post-traumatic stress reactions or PTSD. Every woman who tells us she has already attempted suicide has PTSD. What women describe may not meet the exact criteria in the Diagnostic and Statistical Manual IV (DSM IV) but nevertheless their condition is serious and disabling – and this difference in pattern of symptoms in postpartum cases from 'classic' PTSD has been confirmed in two prospective studies.[5,6]

It should not be thought that this is a problem that only women in developed countries have the luxury of worrying about. Descriptions of westernised birth care in Nepal[7] and Pakistan[8] suggest that damaging emotional effects might be exported as easily as active management of labour and episiotomies. Poor families, already under stress, need protection from trauma even more than the rich. This is a public health issue for us all.

Failures of diagnosis

Most women who come to us have not had their birth trauma diagnosed. If they are being treated, it is solely for postnatal depression, and we have clients two or three years after delivery, still on antidepressants, who have not moved on and may even be worse.

One researcher suggests that recognition of a stressor may depend as much upon social awareness and interpersonal qualities as clinical expertise. Professional practices are embedded within wider, value-laden cultural contexts, and this is evident in the traumas that are neglected. The literature also fails to include the social and political contexts within which trauma occurs, is recognised, defined and processed.[9]

We suggest four reasons for failures of diagnosis:

1. A lack of awareness on the part of GPs, health visitors, obstetricians and even non-specialist psychiatrists, of PTSD as a postpartum illness. The impression our clients are given is that since most women give birth without severe trauma, those who complain must be psychologically weak or at fault. Many are told by GPs, health visitors and even counsellors attached to general practice, they 'should be grateful for a healthy baby' – as one of our clients reported yet again only last week. There are, of course, some who have no live, or healthy, child.

2. The inadequacies of the widely used Edinburgh Postnatal Depression Scale, which fails to discriminate between depression and PTSD. We suspect that many suicide deaths attributed to postnatal depression were in fact precipitated by PTSD, which is known to have a high suicide risk. In fact, we also see cases of prolonged postnatal depression without apparent PTSD symptoms, where an element of birth trauma is involved.

3. The difficulties that health professionals have in listening to, understanding and believing birth stories that are critical of colleagues' behaviour. PTSD can only arise if there were events or behaviour that caused trauma, and the woman's account of what happened (often witnessed by her partner) can be painful to hear. Any complaints voiced are attributed to postnatal depression or the woman's inadequacy.

4. The shortage of psychiatrists and clinical psychologists who are knowledgeable about PTSD and experienced in treating it. It was a psychiatrist who told a pregnant woman with PTSD from her previous birth to go and visit the labour ward. She almost collapsed and we were able to help her obtain what she now insisted on – a home birth, which fortunately went well. Even those few

professionals who do treat PTSD, while experienced in treating members of the armed forces, police or accident victims, may not understand the crucial differences between their usual patients and postpartum cases.

Patterns of causation

The problem first came to our attention in the early 1970s, when induction of labour with oxytocin became common and in some units rose to 60% of births. As chairman of the Patients Association at the time, I received hundreds of letters about it,[10,11] and also studied those received by an agony aunt. Women who had previously given birth were describing a syndrome that I could only compare with the 'shell shock' I had read about in histories of the First World War, which proved to be prophetic. I telephoned mother and baby psychiatric units up and down the country and asked 'Have your mother and baby admissions gone up?' and always got the same reply: 'it's funny you should mention that…' But there were differences in the pattern of stories received from different areas. Women who had been cared for in high-tech units by midwives with long experience of giving individual care in home births were better supported and more likely to survive emotionally. What worried me was that with the decline of home births such experience would vanish and women would have a combination of a high-tech birth with a high-tech midwife. Increasingly, my colleagues and I at AIMS became interested not just in maternal morbidity but total family morbidity, and its obverse – promoting good family health, which remains our concern to this day.

We find that patterns of causation have changed as the pattern of obstetric and midwifery care has altered. Following the rise in induction complaints, we then saw more frequent mention of amniotomy (especially early amniotomy). Augmentation of labour with oxytocin and later induction with prostaglandins were often described as creating non-physiological patterns of labour and levels of pain that were very different from labours women had previously experienced. Although epidurals are now more widely used to control pain, when they do not work, or are not topped up appropriately, more problems can follow. A number of women with birth trauma have told us they had an epidural, which they had accepted only because they felt their chance of controlling birth interventions was nil. In our more recent cases, the ratio of midwifery-to-doctor incidents mentioned has increased. We suspect that changes in midwifery training, shortages of midwifery staff, pressures of work and management reluctance to pay for senior staff grading may be having adverse effects.

We virtually never see trauma cases that result from intervention alone. There is always an element of staff behaviour (or perceived behaviour).

It is not just treatment of the mother but also treatment of the child. Postnatal care, failure to treat mother and baby as a dyad, unnecessary removal of, prolonged separation from, or unwanted treatment of the newborn have also appeared in accounts relayed to us by women with PTSD.

Effects on the family

To describe how serious the effects may be would take longer than the space allowed for this chapter. We have recently commented on avoidance behaviour alone,[12] which may cause families to move to another area to avoid being near a certain hospital, or any hospital. One woman cannot go to the GP's surgery for fear of seeing a white coat or any medical equipment. None of the women can watch any medical television programme. One stopped going to a mothers' group because someone there had the same first name as a midwife she says was responsible; another has to leave a building or a bus if anyone is wearing the same perfume that a particular midwife wore.

We have not had reports of the increased violence reported in American military veterans with PTSD – with one exception. One woman was so angry with her husband that she actually stabbed him and spent the night in police custody. Although we make gentle enquiries about children, we have had not had reports of problems other than those common to postnatal depression and none of violence or serious threats of it. However, most mothers tell us that they worry about possible effects on their children. An Australian study refers to secondary damage to the partner.[7] We know of two families in which both parents have chronic PTSD, and suspect there may be more. One of those families is now worried about a child's behavioural problems at school. They have failed to obtain effective treatment, largely because of their location.

There is, understandably, a high marital breakdown rate. Husbands and partners are often unable to cope with the altered personality, so the sick woman is left to cope with the children. There may also be unique damage to the marriage itself in that the husband often feels guilty for not having intervened. It may be of some consolation when we mention that doctor husbands present have also felt helpless. Some wives tell us that they blame partners for not protecting them, even though they know this to be unfair. Women often also feel guilty for not having protected themselves and their babies.

Subsequent risks

Suicide is not the only risk to life. There may be increased risk in any subsequent pregnancy. Our requests for otherwise unnecessary elective caesarean sections come not from women who are 'too posh to push' but almost entirely from those who want to avoid a repetition of previous trauma – a problem also reported by researchers.[6,13] Each caesarean section increases the risk of placenta praevia, placenta accreta, ruptured uterus and emergency hysterectomy – hazards not only for the mother but for her future children.

There is another group of women, however, who choose home birth however great their risk. They tell us firmly that they would rather die than give birth in hospital again.

Other risks may arise from avoidance of future medical care, including a number of cases of failure to have investigation and treatment in women known to have abnormal cervical smears. Women may also avoid other medical encounters or premises.

Incidence

How common is postpartum PTSD? We are grateful to clinical psychologist Dr Susan Ayers of St George's Hospital Medical School, London, whose doctoral thesis describes a large 'prospective study measuring levels in pregnancy and postpartum'. At a London hospital, she found that 2.8% had PTSD at six weeks postpartum and 1.5% at six months[14] (this could be an underestimate as the 'questionnaire used is a conservative measuring tool, only women expecting normal births were included, and those whose babies died were excluded'). She estimates that her findings could mean 10 000 chronic cases arising annually in the UK. This figure does not, of course, cover shorter-term problems of traumatised women, which may still have serious effects.

Prevention

We differ from Ayers in her recommendation for primary prevention: 'identifying vulnerable women'. She suggests that they might be offered alternative birth procedures or have notes highlighted so that distressing procedures are avoided. This echoes the pattern of sympathetic care provided by obstetrician Helen Allott, which has no doubt been helpful to many women.[15] But whatever the consultant writes on the case notes, promises may not always be kept when a junior doctor is on duty at midnight, and we have seen a few double disasters.

We do not doubt that there are vulnerable women (especially those with a past history of sexual abuse) but we await evidence that they will all wish this to be recorded in notes or that labelling them will necessarily bring benefits. Would this be more effective than treating all women as individuals whose rights and preferences should be respected?

Some of our clients were at risk for other reasons – they have characteristics that some staff members found unattractive and that made them liable to be scapegoated (ethnicity, religion, social status and so on), of which we have seen many examples.[16] Our reports echo the higher than expected number of maternal deaths reported in the latest CEMD in socially excluded groups such as travellers, most of whom had received substandard care. We also receive reports of adverse treatment of women wanting normal births in a culture where this is not approved; at one hospital women providing birth plans have worse outcomes and it is suggested that the reason may be adverse reactions from staff.[17]

The AIMS view of true primary prevention is that actions and behaviour that cause PTSD should be identified and staff should be trained to avoid them. The videotaping of labour and birth now being studied by midwives would be an ideal training tool.

Accounts of women traumatised by emergency care could suggest how changes in staff behaviour before, during and after the event might reduce risk.[18,19] Our quarterly journal would provide many case histories, including one that led to litigation.[20]

As for secondary prevention, we remain sceptical about debriefing. We are concerned not merely about its unproven efficacy and possible adverse effects but also about ethical issues concerning its use as a tool of risk management, which so far have not been addressed.[21] We are also concerned about quality of care. Some of our clients have reported not only useless treatment but damage from both midwife counsellors and therapists attached to GP practices. This is not an area for dabblers – especially those who do not realise when they are getting out of their depth. What some in effect are doing is scraping the scar tissue from a deep wound (especially in those with a history of sexual abuse), finding that they cannot cope, failing to refer on and sending the patient away worse than before. Unfortunately, specialist psychologists and psychiatrists in this area are hard to find in the NHS and so far there are few reassuring data on long-term effectiveness of treatment. That is why prevention is particularly important.

Possible causes

We can only give an assessment based on our impressions from our workload. Level of damage seems to depend on a combination of the woman's vulnerability and the treatment she receives.

Although we do not ask intrusive questions of mothers, it is quite clear that some were more vulnerable than others – particularly those with a history of sexual abuse or previous traumatic births. If a woman says she wants only female staff, or only male staff, this should be respected. She will have a good reason. She may not wish to say why and should not be pressurised into telling. We suspect that some staff members may even see them as targets for abuse.[16]

Sometimes we ask women how they would describe themselves. It is sometimes helpful to have an idea of what a distressed woman was like before the damage occurred. They are usually frank and forthcoming: 'I always was a bit of a wimp', 'I'm the get-up-and-go-for-it type – nothing usually bothers me'. Our impression is that 'vulnerable' women may develop trauma problems after events or staff behaviour that is less likely to have such serious effects on some others. However, we are not prepared to see this develop into victim-blaming and agree with Davis that the potential for stigmatisation is heightened by a focus on individual predisposition.[9]

Since we hear and read hundreds of birth stories a year, the events and behaviour that these mothers describe are only too familiar to us and appear in accounts from others who were only mildly traumatised but are also distressed and angry, and often make formal complaints. They also appear in many research papers on causes of dissatisfaction with maternity care.[22] This suggests that reduction in behaviours that cause PTSD, even if only in the most vulnerable women, is also likely to reduce complaints to both health authorities and professional regulatory bodies, as well as litigation. Similarly, close attention to remedying causes of maternity complaints could reduce the incidence of PTSD.

Women who were severely traumatised complain later than others – typically their complaints arrive around three years after the event, when they feel able to write and describe what happened. Often they can only do this with extensive support and it can be a painful and lengthy process. This delay, of course, makes such complaints more difficult to investigate.

Women who appear to have been psychologically stronger initially are not invulnerable but tend to develop PTSD after events that are apparently more serious to an outsider, for example dramatic cases where lives were clearly at risk and urgent steps had to be taken. Such cases have also been described in Sweden.[23]

What is common to both groups, however, is that regardless of whether pain levels are high, or intervention such as forceps delivery is necessary, the behaviour of staff as described by the woman makes a major difference to the risk. If they are perceived as distant, cold, uncaring, unsympathetic or even cruel, this is associated with a greater likelihood of trauma. This includes body language, which can be of great importance, since labouring and birthing women are hypersensitive to the atmosphere around them.

Staff described in these accounts include not only midwives and obstetricians but also paediatricians and anaesthetists. Our impression from anecdotal evidence is backed by studies from both England and Sweden showing that negative impressions of staff are related to PTSD risk.[22,23] A study on unhappiness after childbirth found that it was related not to interventions *per se* but to interventions that women thought they should not have had.[22] It was to do with power and control. It was also related to the adequacy of information received and feeling of control over what staff were doing. Women who described staff as rushed or bossy had lower emotional wellbeing scores.

Often the picture presented is not of one major event but a series of incidents that prepare the ground by raising anxiety levels and gradually get worse. It is easy to see how both culture of the unit and excessive work levels for the staff could affect risk.

This raises the obvious question – is the woman's impression skewed or are the staff really insensitive or worse? We know that midwives have different patterns of behaviour, from warm and empathetic to distant and authoritarian,[24] so for the woman it is chance as to who is on duty – and many women report different attitudes as staff change shifts. AIMS also notices certain patterns in stories about certain units, and occasionally about certain members of staff. Each maternity unit has its own culture that seems very long-lasting and when the chairman and I share our latest cases, sometimes the listener will instantly identify where the woman had the baby. Our relief was great when a certain midwifery manager retired.

Another factor is lack of consent, and this also features in the findings of Menage[25] and Ryding *et al.*[26] What we find is not merely manipulated consent and lack of consent, but cases where specific refusal is ignored.[27] Once again, very similar accounts of staff behaviour appear in our complaints cases and in accounts of those of women who are traumatised either long- or short-term. Invasion of privacy and the sudden appearance of uninvited observers whom the woman is powerless to exclude are other components in our stories of multicausal damage and also feature in accounts of dissatisfaction with maternity care. We find that invasion of privacy is an increasing cause of complaint in twin births. Unwanted people being present was associated with a three-fold increase in dissatisfaction among multiparous women and two-fold in primiparous women in a large Australian study.[28] We have had a number of references to 'visual rape', especially when women are in the lithotomy position.

Risks of psychiatric records

Lastly I must mention our latest problem, which is rapidly increasing. The CEMD suggests that midwives should take and record psychiatric histories for all pregnant women. We share the concern that a history of postpartum psychosis, with its high risk of recurrence, was wrongly recorded as postnatal depression in the case notes of some maternal suicides, but we beg you to proceed cautiously on this. First, we know that women fear that such histories could adversely affect their care in pregnancy and labour, and we have considerable evidence that their fears can be justified. We are also afraid that some obstetricians may feel empowered to perform forced caesarean sections if the woman is classified as 'mentally ill'. Third, women fear adverse effects on future employment. Fourth – and most important of all – they increasingly fear the intervention of social workers and losing their children. This is no idle fear and such intervention has increased. The number of care orders has risen dramatically, without evidence of need.[29] We worked recently with two other organisations to help a mother with severe but curable postnatal depression to prevent her baby from being taken away and adopted. We had to accompany her every time the social worker called because each visit left her suicidal. I note that two suicides in the latest CEMD were apparently precipitated by mothers' fears of losing their children.[2] The Government's drive to increase adoption figures and to facilitate rapid adoptions is having horrendous effects when crudely interpreted by ill-trained social workers. Two of our families have had post-traumatic stress reactions as a result of needless social work invention, yet there seems little recognition of the potential danger in the sensitive period following birth. Too little attention is paid to the traumatogenic actions of official agencies.[9]

We now receive calls asking about the safety of St John's Wort (hypericum perforatum) for depression during pregnancy and breastfeeding. Women are choosing this herbal remedy because they can buy it over the counter at the health-food shop – they do not even have to go to a chemist – and there will be no entry on their case notes. While it has been shown to be an effective remedy for mild and moderate depression, we worry about women with serious and prolonged illness not receiving good medical care. Professionals underestimate the effectiveness of the community grapevine at dispersing information about lack of confidentiality in health records (especially now that they are linked with social services) and fears of child protection allegations. We ourselves are concerned at the lack of evidence of benefit for social work intervention[30] and our own growing experience of serious and prolonged damage to families when such interventions are made.[31]

A consumer wish-list

We at AIMS would not presume to tell the Royal College of Obstetricians and Gynaecologists what they should recommend, but we can say what we would like to see. Much of childbirth trauma is iatrogenic and could be avoided. Therefore we need:

1. A recognition that mental health outcomes are an essential component of maternity care and should be measured. We believe that some maternity units and styles of care offer greater mental safety than others but at present we cannot prove it.
2. Research on staff attitudes, behaviours and procedures that women describe as preceding the onset of post-traumatic stress reactions or PTSD.
3. Training of all staff and students who come into contact with labouring or newly delivered women on their sensitivity, as well as psychological and spiritual aspects of giving birth.
4. Adjustment of the Edinburgh postnatal depression scale to discriminate between depression and traumatic reactions.
5. Research on the differences between PTSD that follows childbirth and PTSD following exposure to battle, fire, accidents etc., on which most of the research is based.
6. Wider availability of specialist maternity psychiatric services, including mother and baby units.

References

1. Texeira J, Fisk N, Glover V. Association between maternal anxiety in pregnancy and increased uterine artery resistance index: cohort based study. *BMJ* 1999;318:153–6.
2. Drife J, Lewis G, editors. *Why Mothers Die 1997–99. The Confidential Enquiries into Maternal Deaths in the United Kingdom.* London: RCOG Press; 2001. p. 13.
3. Simkin P. Just another day in a woman's life? Part II: Nature and consistency of women's long-term memories of their first birth experiences *Birth* 1992;19:64–81.
4. Beech B, Robinson J. Nightmares following childbirth. *Br J Psychol* 1985;147:586.
5. Ayers S. Post-traumatic stress disorder following childbirth [PhD thesis]. London: University of London; 1999.
6. Creedy DK, Shochet IM, Horsfall J. Childbirth and the development of acute trauma symptoms: incidence and contributing factors. *Birth* 2000;27:104–11.
7. Carla B. A questionable legacy: hospital birth in Nepal. *Br J Midwifery* 2001;9:103–6.
8. Brady M, Shotton E. Midwifery in Sahiwal, Punjab, Pakistan. *Br J Midwifery* 1995;3:387–90.
9. Davis H. The psychiatrization of post-traumatic distress: issues for social workers. *Br J Social Work* 1999;29:755–7.
10. Robinson J. Elective induction of labour. *Lancet* 1975;1:1088.
11. Robinson J. Why mothers fought obstetricians. *Br J Midwifery* 1995;3:557–8.
12. Robinson J. Post-traumatic stress disorder: avoidance behaviour. *Br J Midwifery* 2001;9:775.
13. Ryding E. Investigation of 33 women who demanded a cesarean section for personal reasons *Acta Obstet Gynecol Scand* 1993;72:280–5.
14. Ayers S, Pickering A. Do women get posttraumatic stress disorder as a result of childbirth? A prospective study of incidence. *Birth* 2001;28:111–18.
15. Allott H. Picking up the pieces: the post-delivery stress clinic. *Br J Midwifery* 1996;4:534–6.
16. Robinson J. Scapegoats. *Br J Midwifery* 2002;10:278.
17. Jones MH, Barik S, Mangune H, Jones P, Gregory SJ, Spring JE. Do birth plans adversely affect the outcome of labour? *Br J Midwifery* 1998;6:38–41.
18. Williams S. Post-traumatic stress: a personal experience. *Br J Midwifery* 1996;4:528–30.
19. Robinson J. Do a caesarean and I'll sue! *Br J Midwifery* 1997;5:502.
20. Spear C. A legal precedence. *AIMS Journal* 1997;9:15–18.
21. Robinson J. Dangers of debriefing. *Br J Midwifery* 1998;6:251.
22. Green J, Coupland V, Kitzinger J. *Great Expectations: A Prospective Study of Women's Expectations and Experience of Childbirth.* Hale, Cheshire: Books for Midwives; 1998.
23. Ryding E, Wijma K, Wijma B. Post traumatic stress reactions after emergency cesarean section. *Acta Obstet Gynecol Scand* 1997;76:856–61.
24. Menage J. Post traumatic stress disorder in women who have undergone obstetric and/or gynaecological procedures. *J Reprod Infant Psychol* 1993;11:221–8
25. Ryding E, Wijma K, Wijma B. Predisposing psychological factors for post-traumatic stress reactions after emergency cesarean section. *Acta Obstet Gynecol Scand* 1998;77:351–2.
26. McCrea BH, Wright ME, Murphy-Black T. Differences in midwives' approaches to pain relief in labour. *Midwifery* 1998 14:174–80.
27. Robinson J. Intimate examinations: the complexities of consent. *Br J Midwifery* 2001;9:708–9.
28. Brown S, Lumley J. Satisfaction with care in labor and birth: a survey of 790 Australian women. *Birth* 1994;21:4–13.
29. Beckett C. Critical commentary: the great care proceedings explosion. *Br J Social Work* 2001;31: 493–501.
30. Macdonald G. Social work: beyond control? In: Maynard A, Chalmers I, editors. *Non-random Reflections on Health Services Research.* London: BMJ Publishing Group; 1997. p. 122–46.
31. AIMS Evidence submitted to the Climbié Enquiry. March 2002. Association for Improvements in the Maternity Services, Surbiton.

Chapter 27

Adverse psychological outcomes of care in pregnancy: the role of health professionals

Theresa M Marteau and Esther Maissi

Introduction

The aim of antenatal care is to provide medical care and psychological support to help parents have healthy babies while keeping the risks of adverse maternal outcomes, including death, to a minimum. While many parents achieve such outcomes, some experience adverse psychological outcomes that, in part, stem from a failure of this care. The most frequently documented psychological problems in pregnancy stem from extreme responses to the uncertainty inherent in the outcomes of pregnancy, reflecting either an excessive concern with fetal wellbeing or giving birth or the converse, a belief that a healthy child and an uneventful labour are certain outcomes of the pregnancy. This chapter focuses upon these most frequently documented adverse psychological outcomes of pregnancy care and considers the role that health professionals may play both in contributing to these and in preventing or minimising them. The first part of this chapter considers how health professionals' behaviour can influence these outcomes, for worse and for better. Effective and sensitive communication is identified as the main way of achieving the latter. The second part of the chapter considers the causes of ineffective communication and how these might be overcome. The final section considers the central uncertainties that need researching to ensure that policies in this area can become strongly evidence-based in the near future.

Anxiety in pregnancy

Much of the anxiety experienced by women during pregnancy reflects fears surrounding the wellbeing of the fetus and giving birth.[1–3] Some of this concern is appropriate. About one to two percent of fetuses have significant developmental or health problems. In addition, childbirth itself is accompanied by a small risk of death for both mother and child. For some women, however, concern about these possibilities can result in extremely high levels of anxiety, leading sometimes to clinical states of anxiety or depression.

While uncertainty remains over the extent to which sustained, high levels of anxiety affect clinical outcomes in pregnancy, they are certainly associated with preterm delivery,[4] longer labour[5] and a higher rate of complications during labour.[6] Such anxiety levels also have the potential to adversely affect a mother's relationship with her baby,[7] as well as to increase her vulnerability to clinical levels of anxiety and depression postpartum.

This section considers first the anxiety associated with fetal abnormalities and then the anxiety associated with childbirth.

Anxiety associated with fetal abnormality

Raised general levels of anxiety and specific concerns have most often been documented in women who are informed that they have an increased risk of having a baby with a fetal abnormality. This may follow serum screening for Down syndrome,[8] the detection of soft markers on ultrasound examination,[9] identification of parents as carriers for cystic fibrosis[10] and diagnosis of gestational diabetes.[11] It may also follow from comments made during routine clinical examinations expressing, for example, uncertainty about the rate of fetal growth. When tests reveal an increased risk of a problem, anxiety often returns to normal levels following further testing in which no abnormality is revealed.[12,13] This, however, is not always the case: for some women, anxiety and concerns remain even after the birth of an unaffected child.[13,14]

A small proportion of those undergoing diagnostic testing will receive an abnormal test result. This news is invariably received with shock and distress, as is evident in vivid personal accounts from women who have been in this situation.[15,16] These levels of distress dissipate, although there is wide variability in how rapidly this occurs. While knowing about an abnormality during pregnancy is associated with shock and distress, it can also facilitate adjustment to the birth of an affected child for parents who decide to continue with the affected pregnancy. For example, parents given an antenatal diagnosis of a cleft lip and palate felt prepared for the birth and were more satisfied with their counselling than those for whom the diagnosis was made postnatally.[17]

Preventing anxiety associated with providing risk information

The way in which people respond to any situation depends on its characteristics, as well as what they bring to it by way of coping resources.[18] Responses to risk information in pregnancy are thus a function of the information that a woman is given and of the emotional support that she receives from health professionals providing her care, as well as her own emotional and social resources. Pregnant women may be particularly sensitised to threatening information, as part of a biological preparedness for protecting the fetus,[19] thus making them highly responsive to information that to others may seem completely benign. This suggests that the way in which risk information is presented has the potential for great harm as well as great benefit for pregnant women compared with non-pregnant populations.

Experimental studies from screening conducted outside of antenatal care suggest how some of the high anxiety levels arising from detection of increased health risks may be prevented or reduced by provision of detailed information about their meaning when giving test results.[20] There is, however, no experimental evidence to show that anxiety following identification of increased risk is avoided if pre-test knowledge is high. A survey of ultrasonographers identified that the main factor causing difficulties to them when giving bad news was that the patient was not expecting it.[21] Views, however, are divided as to whether it is appropriate to spend resources and risk worrying many pregnant women by preparing them all for an adverse outcome that would affect only a few.[21,22] Good experimental evidence is needed to inform this debate.

Despite the absence of such evidence, reflecting the evidence that exists on the positive clinical and psychological outcomes of preparation for surgery,[23] as well as ethical guidelines that emphasise the importance of informed consent, there is a consensus that women do need to be informed about the pros and cons of all procedures, including screening, before deciding whether to undergo them.[24,25] There is, however, no consensus or evidence as to how such information should be presented in order to achieve informed choices. There is little evidence concerning the relative effectiveness of different numerical or verbal expressions in communicating uncertainty and facilitating decision-making in healthcare contexts.[26] Among numerical expressions, understanding of chance is enhanced when it is presented using frequencies rather than probabilities.[27] While decisions are affected by whether chance is presented in terms of absolute or relative risks,[26,28,29] the impact of these different expressions of chance upon understanding and subsequent anxiety has not been studied.

The medium in which information before testing is most effectively conveyed has been the focus of several studies in antenatal care. Experimental studies have been conducted to evaluate the effectiveness of leaflets compared with videos[30,31] and interactive software,[32] as well as individual consultations compared with group sessions.[30,33] The aims of these studies have varied and have included increasing knowledge[31,32] and informed choice[34] and reducing anxiety.[30,33] The results of these studies have been equivocal. Generally, well-written leaflets have been found to be as effective as more complex technologies.[30,32]

There has been little research on the impact of information given face-to-face in consultations. Such information is sometimes inaccurate[35] and sometimes partial, directing women towards interventions in pregnancy.[35,36] Evidence that information given by health professionals may have far greater impact than information presented in other media appears in a small descriptive study of women informed of a soft marker detected during a routine anomaly scan. Analyses of tape-recordings of these scans showed that women told during the scan that the baby would probably be all right were significantly less anxious and worried about their babies than those not told this.[37] Experimental studies are now needed to determine the causal link between providing reassurance and reducing anxiety and to ensure that this does not undermine adjustment in the two to six percent of parents for whom a soft marker is indicative of a chromosome abnormality in the baby.[38]

Perhaps one of the most important aspects of care provided after identification of increased risk or the diagnosis of a fetal abnormality is the provision of full and accurate information about the condition diagnosed and the range of options available. The information given at this stage is regrettably sometimes incomplete or inaccurate. This seems to be particularly the case following the diagnosis of less common conditions. Interviews with parents after they had been informed of a diagnosis of a sex chromosome anomaly, following diagnostic testing for Down syndrome, revealed enormous parental distress at the diagnosis by health professionals ignorant of the condition.[39] Given that such information seems to influence parents' decisions about whether to terminate an affected pregnancy,[40–42] it is vital to invest greater effort in training health professionals in how to provide full and accurate information about the conditions for which testing is available.

In summary, the limited evidence to date suggests no evidently superior medium for informing women about the myriad of tests that they will be offered during pregnancy. More important is the service within which they are incorporated. Thus, while written information was as effective as interactive software in one hospital, in a series of other hospitals, written information was ineffective at helping women to make informed choices. This suggests that antenatal clinics do not have to invest in expensive technologies to impart information. Rather, the investment needs to be made in the health professionals providing the services, in particular training them to provide information in an effective and sensitive manner, as discussed in the final section of this chapter.

Fear of childbirth

While fear of childbirth is common, it is estimated that for around six to ten percent of pregnant women these fears are extreme and, in their most extreme form, result in tokophobia, a phobic avoidance of childbirth.[43,44] Those with a form of this condition who become pregnant may then request a caesarean section, and there are poor outcomes for women denied this.[43] For some women, no cause is evident, for some it follows a traumatic delivery and for others it is a symptom of depression. Strong fear of birth is more common in women with high levels of general anxiety and lack of social support, particularly from partners.[5]

Reducing fear of childbirth

Many women fear childbirth. In recognition of this, antenatal classes, with their focus on preparation for birth, have become incorporated into routine care in the UK and elsewhere. However, there is little evidence showing that participation in these classes either reduces distress or increases satisfaction with labour.[45] Continuity of care and community-based care have been found in randomised trials to improve women's satisfaction with the birth,[46] as well as to result in fewer adverse maternal and neonatal outcomes,[47,48] including lower caesarean rates.[49] It is unclear which aspects of continuity of care or community-based care are essential in producing these effects.[50]

While such practices may achieve their effects in part by reducing fear of childbirth, more intensive interventions are probably required for pregnant women who suffer from extreme fear of labour. The one experimental study conducted to date showed an advantage of five as opposed to two sessions of anxiety management for reducing anxiety about birth, as well as for reducing the amount of time in labour.[5] It did not, however, reduce the rate of caesarean deliveries, which were a minority in both groups, suggesting that the less intensive intervention may be an effective one. These results are consistent with descriptive studies in those areas that find psychological interventions or support are associated with improved clinical and psychological outcomes in women fearing childbirth. Bewley and Cockburn[51] suggest that, in the light of current evidence, optimal outcomes for such women involve early detection of such a fear and prompt referral for anxiety management.

False reassurance

For more than two decades, anxiety was considered the most common problem to arise from antenatal care. There is, however, growing recognition of the problems arising from false reassurance in pregnancy; that is, the belief that a healthy child is a certain outcome. Estimates of how common false reassurance is varies from over 50% of women being falsely reassured about screening tests to fewer than 6%.[52–54] We are unaware of any research documenting the frequency of false reassurance about labour or its adverse effects. There is some evidence that false negative results may have had a large legal impact based on reports in the UK and the USA, largely stemming from a failure of those running such programmes to ensure that participants understood the residual risks inherent in a low-risk or negative test result.[55]

Awareness in pregnancy of residual risks of adverse outcomes may facilitate subsequent adjustment to the birth of a child with a disability. Evidence to support this comes from a retrospective study of parents with children with Down syndrome. The parents' adjustment to having a child with Down syndrome appeared to be slightly undermined for those in whom screening had failed to detect the affected child, compared with adjustment of parents either not offered or who declined testing.[56] Overall, parents adjusted well to having a child with Down syndrome, regardless of screening history. However, compared with mothers who had declined screening, mothers who had received a false negative result on screening had more negative attitudes towards their children, while the fathers reported higher levels of parenting stress. Twenty-eight percent of parents receiving a false negative result (compared with 13% of parents not offered testing and none of those declining testing) blamed health professionals or the healthcare system in general for the birth of their affected child. Such blame often reflected unrealistic expectations of screening resulting in false reassurance following a negative or low-risk result.

Preventing false reassurance

False reassurance stems largely from unrealistic expectations of screening and the failure of those providing screening programmes to provide information to alter these expectations.[57] There is wide variation in the reporting of normal or low-risk results,[58] with a few centres not reporting such results at all. When they are reported, the terms used to convey their meaning range across a variety of verbal and numerical expressions. The one experimental study in this area found that using a number to convey residual risks was more effective than just using the term 'low-risk'.[52] There is growing evidence from a number of areas that such numbers are most effectively presented using natural frequencies rather than proportions or percentages.[27,59,60] Thus, the women were more likely to understand the probability that a pregnancy was affected by Down syndrome when it was presented as a frequency (8.9/1000) than as a proportion (one in 112).[60]

It is possible that understanding the residual risk inherent in a negative test result before undergoing one may also increase the likelihood that women are not falsely reassured once they receive such a test result.

Targeting women vulnerable to adverse psychological outcomes in pregnancy

Some women are particularly vulnerable to anxiety in pregnancy, either in response to learning about increased risks of fetal abnormality or in anticipation of labour. These include women with high levels of general anxiety or depression[61] and those with low levels of social support.[5,40] Women with low levels of education know least about the antenatal care they are offered,[31,52] which makes them vulnerable to anxiety and false reassurance born of inappropriate expectations of their care. Identifying these vulnerable women and providing them with information in a form that they understand, as well as emotional and social support, is likely to be an efficient use of antenatal care resources.

Achieving sensitive and effective communication

As discussed above, experimental and descriptive studies conducted in antenatal care and elsewhere suggest that anxiety and false reassurance in pregnancy may be prevented or minimised by sensitive and effective communication. The evidence for this, however, is still quite weak, reflecting an absence of evidence rather than evidence of absence of effect. While evidence is gained concerning the precise ways in which different types of communication and support are effective for achieving different outcomes, there is a growing consensus that communication between healthcare professionals and pregnant women could be improved. Before considering how this might be achieved, it may be instructive to consider some of the barriers to effective communication.

Understanding ineffective communication

There are several barriers to achieving effective communication. These include time, as well as a range of beliefs and attitudes held by health professionals as to the consequences of communication and their own skills.

Time

In antenatal care, there have been many calls for more time to be made available for listening to women and explaining care to them, particularly in the context of technological developments.[8,21,22] There is now good evidence from primary care that longer consultations are associated with better clinical and psychological outcomes for patients.[62] Such evidence is now needed for antenatal care.

Beliefs about communication

There is evidence of negative attitudes among obstetricians and midwives towards communicating fully with women about different aspects of their antenatal care. These attitudes stem, in part, from a fear that presenting options fully may result in women selecting options that could expose the health professional to a risk of litigation, particularly when the option selected is a non-interventionist one.[63] Other attitudes that may undermine effective communication relate to the value health professionals place on communicating with patients. Research into medical students' communication skills showed that those selecting hospital-based specialties as opposed to general practice gave lower ratings to the relevance of communication skills to the practice of medicine.[64] Placing a low value on communicating with patients may stem from a lack of awareness of the positive impact that such communication may have upon clinical as well as psychological outcomes. A further barrier to improving communication with pregnant women may be a misplaced confidence in existing communication skills. This same study of medical students referred to above provided evidence that students with poorer communication skills had the greatest confidence in their ability to communicate effectively, a confidence–competence gap also documented for resuscitation skills in physicians.[65]

Towards effective communication

Achieving effective communication requires interventions on several different levels, within written protocols and training.

Written protocols

As part of developing written protocols, it is necessary to identify the multidisciplinary team involved in providing different components of antenatal care, to ensure that the protocols fully reflect their perspectives. For example, in relation to prenatal screening programmes, it is important to involve paediatricians as well as obstetricians, and clergy as well as counsellors.[66] In relation to fear of childbirth, it is important to identify clinical psychologists and psychiatrists with skills in managing tokophobia, as well as anxiety and depression in pregnant women.

Training

All health professionals involved in providing antenatal care require some general training in communication skills, as well as specific training in the presentation of risk information. Such training is currently neither mandatory nor evidence-based. Training in general communication skills involves teaching active listening, as well as skills in presenting complex information. While such training is not aimed at turning antenatal staff into psychotherapists,[67] it should be aimed at providing some basic counselling skills, essential for any clinical work. There is some evidence that it is more effective if it involves personalised feedback of skills.[68,69] Feedback is particularly important in reducing the gap between confidence to communicate effectively and actual ability to do so. Training in communication needs to be mandatory for, without this, those failing to attend are those who are the least skilled communicators.[70]

As well as these basic communication skills, such training needs to address health professionals' beliefs about the consequences of their communication with pregnant women. It needs to recognise tensions that health professionals experience in providing risk information,[22] as well as negative attitudes towards giving risk information.[63,71] Such training also needs to incorporate ways of responding to requests for non-medically indicated caesarean sections arising from fears of vaginal deliveries.[51]

As part of continuing training and support, it is important that clinical staff at all grades are provided with expert support, comprising both clinical and psychological expertise. This may take the form of regular groups, jointly facilitated by outsiders with the appropriate expertise.

Costing time

The amount of time required to counsel patients about the care that they are offered is rarely included in estimates of their true costs. This raises the question of why time is discounted in this way. As evidence of the adverse psychological, clinical and economic consequences of poor communication accumulates, so the need to cost time, a necessary resource for effective communication, may be recognised.

Evidence gaps

Two core questions could readily provide the basis for research over the next ten years aimed at preventing adverse psychological outcomes of antenatal care:

1. How is uncertainty about the wellbeing of the fetus, the pregnancy and the birth most effectively provided to all women, to minimise anxiety and false reassurance, as well as to facilitate informed choices?
2. What are the most effective ways of managing clinical levels of anxiety concerning fetal wellbeing and childbirth?

One aspect of the first question where evidence is lacking concerns the differential effectiveness of interventions across literacy levels and cultural groups. About 20% of the UK population is functionally illiterate. Indeed, some people speak languages for which there is no written form. Women with lower levels of education know less about prenatal screening tests and are more likely to be falsely reassured following prenatal screening,[31,52] which partly reflects the ineffectiveness of current methods of conveying information. Interventions that can be effective for all women need to be designed, and studies need to have sufficient statistical power to detect subgroup effects.

More evidence is needed as to the most effective ways of communicating about the conditions detected during pregnancy.[72] Evidence from descriptive studies suggests that the way in which such information is conveyed has a significant influence on whether or not pregnancies are terminated.[40–42] There are no data regarding the emotional consequences of the decisions made following different information about the condition diagnosed.

More experimental evidence is needed as to the most effective ways of managing women with high levels of fear about childbirth.[51] Such management involves effective screening, as well as effective interventions. Information, support and cognitively based anxiety management techniques were each included in the one trial reporting to date. This trial needs repeating in other centres, and the precise nature of the components and their relative contribution to success needs to be delineated. The roles of midwives and obstetricians, as well as the mental health specialisms of clinical psychologists and psychiatrists, also need to be determined.

Conclusion

While the health outcomes for everyone, including pregnant women, are better than ever before, concern over risks is more acute than ever before, a paradox inherent in the 'risk society', as well as the generation of uncertainty as opposed to certainty that accompanies scientific knowledge.[73,74] Placed in this cultural context, there is some evidence that excessive concern in pregnant women can be mitigated by the way in which care is provided. Similarly, false reassurance, which feeds into an increasingly litigious society, can be reduced or avoided by the way in which information is given. There are several significant barriers to achieving effective and sensitive communication at all stages of antenatal care, including insufficient time to communicate with women, as well as the attitudes of health professionals towards their communication skills and the impact of effective communication. While few would dispute the need for resources to ensure that any medical or surgical interventions offered are reliable and clinically safe, a consensus is less evident concerning the need for resources to ensure that the care provided is psychologically safe.

The words selected to communicate about the uncertainties inherent in pregnancy and childbirth have immense power. Their power both to harm and to prevent harm are frequently underestimated. Acknowledgement of this should form the basis for ensuring that those charged with providing antenatal care are trained in listening to patient concerns and communicating uncertainty in a sensitive and effective manner.

Acknowledgements

Theresa Marteau is funded by the Wellcome Trust. We are grateful to Susan Bewley and Lyn Chitty for comments on an earlier draft of this manuscript.

References

1. Royal College of Midwives. *Preparation for Parenthood*. Taunton: Barnicotts Ltd; 1966.
2. Yali AM, Lobel M. Coping and distress in pregnancy: an investigation of medically high risk women. *J Psychosom Obstet Gynaecol* 1999;20:39–52.
3. Melender HL, Lauri S. Fears associated with pregnancy and childbirth – experiences of women who have recently given birth. *Midwifery* 1999;15:177–82.
4. Austin MP, Leader L. Maternal stress and obstetric and infant outcomes: epidemiological findings and neuroendocrine mechanisms. *Aust N Z J Obstet Gynaecol* 2000;40:331–7.
5. Saisto T, Salmela-Aro K, Nurmi JE, Kononen T, Halmesmaki E. A randomized controlled trial of intervention in fear of childbirth. *Obstet Gynecol* 2001;98:820–6.
6. Da Costa D, Dritsa M, Larouche J, Brender W. Psychosocial predictors of labor/delivery complications and infant birth weight: a prospective multivariate study. *J Psychosom Obstet Gynaecol* 2000;21:137–48.
7. Reading AE, Cox DN, Sledmere CM, Campbell S. Psychological changes over the course of pregnancy: a study of attitude towards the fetus/neonate. *Health Psychol* 1984;3:211–21.
8. Green JM. Serum screening for Down's syndrome: experiences of obstetricians in England and

Wales. *BMJ* 1994;309:769–72.
9. Baillie C, Hewison J, Mason G. The psychological costs of screening for aneuploidy by ultrasonography and maternal serum screening. *Br J Obstet Gynaecol* 1998;105 Suppl 17:26.
10. Miedzybrodzka Z, Hall M, Mollison J, Templeton A, Russell I, Dean J, *et al.* Antenatal screening for carriers of cystic fibrosis: randomised trial of step-wise vs. couple screening. *BMJ* 1995;310:353–7.
11. Kerbel D, Glazier R, Holzapfel S, Young M, Lofsky S. Adverse effects of screening for gestational diabetes: a prospective cohort study in Toronto, Canada. *J Med Screen* 1997;4:128–32.
12. Beeson D, Golbus MS. Anxiety engendered by amniocentesis. *Birth Defects Orig Artic Ser* 1979;15:191–7.
13. Marteau TM, Johnston M, Shaw RW, Michie S, Kidd J, New M. The impact of prenatal screening and diagnostic testing upon the cognitions, emotions and behaviour of pregnant women. *J Psychosom Res* 1989;33:7–16.
14. Griffiths MD, Gough MH. Dilemmas after ultrasonic diagnosis of fetal abnormality. *Lancet* 1985;1:623–4.
15. Statham H. Cold comfort. *The Guardian* 1987;12 March:26.
16. Brown J. The choice: a piece of my mind. *JAMA* 1989;262:2735.
17. Davalbhakta A, Hall PN. The impact of antenatal diagnosis of the effectiveness and timing of counselling for cleft lip and palate. *Br J Plast Surg* 2000:53:298–301.
18. Mischel W. Toward a cognitive social learning reconceptualization of personality. *Psychol Rev* 1973;80:252–83.
19. McNally RJ. Preparedness and phobias: a review. *Psychol Bull* 1987;101:283–303.
20. Shaw C, Abrams K, Marteau TM. Psychological impact of predicting individuals' risk of illness: a systematic review. *Soc Sci Med* 1999;49:1571–98.
21. Simpson R, Bor R. 'I'm not picking up a heart-beat': Experiences of sonographers giving bad news to women during ultrasound scans. *Br J Med Psychol* 2001;74:255–72.
22. Williams C, Alderson P, Farsides B. Dilemmas encountered by health practitioners offering nuchal translucency screening: a qualitative case study. *Prenat Diagn* 2002;22:216–20.
23. Johnston M, Vogele C. Benefits of psychological preparation for surgery: a meta-analysis. *Ann Behav Med* 1993;15:245–56.
24. General Medical Council. *Seeking Patients' Consent: The Ethical Considerations*. London: GMC; 1999.
25. Andrews LB, Fullarton JE, Holtzman NA, Motulsky AG, editors. *Assessing Genetic Risks: Implications for Health and Social Policy*. Washington DC: National Academy Press; 1994.
26. Edwards A, Elwyn G, Covey J, Matthews E, Pill R. Presenting risk information – a review of the effects of 'framing' and other manipulations on patient outcomes. *J Health Commun* 2001;6:61–82.
27. Gigerenzer G, Hoffrage U. How to improve Bayesian reasoning without instruction: frequency formats. *Psychol Rev* 1995;102:684–704.
28. Misselbrook D, Armstrong D. Patients' response to risk information about the benefits of treating hypertension. *Br J Gen Pract* 2001;51:276–9.
29. Nexoe J, Gyrd-Hansen D, Kragstrup J, Kristiansen IS, Nielsen JB. Danish GPs' perception of disease risk and benefit of prevention. *Fam Pract* 2002;19:3–6.
30. Michie S, Smith D, McClennan A, Marteau TM. Patient decision-making: an evaluation of two different methods of presenting information about a screening test. *British Journal of Health Psychology* 1997;2:317–26.
31. Hewison J, Cuckle H, Baillie C, Sehmi I, Lindow S, Jackson F, Batty J. Use of videotapes for viewing at home to inform choice in Down syndrome screening: a randomised controlled trial. *Prenat Diagn* 2001;21:146–9.
32. Graham W, Smith P, Kamal A, Fitzmaurice A, Smith N, Hamilton N. Randomised controlled trial comparing effectiveness of touch screen system with leaflet for providing women with information on prenatal tests. *BMJ* 2000;320:155–60.
33. Thornton J, Hewison J, Lilford RL. Vail A. A randomised trial of three methods of giving information about prenatal testing. *BMJ* 1995;311:1127–30.
34. O'Cathain A, Walters SJ, Nicholl JP, Thomas KJ, Kirkham M. Use of evidence based leaflets to promote informed choice in maternity care: randomised controlled trial in everyday practice. *BMJ* 2002;324:643.
35. Marteau TM, Slack J, Kidd J, Shaw RW. Presenting a routine screening test in antenatal care: Practice observed. *Public Health* 1992;106:131–41.
36. Royal College of Obstetricians and Gynaecologists. Clinical Effectiveness Support Unit. *National Sentinel Caesarean Section Audit Report*. London: RCOG Press; 2001.
37. Watson MS, Hall S, Langford K, Marteau TM. Psychological impact of the detection of soft markers

on routine ultrasound scanning: a pilot study investigating the modifying role of information. *Prenat Diagn* 2002;22:569–75.

38. Chitty LS. Ultrasound screening for fetal abnormalities. *Prenat Diagn* 1995;15:1241–57.
39. Abramsky L, Hall S, Levitan J, Marteau TM. What parents are told after prenatal diagnosis of a sex chromosome abnormality: interview and questionnaire study. *BMJ* 2001;322:463–6.
40. Robinson JO, Hibbard BM, Laurence KM. Anxiety during a crisis: emotional effects of screening for neural tube defects. *J Psychosom Res* 1984;28:163–9.
41. Holmes-Siedle MN, Rynanen M, Lindenbaum RH. Parental decisions regarding termination of pregnancy following prenatal detection of sex chromosome abnormality. *Prenat Diagn* 1987;7:239–44.
42. Marteau TM, Nippert I, Hall S, Limbert C, Reid M, Bobrow M, *et al.* Outcomes of pregnancies diagnosed with Klinefelter syndrome: the possible influence of health professionals. *Prenat Diagn* 2002;22:562–6.
43. Hofberg K, Brockington IF. Tokophobia: an unreasoning dread of childbirth. *Br J Psychiatry* 2000;176:83–5.
44. Jolly J, Walker J, Bhabra K. Subsequent obstetric performance related to primary mode of delivery. *Br J Obstet Gynaecol* 1999;106:227–32.
45. Spiby H, Henderson B, Slade P, Escott D, Fraser RB. Strategies for coping with labour: does antenatal education translate into practice? *J Adv Nurs* 1999;29:388–94.
46. Waldenstrom U, Brown S, McLachlan H, Forster D, Brennecke S. Does team midwife care increase satisfaction with antenatal, intrapartum, and postpartum care? A randomized controlled trial. *Birth* 2000;27:156–67.
47. Rowley MJ, Hensley MJ, Brinsmead MW, Wlodarczyk JH. Continuity of care by a midwife team versus routine care during pregnancy and birth – a randomized trial. *Med J Aust* 1995;163:289–93.
48. Biro MA, Waldenstrom U, Pannifex JH. Team midwifery care in a tertiary level obstetric service: a randomized controlled trial. *Birth* 2000:27:168–73.
49. Homer CSE, Davies GJ, Brodie PM, Sheehan A, Barcley LM, Wills J, *et al.* Collaboration in maternity care: a randomised controlled trial comparing community-based continuity of care with standard hospital care. *BJOG* 2001;108:16–22.
50. Johanson R, Newburn M, Macfarlane A. Has the medicalisation of childbirth gone too far? *BMJ* 2002;324:892–5.
51. Bewley S, Cockburn J. Responding to fear of childbirth. *Lancet* 2002;359:2128–9.
52. Marteau TM, Saidi G, Goodburn S, Lawton J, Michie S, Bobrow M. Numbers or words? A randomised controlled trial of presenting screen negative results to pregnant women. *Prenat Diagn* 2000;20:714–18.
53. Smith DK, Shaw RW, Marteau TM. Informed consent to undergo serum screening for Down syndrome: the gap between policy and practice. *BMJ* 1994;309:776.
54. Whynes DK. Receipts of information and women's attitudes towards ultrasound scanning during pregnancy. *Ultrasound Obstet Gynecol* 2002;19:7–12.
55. Petticrew MP, Sowden AJ, Lister-Sharp D, Wright K. False-negative results in screening programmes: systematic review of impact and implications. *Health Technol Assess* 2000;4:1–120.
56. Hall S, Bobrow M, Marteau TM. Psychological consequences for parents of false negative results on prenatal screening for Down's syndrome: retrospective interview study. *BMJ* 2000;320:407–12.
57. Cockburn J, Redman S, Hill D, Henry E. Public understanding of medical screening. *J Med Screen* 1995;2:224–7.
58. Allanson A, Michie S, Marteau TM. Presentation of screen negative results on serum screening for Down syndrome: variations across Britain. *J Med Screen* 1997;4:21–2.
59. Grimes DA, Snively GR. Patients' understanding of medical risks: implications for genetic counseling. *Obstet Gynecol* 1999;93:910–4.
60. van Vliet HA, Grimes DA, Popkin B, Smith U. Lay persons' understanding of the risk of Down's syndrome in genetic counselling. *BJOG* 2001;108:649–50.
61. Farmer AJ, Doll H, Levy JC, Salkovskis PM. The impact of screening for type 2 diabetes in siblings of patients with established diabetes. Unpublished data.
62. Freeman GK, Horder JP, Howie JGR, Hungin AP, Hill AP, Shah NC, *et al.* Evolving general practice consultation in Britain: issues of length and context. *BMJ* 2002;324:880–2.
63. Stapleton H, Kirkham M, Thomas G. Qualitative study of evidence based leaflets in maternity care. *BMJ* 2002;324:639.
64. Marteau TM, Humphrey C, Matoon G, Kidd J, Lloyd M, Horder J. Factors influencing the communication skills of first year clinical medical students. *Med Educ* 1991;25:127–34.
65. Marteau TM, Wynne G, Kaye W, Evans TR. Resuscitation: experience without feedback increases

confidence but not skill. *BMJ* 1990;300:849–50.

66. Royal College of Obstetricians and Gynaecologists, Royal College of Paediatrics and Child Health. *Fetal Abnormalities – Guidelines for Screening, Diagnosis and Management. Report of a Joint Working Party of the RCOG and the RCPCH*. London: RCOG Press; 1997.
67. Raphael-Leff J. Psychodynamic understanding: its use and abuse in midwifery. *Br J Midwifery* 2000;8:686–8.
68. Maguire P, Fairburn S, Fletcher C. Consultation skills of young doctors. 1. Benefits of feedback training in interviewing as students persist. *BMJ* 1986;292:1573–6.
69. Smith DK, Shaw RW, Slack J, Marteau TM. Training obstetricians and midwives to present screening tests: evaluation of two brief interventions. *Prenat Diagn* 1995;15:317–24.
70. Michie S, Marteau TM. Non-response bias in prospective studies of patients and health care professionals. *International Journal of Social Research Methodology* 1999;3:203–12.
71. Oliver S, Rajan L, Turner H, Oakley A, Entwistle V, Watt I, *et al.* Informed choice for users of health services: views on ultrasonography leaflets of women in early pregnancy, midwives, and ultrasonographers. *BMJ* 1996;313:1251–3.
72. Marteau TM, Dormandy E. Facilitating informed choice in prenatal testing: how well are we doing? *Am J Med Genet* 2001;106:185–90.
73. Beck U. *Risk Society: Towards a New Modernity*. London: Sage Publications; 1992.
74. Peat FD. *From Certainty to Uncertainty: The Story of Science and Ideas in the Twentieth Century*. Washington DC: Joseph Henry Press; 2002.

Chapter 28

Psychiatric causes of maternal death

Margaret Oates

Introduction

The Confidential Enquiries into Maternal Deaths (CEMD) reporting on the triennium 1997–99[1] found suicide to be the leading cause of maternal death in the UK. This finding may surprise those who read Chapter 11, 'Psychiatric causes of death', in which suicide is described as the second leading cause overall (leading cause of indirect deaths), based on cases reported to the CEMD.

Under-ascertainment has been a problem for all Confidential Enquiries and bedevils suicide research. The problem with psychiatric causes of death is compounded by the relatively recent attention paid to them. Psychiatric causes of death have only been separately assessed and included in the CEMD since 1994–96. It is therefore likely that many cases of suicide, in particular, have not been reported to the CEMD. This is particularly likely to have happened if a suicide occurred many months after delivery ('late' late deaths) or if a postmortem did not reveal a previously lost pregnancy. The new Office for National Statistics (ONS) Linkage Pilot Study, which links death certificates with birth certificates in the previous year, allows for a much higher degree of ascertainment than relying upon cases reported to the CEMD. A further 200 cases were identified in this way, of which 59 were probably psychiatric. These 59 cases, which included 40 suicides, eight open verdicts and 11 accidental overdoses of illicit drugs, were not reported to the CEMD. Therefore insufficient details were available at the time of the preparation of this triennium's report to allow them to be included in the analysis. However, the details that were available confirm that all of the 'ONS cases' were late deaths (after 42 days) and that one of the most important findings of this CEMD, the violent nature of the suicides, was true for these cases as well. If the non-reported 'ONS cases' are added to the reported suicides, suicide is the leading cause of maternal death.

Subsequent Enquiries will seek to address these problems. The data capture form will be altered to include psychiatric information and active requests will be made from psychiatric services to supply information. In future, the ONS linkage system will be used to pursue information for the enquiry.

The concern of the psychiatric assessor is that, if more detail had been available at the time of the Enquiry, this might have altered some of the findings and certainly the statistics. However, if the CEMD is regarded as a national audit of maternal deaths, with the standard to be monitored that women should not die, then the themes that emerge and the patterns of suboptimal care that contributed to the death are not invalidated by only considering half of the psychiatric morbidity associated with childbirth. Valid lessons are still to be learned.

The definition of a psychiatric death

A psychiatric maternal death is one in which the psychiatric condition was a major contributor or cause of death and where the death would not have occurred if the woman had not been suffering from a psychiatric disorder. Under the conventions of the CEMD, all psychiatric deaths are classified as indirect or coincidental.

An argument could be made for regarding suicide in a woman suffering from puerperal psychosis or severe postnatal depression as a direct maternal death. However, it is by no means widely accepted that such illnesses are directly caused by childbirth. Neither the International Classification of Diseases, tenth edition (ICD10) nor DSM IV recognise puerperal psychosis or postnatal depression as specific disorders. Therefore the convention remains.

The decision as to whether a case met these criteria was made by the Director of the Enquiry. However, where doubt existed consensus was reached with the psychiatric assessor. Cases were also referred between assessors where there were concerns that there was a psychiatric contribution to the death.

Although the majority of deaths were caused by suicide, not all were (Table 28.1). Other deaths included women with alcohol abuse, one of whom died from inhalation of vomit when intoxicated, and another case of intoxication masking a fatal ectopic pregnancy. A mentally ill woman was murdered by her schizophrenic husband and two, perhaps three, deaths were caused by pulmonary embolism in hospitalised women with puerperal psychosis. The pulmonary emboli were probably related to the antipsychotic medication that they were receiving. However, the majority of the non-suicide psychiatric deaths were in women who were drug-abusing who died from an accidental overdose of heroin.

Table 28.1. Causes of death, Confidential Enquiries into Maternal Deaths 1997–99[1]

	Pregnant	Early	Late	Total
Suicide	6	6	16	28
Illicit drugs overdose	2	0	6	8
Other				6
Pulmonary embolus		1	1	
Adverse drug reactions		1		
Murder		1		
Alcohol-related	2			
Total	10	9	23	42

The methodology

All available information was used to obtain as complete a picture as possible of the antecedents to the woman's death. The sources included not only the data capture form but also reports from psychiatric services, letters from general practitioners and evidence given to the coroner's court (which sadly included, in many cases, statements from the family and suicide notes). Categorical data, including age, ethnicity, parity, diagnosis, psychiatric history and service usage, current psychiatric treatment, method of suicide and the gestational age of the pregnancy or weeks following delivery were collected. Composite summaries of each individual case were made. A textual analysis was performed to extract the minimum number of recurring themes that adequately described all the data.

Finally, recommendations, which were grounded in the data, were made. As with all the CEMD recommendations, these specific psychiatric recommendations involve areas of service provision, education and training, booking and antenatal as well as postpartum care. These will result in new standards that can be measured in future CEMD reports, thereby 'closing the loop'. The detailed findings described in Chapter 11 (p. 165) of the CEMD report for 1997–99[1] are summarised below.

Psychiatric disorders are known to have caused or contributed to 12% of maternal deaths reported to the CEMD, 10% of which were due to suicide.
Although the number of cases reported to this Enquiry suggests that death from mental illness is the second leading cause of maternal mortality, the ONS Linkage Pilot Study has shown that a large number of deaths were not reported and, when these are included, then deaths from psychiatric causes would be the leading cause of maternal death.
Women who have had a past episode of severe mental illness have a one in two to one in three chance of recurrence following the birth of their child.
From the cases reported to this Enquiry, the risk of suicide is one per 100 000 maternities but if all the cases recently identified had been included the risk is two per 100 000 maternities.
Suicides in this group of women are characterised by their violent nature.
There are marked social class differences between suicide and the other causes of maternal death.
All the women who died from substance misuse were severely socially disadvantaged.
Progesterone is not an effective treatment for depressive illness.

These key findings inform the recommendations. However, some of these findings contrast sharply with conventional clinical wisdom in both obstetrics and psychiatry and merit further discussion.

Suicide is the leading cause of maternal death

This may surprise many clinicians. Suicide research over the last 40 years has consistently found that the suicide rate in women is lower than that in men, is decreasing at a greater rate than in men and is lowest of all in pregnancy and in the two years following birth.[2,3] However, despite the apparently protective effect of maternity on suicide in women, some authors have suggested[5] that certain subgroups of pregnant and postpartum women may be at an elevated risk. These include young socioeconomically deprived women and women suffering from serious mental illness in the immediate postpartum period. The findings of the CEMD would support this latter view.

If all cases of suicide (both reported to the CEMD and found through ONS linkage) are included, then the suicide rate in this triennium would appear to be 2/100 000 births. This is in contrast to the current suicide rate among women of 3.4/100 000.[6] The incidence of postpartum mental illness, admission rates to psychiatric hospital following delivery and contact with psychiatric services have long been established.[7,9] It is therefore possible to estimate the number of women suffering from severe postnatal depression and puerperal psychosis, as well as the number in contact with psychiatric services or admitted to hospital during this triennium. An established incidence of 2/1000 deliveries for puerperal psychosis gives an estimated suicide rate for puerperal psychosis of 2/1000 sufferers. Approximately 2% of all women delivered make contact with psychiatric services with a new episode of psychiatric illness in the postpartum year, giving an estimated suicide rate of 0.3/1000 for postpartum psychiatric contacts. These findings suggest that the protective effect of pregnancy, the postpartum period and the presence of young children may be diluted by the presence of serious mental illness.

Violent methods of suicide

Again, research findings consistently suggest that there are differences between the genders in the method of suicide. Women have been shown to be less likely to die violently than men and more likely to die from an overdose, particularly from analgesic or psychotropic medication.[3,6] In stark contrast to these findings, of those suicides reported to the CEMD only three women died from an overdose of medication (one an over-the-counter preparation and two psychotropic drugs). The remainder, 86%, died violently mostly from jumping from a height or by hanging but a few from stabbing and gunshot wounds (see Table 28.2). The currently available details on the 'ONS cases' confirms these findings.

Table 28.2. Method of suicide, Confidential Enquiries into Maternal Deaths 1997–99[1]

	Pregnant	Early	Late	Total
Jumping from height	0	4	1	5
Hanging	4	0	6	10
Stabbing (cutting throat)	1	1	2	4
Burning	0		1	1
Gunshot	0	1	1	2
Drowning			1	1
Road traffic accident			1	1
Illicit drugs overdose	1	0	2	3
Unknown			1	1
Total	6	6	16	28

The manner of these deaths tells clearly of the unequivocal intention to die, in keeping with the serious nature of the underlying illness.

Sociodemographic characteristics

In contrast to maternal deaths from physical causes and from substance misuse, maternal suicides were distinctive by being relatively socially advantaged and married. Many were professional women living in comfortable circumstances and a worrying number were health professionals. Most had apparently supportive relationships. This confirms findings in previous suicide research[2] that female suicide is less strongly associated with factors such as unemployment, poverty, adversity, single status and divorce than is male suicide.

Serious mental illness and the risk of recurrence

In all but six cases of maternal psychiatric death (86%), there was enough information to make a psychiatric diagnosis (Table 28.3). Overall, 56% of maternal psychiatric deaths were suffering from serious mental illness, psychosis or severe depressive illness. Of those women who died from suicide, in all but four cases a psychiatric diagnosis could be made (86%). Of the suicides, 68% have a diagnosis of serious mental illness.

In keeping with the known presentation and clinical features of severe postpartum mental illness, all the early suicides (under 42 days after birth) fell into the category of severe mental illness. All the early deaths were characterised by comfortable social circumstances, married status and an early abrupt-onset psychotic illness, usually within days of childbirth.

Also in keeping with our knowledge of postpartum illness was the frequency with which these women, particularly the early deaths, had a psychiatric history (Table 28.4). Almost half of all the suicides (46%) had a psychiatric history of an illness of a severity that had warranted contact with psychiatric services. Of these women, half had been admitted to a psychiatric hospital following a previous childbirth.

Table 28.3. Diagnosis and cause of death, Confidential Enquiries into Maternal Deaths 1997–99[1]

Probable diagnosis	Suicide	Illicit drugs overdose	Other	Total
Puerperal psychosis Depressive psychosis	7	0	3	10
Severe depression	10	Not ascertainable	0	10
Obsessive compulsive disorder	2	0	0	2
Eating disorder	0	0	1	1
Bereavement reaction	1	0	0	1
Substance misuse	1	6	0	7
Alcohol misuse	2	Not ascertainable	2	4
Personality disorder	1	Not ascertainable	0	1
Not ascertainable	4	2	0	6
			Total	42

Table 28.4. Previous contact with psychiatric services for deaths from psychiatric causes, Confidential Enquiries into Maternal Deaths 1997–99[1]

When death occurred	Previous postpartum contact	At other times	Total (all contacts)
Pregnancy	0	3	3
Early > 42 days postpartum	5	2	7
Late > 42 days postpartum	4	4	8
Total	9	9	18

It has long been known that women with a history of serious mental illness face a risk of recurrence of that illness following childbirth,[7] most recently estimated at between one in three and one in two.[10]

For half of the women who died from suicide, therefore, the risk of recurrence of their illness could have been predicted at booking clinic. In most cases it was not. In those few where the previous illness had been identified, it was in all cases described as postnatal depression or its acronym 'PND'. There was no apparent awareness on the part of maternity staff of the nature or severity of the previous illness, nor of its high risk and timing of recurrence. In only one case was any plan for proactive management put in place. In this case, despite a previous puerperal psychosis with an onset on day five, this woman was given an outpatient appointment for day 14 following her next baby. She killed herself on day six. It was also clear, despite the predictability of the illnesses, that these deaths had taken both general practitioners and psychiatrists by surprise. Some of their letters to the coroner revealed a mistaken belief that 'good social support' and being well in pregnancy made a recurrence of the illness less likely.

Almost half of the women who died from suicide therefore might not have died if their history had been accurately identified and if plans for proactive management had been put in place. At the very least, they should have received close surveillance for the maximum period at risk following delivery and perhaps prophylactic medication. The findings of the CEMD also highlight the importance of not using the term postnatal depression or 'PND' as a generic term for all types of mental illness, with an assumption of psychosocial aetiology and of management.

All those working in obstetrics and psychiatry need to be reminded that a minority of women suffers from severe illnesses of sudden onset in the early puerperium that require robust and specialist management. They also need to be reminded of the high rate of recurrence in subsequent pregnancies and that the timing and severity of the illnesses are likely to be as before. It is also pertinent to remind practitioners that women who have suffered from severe non-postpartum illness may become pregnant and they too face a similar risk of recurrence or relapse following childbirth. It follows therefore that asking for information specifically about the history of serious mental illness is as essential as asking the more accepted questions about diabetes and epilepsy at the booking clinic.

Management as well as detection

Over the last ten years, initiatives to identify women suffering from postnatal depression in the community have become widespread in the UK. These have mainly involved midwives and health visitors by increasing their awareness of postnatal depression and by the widespread use of screening tools such as the Edinburgh Postnatal Depression Scale.[11,12] The identification of postnatal depression and the development of treatment protocols in primary care is now part of the National Service Framework for Mental Health.[13] By implication, the problem of postpartum mental illness is seen as one predominately to be managed in primary care. Despite considerable research interest in puerperal psychosis for many decades and the recent publication of national guidelines on the provision of services for women suffering from severe perinatal psychiatric disorder,[14] there has been much less national emphasis on the service provision for those suffering from serious mental illness in relation to childbirth and the increasingly prominent problem of women with existing serious mental illness who become pregnant.[15] There are few specialist mother-and-baby units in the UK and even fewer trusts that provide specialist liaison psychiatry services to maternity units or community mental health teams.[13] The findings of the CEMD confirm this. None of the women who died either from suicide or from other psychiatric causes had been seen by a specialist community mental health team and none of the women who were admitted during the index pregnancy nor any of those who had been admitted previously following childbirth had been admitted to a mother-and-baby unit. In other words, all the women who had been admitted to a psychiatric hospital following childbirth, either currently or in the past, had been separated from their babies. The impact that this had on their management and suicide risk can only be imagined.

Of all the women who died (from suicide and other causes), 85% had had their psychiatric problems identified and were receiving treatment. Almost half of all the suicides were being seen by psychiatric services (46%) (Table 28.5).

For the women who died, therefore, the way in which they were managed rather than the identification of the disorder was the problem.

Conclusions

The findings that suicide is now the leading cause of maternal death and that the profile of postpartum women who kill themselves is different from that of other women and men are new. They should inform psychiatric practice, particularly in regard to risk

Table 28.5. Current psychiatric contact, Confidential Enquiries into Maternal Deaths 1997–99[1]

Highest level of psychiatric care provided	Index maternity
Inpatient	9
Outpatient/community mental health team	9
Referral but not seen	4
General practitioner treatment only	6
Substance misuse service	5
No contact	3
Unknown	3

assessment. The finding that a psychiatric history, postpartum or otherwise, predicts a high risk of recurrence following delivery is not new. It is consistent with research findings over many years. That it should apparently have had such little impact on psychiatric or obstetric practice is concerning. Unique among the known antecedents of psychiatric illness, childbirth comes with nine months' warning, which is ample time for the risk to be detected and management plans to be put in place. These findings should also inform psychiatric and obstetric practice. The suggestion that the widespread acceptance of postnatal depression might have a counterproductive effect on those suffering from severe mental illness was unexpected and indicates that differential diagnosis is as important in psychiatry as it is in other medical specialties.

The CEMD findings discussed have informed the following recommendations:

- Protocols for the management of women who are at risk of a relapse or recurrence of a serious mental illness following delivery should be in place in every trust providing maternity services.
- Enquiries about psychiatric history, its severity, the care received and clinical presentation should be made routinely in a systematic and sensitive way at the antenatal booking clinic.
- The term 'postnatal depression' or 'PND' should not be used as a generic term for all types of psychiatric disorder. Details of the previous illness should be sought and recorded in line with the recommendations above.
- Women who have a history of serious psychiatric disorder, postpartum or non-postpartum, should be assessed by a psychiatrist in the antenatal period and a management plan should be instituted with regard to the high risk of recurrence following delivery.

Women who have suffered from serious mental illness either following childbirth or at other times should be counselled about the possible recurrence of that illness following further pregnancies.

Future developments: specialisms and managed care networks

Women with serious mental health problems complicating pregnancy and childbirth require specialist psychiatric teams to manage their conditions. Such teams are justified by the specialist knowledge, skills and resources necessary for the management of these women. Only a small number will present every year to locality teams (primary healthcare centres and community mental health teams), which is insufficient to warrant special staffing and to allow for the development of skills. However, on a district-wide basis there will be sufficient numbers to justify specialist teams and to provide the critical mass necessary for the development of skills and to be cost-effective. It is not only the distinctive clinical features of psychiatric conditions themselves that merit the specialist attention but, more importantly, the presence of a baby and the maternity context. Community mental health teams would have difficulty in prioritising these clients within their service and in understanding the different language and procedures of maternity services and relating to different professional groups. These arguments and the supporting evidence are to be found in the Royal College of Psychiatrists' recommendations for perinatal mental health services. Similar recommendations are also to be found in the Scottish Maternity

Services Frameworks and, we hope, in the National Service Framework for Child and Maternity Services for England and Wales. However, they are yet to be widely found in the UK.

It is a Utopian fantasy that, even if there were a specialist perinatal mental health service in every maternity trust area, they would be able to deal with all the mental health problems associated with childbirth, nor indeed should they. The majority of postnatal mental health problems can be well managed in primary care and commonplace emotional reactions to pregnancy and delivery should be within the skills of midwives and obstetricians themselves. Primary care and maternity services therefore need assistance to refer those women in need of specialist services appropriately and help in increasing their capacity and competence to treat minor psychiatric disorder themselves.

Managed care networks

When groups of patients or certain conditions involve many different specialties and professions across different trusts and organisations, the best way forward for managing their conditions is to develop managed clinical networks (MCN).[8] These have already made an impact in many medical specialties and are championed by the Department of Health both in England and in Scotland. The development of MCNs for cancer services is now a government requirement and MCNs exist in neurology for stroke, vascular services and diabetes as well as breast cancer. However, there are no examples of MCNs as yet in psychiatry.

An MCN is a formal and managed group of health professionals who work together in a coordinated manner, unconstrained by existing organisational or professional boundaries, to ensure the best management of a group of patients. One person is appointed to have overall responsibility for the operation of the clinical network by either a trust or by a health commissioner. The MCN has a clearly mapped-out structure, which sets the points at which the service is to be delivered and the connections between these points. The network identifies gaps in service provision. It agrees to develop and adhere to evidence-based treatment guidelines and develops integrated care pathways (patient journeys) so that it is clear to all which patients and which conditions should be managed, at which level of service provision, and which need to be referred on. It incorporates in its integration and in its practice guidelines all levels of care provision – primary, secondary and tertiary – and must involve patient representation.[4] A broadly similar strategy is recommended by the Royal College of Psychiatrists, which is that perinatal mental health strategy groups should be set up in each maternity trust area. Both the commonplace mild-to-moderate conditions known as postnatal depression and the rarer severe mental illnesses are well suited to this way of developing services and managing conditions. Effective management will involve general practitioners, midwives, health visitors, obstetricians and psychiatrists and community psychiatric nurses. The majority of women will be treated in primary care, a smaller number in secondary care and a few will require inpatient treatment in tertiary mother-and-baby units. Unless these different professional groups and organisations can work effectively together in reality instead of merely copying correspondence to each other, seriously ill women will continue to fall between organisations and suffer avoidable morbidity and on occasion die.

Summary

Suicide is a rare event, particularly in women. Maternal death is also a rare event. Nonetheless, suicide is currently the leading cause of maternal death. Some of these women's deaths were probably not predictable and others were probably not preventable. Some died despite receiving high-quality care. However, approximately half of the women who died following delivery were suffering from serious mental illness. For half of these, their deaths might have been prevented if systems had been in place for the identification of women at high risk of serious mental illness and if protocols had been in place for the proactive management of their postpartum period. For the others, better management of their acute postpartum conditions might have improved the outcome.

It is hoped that these recommendations will save the lives of some women but also improve the care of the majority of women with mental health problems associated with childbirth.

References

1. Drife J, Lewis G, editors. *Why Mothers Die 1997–1999. The Confidential Enquiries into Maternal Deaths in the United Kingdom.* London: RCOG Press; 2001.
2. Qin P, Agerbo E, Westergard-Nielsen N, Eriksson T, Mortensen PO. Gender differences in risk factors for suicide in Denmark. *Br J Psychiatry* 2000;177:546–50.
3. Hawton K. Sex and suicide. Gender differences in suicidal behaviour. *Br J Psychiatry* 2000;177:484–5.
4. Holmes J, Langmaack J. Managed clinical networks – their relevance to mental health services. *Psychiatric Bulletin* 2002;26:161–3.
5. Appleby L. Suicidal behaviour in childbearing women. *International Review of Psychiatry* 1996;8:107–15.
6. Schapira K, Linsley KR, Linsley JA, Kelly TP, Kay DK. Relationship of suicide rates to social factors and availability of lethal methods. *Br J Psychiatry* 2001;178:458–64.
7. Kendell RE, Chalmers KC, Platz C. Epidemiology of puerperal psychoses. *Br J Psychiatry* 1987;150:662–73.
8. Kunkler IH. Managed clinical networks: a new paradigm for clinical medicine. *J R Coll Physicians Lond* 2000;34:230–3.
9. Oates M. Psychiatric services for women following childbirth. *International Review of Psychiatry* 1996;8:87–98.
10. Wieck A, Kumar R, Hirst AD, Marks NM, Campbell IC, Checkley SA. Increased sensitivity of dopamine receptors and recurrence of affective psychosis after childbirth. *BMJ* 1991;303:613–16.
11. Leverton TJ, Elliot SA. Is the EPDS a magic wand? 1 A comparison of the EPDS and health visitor report as predictors of diagnosis on the present state examination. *Journal of Reproductive and Infant Psychology* 2000;18:279–95.
12. Elliot SA, Leverton TJ. Is the EPDS a magic wand? 2 Myths and the evidence base. *Journal of Reproductive and Infant Psychology* 2000;18:297–307.
13. Department of Health. *A National Service Framework for Mental Health.* London: DoH; 1999.
14. Royal College of Psychiatrists. *Perinatal Maternal Mental Health Services. Recommendations for Provision of Services for Childbearing Women.* Council Report CR88. London: Royal College of Psychiatrists; 2000.
15. Howard L, Kumar R, Thornicroft G. Psychosocial characteristics of mothers with psychiatric disorders. *Br J Psychiatry* 2001;178:427–32.

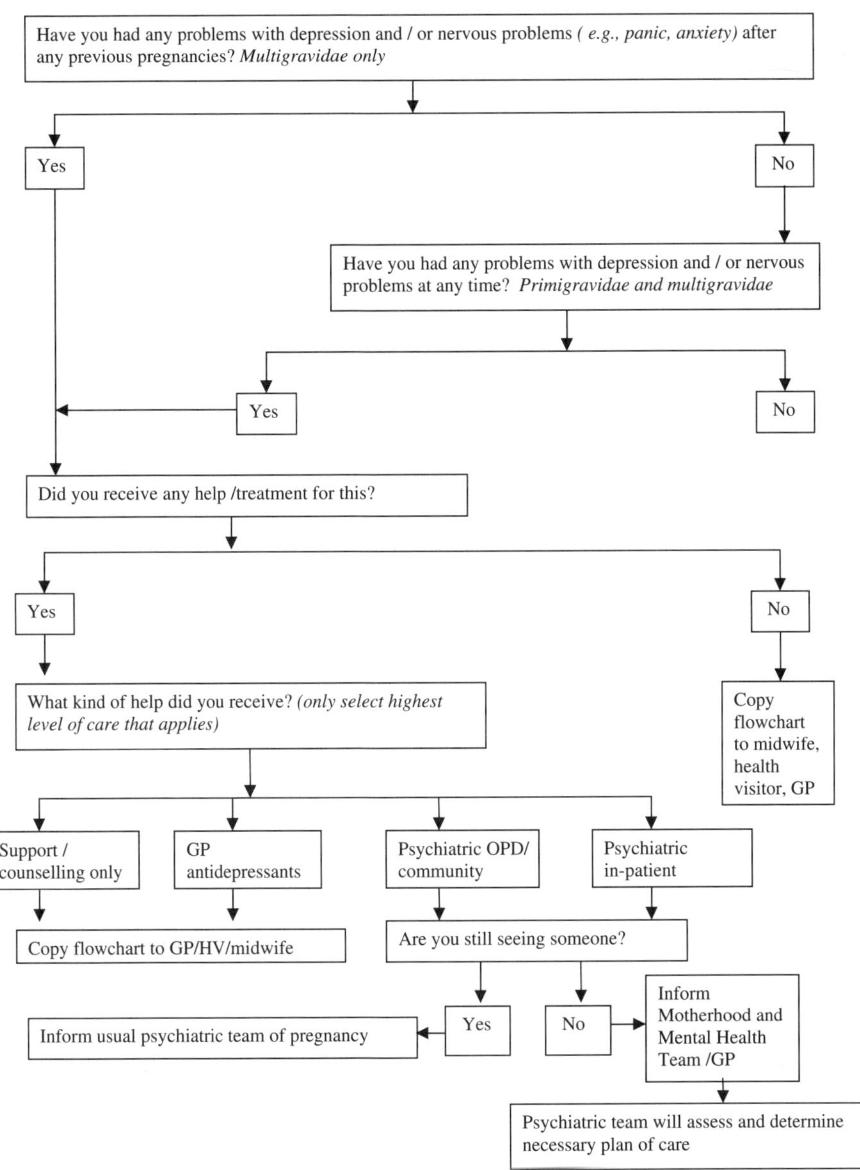

Figure 28.1. Nottingham Booking Clinic Algorithm for detection of women at risk of recurrence of serious postpartum mental illness; HV = health visitor; OPD = outpatient department

Chapter 29

Debriefing after childbirth

Tina Lavender

Introduction

The introduction of the *Changing Childbirth* report in the UK in 1993[1] caused the midwifery profession to re-evaluate the provision of maternity care. Although the main emphasis of the report was on consideration of the maternity service as a complete entity, it focused on antenatal and intrapartum care in particular. Except for limited recognition that postnatal continuity was important, the report made little reference to postnatal health. Although it is a statutory requirement to provide postnatal care,[2] this is interpreted locally and many different models of service provision have arisen. It is even interpreted differently by individual midwives within the same service.

Recently, there has been a small cluster of studies evaluating postnatal care.[3–5] However, these trials have concentrated primarily on the physical aspects of the care. One aspect that has received comparatively little interest is the psychological care of women in the postnatal period. There is, however, a growing expectation that birth should not only result in a healthy mother and baby but also be a rewarding psychological experience.[6] Importantly, health professionals have begun to appreciate psychological morbidity and relate it to postnatal outcomes such as breastfeeding and bonding.[7] Furthermore, a recent cluster randomised trial found that redesigning care so that it is midwife-led, flexible and individualised could help to improve women's mental health and reduce depression at four months.[8] It therefore seemed important that health professionals search for ways to reduce psychological morbidity in the postnatal period. As a consequence, postnatal debriefing has become a fashionable aspect of postnatal care.

What is debriefing?

'Debriefing is a psychological treatment intended to reduce the psychological morbidity that arises after exposure to trauma'.[9] Debriefing traditionally implies a structured intervention in which the process encourages the recollection of the event followed by some form of emotional processing.[10,11] The belief that debriefing helps psychological recovery following traumatic experiences has led to an expansion of debriefing programmes in various situations in society such as after disasters, for emergency services staff and following trauma and violence.[12-14]

Debriefing has two main purposes – to reduce psychological distress following a traumatic event and to prevent the development of a psychiatric disorder.

What is postnatal debriefing?

Despite the fact that many women find childbirth to be a fulfilling experience, it is nevertheless often a life-changing event that can be a traumatic experience.[15] A natural consequence of this is the maternal need to reflect on the experience and discuss the event with others, either professionals or lay people. Evidence exists to support the claim that women like to discuss their labours.[16] Similarly, evidence suggests that providing women with the opportunity to integrate and make sense of their birth experience is beneficial in strengthening psychological process.[17]

'Debriefing' is a frequently used term in obstetrics that has several definitions.[18] However, the degree of interest in 'debriefing' may have contributed to a growing interest in the women's psychological needs in the postnatal period. The term 'debriefing', in maternity services, is usually used to describe the process whereby women are facilitated to discuss their labour on a one-to-one basis with a midwife or obstetrician in an attempt to make sense of their experience. However, as discussed by Wessely,[19] labour is not an abnormal event and therefore it may be inappropriate to use criteria that are applied in the discipline of psychiatry. Furthermore, a process that medicalises the distress may in fact be more harmful than beneficial.

Consumers have voiced concerns that dissatisfied customers who are 'debriefed' may be less likely to complain. This, they believe, encourages a woman to accept events that have happened, thus discouraging professionals from admitting that care may have been 'faulty'.[20] Debriefers thus become 'shock absorbers' for the institutions rather than acting in the interest of the woman.

Does postnatal debriefing have a positive effect on psychological morbidity?

Despite the limited available evidence for postnatal debriefing, authors continue to promote it as an important aspect of postnatal care.[6] Furthermore, this limited evidence has not prevented the incorporation of debriefing services into maternity units across the country. A survey of the prevalence of debriefing-type interventions in maternity units in England and Wales demonstrated that such services are widespread.[21] In this survey, it was found that 36% of units had formal arrangements in place for debriefing and a further 26% had plans to introduce services.

However, as with any intervention, its safety and efficacy needs to be evaluated before implementation and the most appropriate way is by carrying out a randomised controlled trial. However, there is a notable lack of methodologically sound research into the impact of post-childbirth interventions on psychological outcome.

A recently updated systematic review of debriefing identified 11 trials that focused on people exposed to a traumatic event.[22] Eight of the studies involved participants following accidental or violent injuries. Two studies involved women following childbirth and one study involved women following miscarriage. All trials consisted of a single intervention session, which involved emotional processing, recollection and normalisation of emotional reaction. Following this review, the authors concluded that a single session of individual debriefing did not reduce psychological distress or prevent the onset of post-traumatic stress disorder. Those who received the intervention showed no significant short-term (three to five months) reduction in the risk of PTSD (OR 1.22; 95% CI 0.60–2.46). One trial actually reported a significantly increased risk of PTSD in those receiving debriefing (OR 2.88; 95% CI 1.11–7.53). There was also no evidence that debriefing reduced general psychological morbidity, depression or anxiety.

Of the 11 trials included in the review, only three were related to obstetrics and gynaecology. In the gynaecological study,[23] psychologists debriefed women at home two weeks after a miscarriage. Although the women found the process helpful in terms of having someone to listen to them, there were no differences in outcomes (Hospital Anxiety and Depression Scale; Impact of Events Scale) at four months.

Two trials included postnatal women.[24,25] However, because the intervention in the two obstetric studies was 'patient-led', comparison with other studies was problematic. These studies were therefore excluded from analysis. Furthermore, although the two obstetric studies had similar interventions, which included a midwife one-to-one session and a woman-led discussion, they differed in several other ways, making comparisons difficult.

Lavender and Walkinshaw[24] conducted a randomised controlled trial of 140 primigravid women, whereby participants were allocated to receive either a psychological intervention or the usual hospital care. Participants were those who had progressed through an uncomplicated labour that resulted in a normal spontaneous birth. The intervention included a one-to-one session with a research midwife who discussed both positive and negative aspects of the childbirth experience, answered questions when asked and referred to the hospital notes when appropriate. These sessions occurred within one week of delivery on the postnatal ward in single en-suite rooms. The main outcome measure was the Hospital Anxiety and Depression (HAD) scale administered by postal questionnaire three weeks post delivery. The findings of this study were that women who received the intervention of debriefing were less likely to have high anxiety ($P < 0.0001$) and depression scores ($P < 0.0001$) after delivery when compared with the control group.

Small *et al.*[25] conducted a randomised controlled trial of 1041 women. Unlike the previous study, they included only women following an operative delivery. Again, the intervention involved debriefing by midwives before hospital discharge and the participating woman led the discussion. The main outcome measures were maternal depression (score ≥ 13 on the Edinburgh Postnatal Depression Scale, EPDS) and overall maternal health status (Short-form 36 questionnaire) at six months. This study found no significant differences in EPDS between the trial arms. Moreover, women allocated to debriefing had poorer health status on seven of the eight SF-36 subscales, although the difference was significant only for role functioning (emotional) (mean 73.32 versus 78.98, t = –2.31; 95% CI –10.48 to –0.84).

There is anecdotal evidence to suggest that debriefing by midwives was valued by the women who experienced it[26–28] and evidence from a large qualitative study[29] supports this view. Many women commented on the lack of information they received following the delivery of their baby. Although the women were questioned on the second postnatal day, they were already seeking answers to questions regarding their intrapartum experience. Among the 87 (21%) women who commented on postnatal information, a consensus was reached that postnatal psychological support was lacking:

'Someone should talk to you after you have had your baby because, although my midwife was very good when I was in labour, I would have liked to have asked her about what went on. My labour went fine, I think, because I had a normal delivery but it would just have been nice to talk to the midwife about the labour'.

Personal examples of debriefing

During the study by Lavender and Walkinshaw,[24] the 'debriefing' sessions varied on an individual basis. Although the examples below may be viewed as anecdotal evidence, they do highlight the difficulties of describing the interactive process. Furthermore, they illustrate the importance of women being given the opportunity to discuss and clarify their experience regardless of whether the labour is considered 'normal' by the practitioner.

Example 1

A married woman aged 35 years and having her first baby entered the labour room with her husband, and was 'excited at the prospect of giving birth'. On reading her case records in the postnatal period, one could see that the woman had a straightforward labour, with no intervention, followed by a normal spontaneous birth. However, when the woman was approached to discuss her labour she burst into tears. The woman had not met the midwife before the labour and was horrified at her attitude towards her. She felt that the midwife was trying to control her and repeatedly talked to her as if she was a child. The woman explained that she felt she was being mentally tortured and likened the events to the horror film 'Misery'. The midwife showed no warmth and towards the end of the first stage when the woman reached out and requested to hold the midwife's hand her request was refused. She was also 'threatened with a doctor' if she didn't 'push harder'. At one point, the woman crawled to the door to shout for someone to 'save' her (the midwife had not informed her of the call bell system). Following the birth, the woman felt too scared to close her eyes as she was having nightmares.

In this case, the debriefer believed it necessary, with maternal consent, to inform a supervisor of midwives and formal action was taken.

Example 2

A 16-year-old woman, supported by her mother, entered the labour room in spontaneous labour to give birth to her first baby. Following a quick and uncomplicated labour, she gave birth to a healthy baby. However, when this woman was asked about her labour she was extremely upset. She had thought that there was something wrong with her and/or the baby because she had received regular vaginal examinations and continuous fetal monitoring. She said that the midwife had offered no explanation for the procedures and she herself was too scared to question the midwife. The woman kept checking the baby 'just in case there was something wrong' that she hadn't been told and she felt that the midwife was withholding information. She described the experience as the worst in her life and felt that she couldn't stop crying.

In this case, a simple explanation of labour appeared to alleviate anxieties.

Example 3

A 25-year-old married woman having her first baby progressed through labour spontaneously with her husband present at all times. During the pregnancy, the couple had attended parent education classes and had devised a birth plan. They had decided that the partner would have an active role by cutting the cord, assisting with delivering the baby's body and massaging his wife's back.

Unfortunately, when the event occurred the partner felt unable to fulfil the role that he had anticipated. Every time they were left alone, he 'panicked' and shouted for the midwife, making his wife more anxious. The woman was very unhappy with her partner and felt extremely angry and 'let down'. She had not spoken to her partner since the birth, although he had visited regularly.

In this case the debriefer discussed labour events with the mother and father independently and together as a couple.

Not all women are given the opportunity to discuss their labour formally. Yet the above examples were resolved through a one-to-one session with a midwife. Without this opportunity, the long-term consequences for the women in the examples might have been considerable.

Recommendations

Practice

It is clear from the literature that authors define 'debriefing' in numerous ways. If this term is to be used in maternity services, a consensus on its definition and use needs to be made. Similarly, as women are also using the term, an exploration of the meaning attached to the word 'debriefing' by women should also be made.

The recommendations outlined in *Making a Difference*[30] should be considered by obstetricians and midwives as outlined below.

- Identify local training needs and facilitate programmes for midwives and obstetricians – i.e. listening skills.
- Ensure that obstetricians and midwives have the time to listen actively to what women say. Elevate the status of listening to women.
- Explore ways to raise the status of what women have to say about the birth experience: supply appropriate link workers, interpreters, special-needs practitioners to enable all women to discuss their experience.

- Put in place appropriate referral mechanisms, i.e. for postnatal depression and domestic abuse.
- Recognise the importance of the emotional wellbeing of women and their partners.
- Offer women the opportunity to discuss their labour experiences.
- Explore and listen to women's views so that they are in a position to influence change and improve maternity services.

Several suggestions have been made to change the current culture of routine task-orientated care. This includes an appropriate assessment of the woman's needs, equal opportunities to access psychological care, the offer of separate community visits to discuss their experience, the documentation of discussions, continual re-evaluation of postnatal care and referral to psychotherapist and/or postnatal support groups as necessary.

There are several possible explanations for women often not appearing to receive appropriate psychological care. Busy workloads, unsociable shifts and heavy case-loads may contribute to women not receiving the psychological care they deserve.

A second explanation is that many midwives have been through nurse training at a time when task-orientated work was the accepted norm. These attitudes are difficult to dispel. We, as a profession, feel guilty if we are talking to a woman, yet performing a dressing or removing sutures may be considered a valuable use of resources. Many midwives can relate to the ward scenario of looking busy when the senior midwife enters the area. Unfortunately, women, too, appear to have developed these same notions. Women can see that midwives are busy and whereas they may call for assistance to bath the baby or check their lochia, they appear to find it more difficult to ask for psychological support.

Research

Before any further randomised controlled trials, qualitative research is urgently needed to explore the issues surrounding postnatal debriefing. This is necessary, given that the impacts of such interventions are poorly understood.[31] Little information is available on the frequency, timing, setting and content of debriefing. Moreover, we need to question who is the most appropriate person to conduct the session and who should be present.

It is debatable which is the most appropriate time for women to discuss their experience. In both obstetric randomised trials, the intervention took place during the first week after the birth. However, as discussed by Wessely,[19] this may have coincided with postnatal depression, which in the Lavender study[24] may have accounted for the high incidence of depression and anxiety in the control group.

A further issue is where the intervention should take place. In the two obstetric randomised controlled trials,[24,25] it took place in the hospital, which may have been more favourable than in the community, as women spoke negatively about the hospital midwives in terms of 'never being able to talk' and the comments showed a sense of frustration when questions were left unanswered. However, this approach does not allow time for reflection away from the clinical setting.

It may be that the ward environment acts as a deterrent in psychological care. In the study by Lavender and Walkinshaw,[24] all the participants had a single postnatal room. Although individual en-suite rooms have several advantages, such as additional privacy, they greatly reduce women's opportunities to discuss their experience with like-minded women.

Another important issue is who should carry out the intervention. There is no evidence within maternity care to indicate whether the woman should know the debriefer or whether it should be an outsider.

Who should receive the intervention is another unanswered question. Should we be targeting specific groups of women and, if so, is there a need to develop predictive tools to highlight those women most likely to benefit? Yet targeting an isolated group (e.g. those who had instrumental deliveries) may cause women within that group to feel more vulnerable, as debriefing assumes that there is a uniform, predictable reaction to trauma. A woman who has given birth with the aid of forceps, for example, may not remember it to be a traumatic event until she is asked to discuss the experience. As discussed by Thompson,[32] 'the mere act of debriefing may sow the seed of doubt'. Recalling the event may be a 'secondary trauma' – attempting to forget may be an adaptive response.[22] Intervention may therefore interfere with an adaptive defence mechanism.

Conclusion

All women deserve appropriate psychological care to meet their needs. Some will already have built support networks and will not feel it necessary to discuss their experience with a professional. Others, however, will welcome being offered some form of social intervention. Interestingly, it appears that when women are offered the opportunity to discuss their labour, they usually do so. This emphasises the need for a service that is proactive in encouraging women to discuss their experience. If the women are not offered this opportunity, it is questionable how many would have requested it. It could, however, be – as suggested by Rose[22] – that the wider culture has changed, rendering debriefing unnecessary. Family and friends may be more aware of the need to discuss the experience.

It appears that women like discussing their childbirth experiences, which may in fact produce a feeling of wellbeing. However, as pointed out by Stallard[33] 'talking about the experience, listening with empathy and facilitating understanding of typical reactions are important but in themselves are not debriefing'. The evidence surrounding debriefing and either short- or long-term morbidity is inconclusive, thus requiring further investigation. The fact that deaths from suicide are not only the leading cause of indirect death, but also the leading cause of maternal deaths overall[34] indicates that this area should be a major concern for midwives and obstetricians.

References

1. Department of Health. *Changing Childbirth*. Report of the Expert Maternity Group London: HMSO; 1993.
2. United Kingdom Central Council. *The Midwives Code of Practice and the Midwives Rules*. London: HMSO; 1998.
3. Marchant S. What are we doing in the postnatal check? *Br J Midwifery* 1995;3:34–8.
4. Bick D, MacArthur C. The extent, severity and effect of health problems after childbirth. *Br J Midwifery* 1995;3:27–31.

5. Morrell CJ, Spiby H, Crowther S. Postnatal social support: counting the cost. *Br J Midwifery* 1997;5:613–14.
6. Axe S. Labour debriefing is crucial for good psychological care. *Br J Midwifery* 2000;8:626–31.
7. Enkin M, Keirse M, Neilson J, Crowther C, Duley L, Hodnett E, *et al. A Guide to Effective Care in Pregnancy and Childbirth.* 3rd ed. Oxford: Oxford University Press; 2000.
8. McArthur C, Winter HR, Bick DE, Knowles H, Lilford R, Henderson C. Effects of redesigned community postnatal care on women's health 4 months after birth: a cluster randomised controlled trial. *Lancet* 2002;359:378–85.
9. Rose S. Psychological debriefing: history and methods. *Counselling* 1997;8:48–51.
10. Mitchell J. When disaster strikes ... the critical incident stress debriefing procedure. *Journal of Emergency Medical Services* 1983;8:36–9.
11. Dyregov A. Caring for helpers in disaster situations: psychological debriefing. *Disaster Management* 1989;2:25–30.
12. Pennebaker JW, Susman JR. Disclosure of traumas and psychosomatic processes. *Soc Sci Med* 1998;26:327–32.
13. Ersland S, Weisaeth I, Sund A. The stress upon rescuers involved in an oil rig disasters 'Alexander I Kielland' 1980. *Acta Psychiatr Scand Suppl* 1989;355:38–49.
14. Shapiro D, Kunkler J. *Psychological Support for Hospital Staff Initiated by Clinical Psychologists in the Aftermath of the Hillsborough Disaster.* Sheffield: Sheffield Health Authority Mental Health Services Unit; 1990.
15. Niven CA. *Psychological Care for Families: Before, During and After Birth.* Oxford: Butterworth-Heinemann; 1992.
16. Marchant S, Garcia J. The need to talk after birth: evaluating new services. In: Alexander J, Roth C, Levy V, editors. *Midwifery Practice. Core Topics 3.* Basingstoke: Macmillan Press; 2000.
17. Ball J. Mothers need nurturing too. *Nurs Times* 1998;84:29–30.
18. Alexander J. Confusing debriefing and defusing postnatally: the need for clarity of terms, purpose and value. *Midwifery* 1998;14:122–4.
19. Wessely S. Commentary: reducing distress after normal childbirth. *Birth* 1998;25:220–1.
20. Robinson J. Dangers of debriefing. *Br J Midwifery* 1998;6:251.
21. Davidson L. Psycho-social interventions in maternity care; the need for evaluation. *BMJ Com* 2000;21 December.
22. Rose S, Bisson J, Wessely S. Brief psychological interventions ('debriefing') for trauma-related symptoms and the prevention of post traumatic stress disorder. *Cochrane Database Syst Rev* 2000;(2):CD000560.
23. Lee C, Slade P, Lygo V. The influence of psychological debriefing on emotional adaptation in women following early miscarriage: a preliminary study. *Br J Med Psychol* 1996;69:47–58.
24. Lavender T, Walkinshaw S. Can midwives reduce postpartum psychological morbidity? A randomised trial. *Birth* 1998;25:215–19.
25. Small R, Lumley J, Donohue L, Potter A, Waldenstrom U. Randomised controlled trial of midwife led debriefing to reduce maternal depression after operative childbirth. *BMJ* 2000;321:1043–7.
26. Charles J, Curtis L. Birth afterthoughts: setting up a listening service. *Midwives Chron* 1994;107:266–8.
27. Smith JA, Mitchell S. Debriefing after childbirth: a tool for effective risk management. *Br J Midwifery* 1996;4:581–6.
28. Westley W. 'Time to talk' listening service. *Midwives* 1997;110:30–1.
29. Lavender T, Walton I, Walkinshaw S. A prospective study of women's views of positive factors contributing to a positive birth experience. *Midwifery* 1999;15:40–6.
30. Department of Health. *Midwifery Action Plan: Making a Difference – The Nursing, Midwifery and Health Visiting Contribution.* London: DoH; 2001.
31. Powell A, Davies HTO. Mixing apples and pears. *BMJ Com* 2000;16 November.
32. Thompson A. Midwife-led debriefing and maternal depression after operative childbirth. *BMJ Com* 2000;8 November.
33. Stallard P. The effectiveness of psychological debriefing: a more sophisticated approach is required. *BMJ Com* 2000;8 November.
34. Drife J, Lewis G, editors. *Why Mothers Die 1997–1999. The Confidential Enquiries into Maternal Deaths in the United Kingdom.* London: RCOG Press; 2001.

Chapter 30

Psychological morbidity

Discussion

Discussion following the papers of Ms Robinson, Professor Marteau, Dr Oates and Dr Lavender

Hall: Could I ask Dr Oates to reiterate the ratio of mother-and-baby beds to population that you stated was required?

Oates: In my chapter, there is a reference to the Royal College of Psychiatrists' Council document.[1] It describes the resource requirements. In general, you need a six-bedded mother-and-baby unit approximately per one to one and a half million of population. The leeway relates to the kind of geographical area. For example, in a densely populated urban area, with a community mental health team, you can probably get away with rather fewer beds. If, however, you have a large geographical area, where people have to stay in hospital rather longer, and travelling distances are long – which I guess you may have in your part of the world – then you will need a slightly higher ratio of beds.

There are also population estimates for consultant sessions, numbers of community psychiatric nurses and so on in this policy document. We know the epidemiology of the condition – this is one of very few disorders for which you can actually work out what you need.

Hall: But providing a service for a dispersed population would present all sorts of difficulties that would not occur within an urban population.

Oates: Absolutely. In this document, we provide various models of service provision, including the suggested model for widely dispersed rural communities over large geographical areas. There are many ways of skinning a cat and the model can be altered for different situations.

Drife: I have a comment first, and then a couple of questions. The theme of having enough time to talk to people came up in a couple of presentations. In the context of gynaecology, last year the Royal College of Obstetricians and Gynaecologists produced a working party report with an arbitrary suggestion of 20 minutes for the length of a gynaecological consultation – which was regarded as ridiculously long by some people.[2] This was the only recommendation by the College that was picked up spontaneously by the most high-ranking people at the NHS Executive and the Department of Health as something that they did not think the College had any business to make recommendations about.

The professional push that is required to provide us with enough time to talk to patients or clients has come from the College and, interestingly, met with dispute from the NHS. Whether that will change with more money being made available in the Budget this afternoon, I do not know. In other words, the College is already 'on the case' in gynaecology, although not in obstetrics.

I have one question for Dr Lavender about who did the debriefing that worked so well. If an empathic person does the debriefing, that might make all the difference, and coming immediately after the event is a good idea. Ms Robinson said in her presentation that initially the Association for Improvements in the Maternity Services (AIMS) received a large number of complaints about high induction rates and intervention rates: when induction rates came down, the complaints were about something else. This made me wonder whether there is a normal distribution of people who are very satisfied and people who complain and, whatever we do, people at one end of that distribution will complain. Is that other people's impression?

Lavender: To answer your first question about who had carried out the debriefing that was done so well, it was me.

On the question about induction, one of the earliest studies that looked at maternal satisfaction and intervention was carried out by Cartwright in 1979.[3] This found that it was not the induction *per se* but the lack of information associated with the intervention that contributed to an increase in maternal dissatisfaction.

Lewis: Ms Robinson, you have told us a little about the nature of the change, but do you have any impression that things are going a little better than when you first started?

Robinson: To be honest, people do not like to complain and they just want to settle down with their children. When you have a new baby, that is the last thing you want to be involved in.

This really is affected by obstetric practice. The induction stuff was horrendous and I have never forgotten it. It was first brought to my attention by *Woman's Hour*, who told me that they were receiving these horrific letters. I had hundreds of them, which I analysed and wrote to *The Lancet* about.[4]

One of the more recent issues has been prostaglandin inductions. The oxytocin went down, but prostaglandins are just as bad and the woman's experience can be horrific. We then had more complaints about ruptured uteri, long before it got into the literature, when the woman had a previous scar, and they introduced a pessary.

I suspect that the information we are receiving about behaviour is a reflection of a shortage of experienced staff, a heavy workload and the fact that inadequately trained midwives are put on to the labour ward without support. These are newly qualified people working without mentors. There is a connection between what we see in the literature and what is worrying women at the time.

There is this question of the difference of pattern seen in different units, as I have pointed out to someone here who works in a unit from which we have an extremely low volume of complaints in relation to workload. We hear certain types of complaint recurring from certain areas. For example, we have far more complaints from Wales about overriding consent and dominant, authoritarian attitudes in labour to women who are trying to refuse procedures. There are clusters. Also, as you move north, where you have a higher percentage of working-class population, women do not argue with obstetricians and obstetricians expect to be obeyed.

I can only say that it is not the case that there is a population out there who will find something to complain about. People very seldom complain about home births, although I have had two cases of post-traumatic stress disorder from home births.

Marteau: Could I add to that comment by suggesting that we think about the slightly broader literature on adjustment to adverse outcomes? We know that when people blame others for an adverse outcome, their psychological adjustment is poorer. There has been a good deal of work aimed at teasing apart the causal nature of that association,[5] and the answer falls somewhere in the middle. There are some people who are more likely to blame others for an adverse outcome, so there is an individual difference there. Also, there are some events that are more likely to lead people to blame others. That is the very general picture given in the literature.

To take a specific example within the context of obstetrics, we looked at parents' adjustments to giving birth to a baby with Down syndrome.[6] We found that, overall, around 20% of those parents blamed others for that adverse outcome. However, blaming was much more common where the parents had gone through screening and been told that everything was all right than where the parents did not have screening and where none of them blamed anyone specific for that adverse event. It is a mixture that is partly to do with the individual but also with the event that they have experienced.

Nelson-Piercy: I have a question for Ms Robinson. Over the last three days, you have made disparaging comments about social workers, counsellors and debriefing. I understand that you must see women for whom those services have not fulfilled their purpose. However, as we were discussing yesterday, many of the issues we have to grapple with include how to stop people from less privileged backgrounds being disenfranchised and how to cope with the huge factor of social disadvantage in the women who die. Do you accept that social services, and debriefing and counselling, work for some women?

Robinson: What I have not seen is evidence. For example, if we look at the trial quoted by Geraldine MacDonald, Professor of Applied Social Work at Bristol University on the only long-term follow-up of 20 years that we know of, based on people randomly allocated or not to a social worker, which was the group that was more likely to have ended up in prison, in care, dropping out of education – a whole range of bad outcomes? It was the group that had been randomly allocated to a social worker.[7]

The statistics indicate that care orders have rocketed and this has been commented upon within the profession. Under the Children Act, social workers are not providing what should be available under Section 17, which is support services. They have switched to policing services – understandably – because of the kind of criticism they receive when something goes wrong, such as the Victoria Climbié case. We gave evidence to that enquiry.

What is more, they are moving far more into contact with *pregnant* women. We are now receiving allegations of antenatal Münchhausen's by proxy. I had to give evidence in one case that this was complete nonsense in a family court. Interestingly enough, two women who had questioned the need for caesarean section were accused of having Münchhausen's syndrome by proxy, which is the opposite to what you would expect, because women with Münchhausen's-by-proxy are those who demand extra services. In this case, they wanted low-tech births and this is now viewed as Münchhausen's by proxy. It is increasing stress in pregnancy, and they are also taking away the babies of breastfeeding women, which may be damaging to the child as well. It is the higher level of intervention that is leading us to ask questions, when we do not have evidence of benefit, and our anecdotal evidence is of harm.

Drife: The problem about the methodology from consumer organisations is that the only story they hear is from the consumer. The only evidence about practice originates from hearsay. Like many of the other professionals around the table, when you hear a comment about a doctor's attitude, you think of the last difficult case that you saw.

Two weeks ago, I spent over an hour in a busy clinic with someone who was not happy. It would not surprise me at all if that person, at the end of the consultation when strenuous efforts had been made to help her, went off and telephoned AIMS, misquoted me and represented me as a fool. The importance of this is not so much my finer feelings, which I am paid to cope with. In the work that this Study Group is trying to do, no support is received from professionals if they are insulted. It is important for this Study Group, in its recommendations, to say that. I would suggest that it is important for consumer representatives to take that message on board too. You obtain co-operation and enhancement of practice by recognising what people are doing and trying to correct it, rather than by unnecessarily confronting them.

Robson: I would like to make a general point, which is mainly directed to Dr Lavender, about the use of off-the-shelf scales to examine pivotal endpoints of childbirth, or any sort of process, many of which we have talked about today.

There is a recurring theme that people fail to demonstrate statistical significance using a scale and then resort to qualitative comments. That is not a criticism, but it may be that we should move away from using off-the-shelf scales. Every single scale that people have talked about has been castigated in some professional area, often because they are looking for examples of 'case-ness' in what is not an absolute threshold. I wonder whether part of the problem is the fact that we are obsessed with off-the-shelf scales that were perhaps not designed to look at the endpoints that we are implementing by looking at debriefing.

Lavender: I totally agree with that. We are actually moving in the direction of greater triangulation of research methods, which gives us a more holistic picture of what is going on.

The status of qualitative research has been elevated and people have seen its usefulness in its own right without having to attach a scale to it. There are still those who want to see the numbers but views are changing. I totally agree with you.

Oates: I would like to say two things. Ms Robinson does not know this, but if people in Nottingham heard me robustly defending social services, they would fall off their chairs. However, uniquely among the people here, I probably spend much of my working life in contact with social workers, because it is necessary for me to do so.

Social services have two legal obligations and we cannot afford to insult them. The first is under the Mental Health Act and they are therefore my close colleagues in assisting in the treatment of mental health patients. Second, as doctors, we have obligations or at least duties of care under the Children Act to act if we believe that a child is at risk of significant harm because their parent is not behaving in a responsible manner. Those instances that Ms Robinson was talking about are actually illegal and they would be subject to allegations of professional misconduct if they were reported to social service agencies.

However, just as we do not damn the whole medical profession for the occasional case that goes before the GMC, we have to be very careful. Some of the most inspired people I have ever met have been social workers. Second, the real art of qualitative research in health is that it must be as robust and disciplined as quantitative research and that it should then inspire quantitative research to raise questions that can only be answered qualitatively. Rating scales with arbitrary cut-off scores are only proxy indicators of problems.

Hands up, in this room, how many people actually know what the ten items are on the Edinburgh post-natal depression scale (EPDS)? How many have actually read it?

Robinson: I have read it, but I could not say that I remember them. [*Several study group members say they have read it.*]

Oates: And yet most of you will quote evidence from papers that have used it, when you do not have a clue what it means! If that is true of the EPDS, it may well be true of other instruments too. People quote studies using scales with no knowledge of them.

Bewley: I would like to raise three brief points about shame, unkindness and debriefing. First, there was a fantastic *BMJ* editorial recently, called 'Shame – the elephant in the room',[8] the emotion that we cannot see because it is so huge. Some of the discussions now are concerned with our pain and embarrassment about the things that go wrong. I would love to see some more studies of blame behaviour by doctors, nurses and midwives. We blame others, including consumer groups. Some of it arises from the positive motivation to do good and the shame when it has not gone well.

My suggestion would then be to think about something to do with a word that has not been used yet, which is 'kindness'. Some of the descriptions we have been hearing are about institutional unkindness. I recall a midwife in my unit who, when a woman was telling her that she had had severe bipolar manic depression and been in hospital, said, 'I won't write that in the notes. You don't want people to know that.' That was stupid, as well as unkind and stigmatising.

Dr Lavender demonstrated the value of kindness because, clearly, she is a very kind person who went to see women afterwards and was empathetic. The unkindness lay in the system by which 90% of midwives who did not even see the woman they had delivered. One reason for choosing a home delivery is that you are more likely to see the midwife who delivered you. The list of all the interventions in women that we call 'normal' look like institutional unkindness and the processing of women on conveyor belts and I found that very sad.

I am also interested in Derek Summerfield's work on war and debriefing and our misguided kindness.[9] We can try to be kind and yet make things worse in the process. We really have to go into this extremely cautiously in terms of 'debriefing', because we are very clumsy. He talks about how communities suffering war experiences have to find their own meanings and explanations. The operative phrase here in 'getting women over childbirth' is women getting over childbirth – maybe by talking to one another and telling their stories.

I loved the picture of the group, which you did not say anything about. I recall my own link midwifery team that I went along to. I was scared when all the women who had been delivered every month met and told their birth stories to each other. When I went and sat there in the background, I was terrified of what they might say. The doctors who came – some of my senior registrars and registrars – said that they learnt more about birth and women's experiences in that one session from hearing their stories than from months of training. They just sat there and listened. The women helped each other, and I would like to see more research on women debriefing one another. Ellen Hodnett from Canada has done some work on units with low caesarean section rates – units that get it right.[10] We need more research into where it goes right, the measures of kindness and ways of looking after staff kindly so that those staff will in turn look after women kindly. We know that birth is a joyful, wonderful thing that mostly makes women, their partners and their families very happy. If we could track what are the elements in professionals and institutions that deliver that kindness, we could be a little more positive and less shameful, and we would probably not argue as much.

References

1. Royal College of Psychiatrists Perinatal Mental Health Services. London Royal College of Psychiatrists Council Report CR88; 2000.
2. Royal College of Obstetricians and Gynaecologists. A blueprint for the future: a working party report on the future structure of the medical workforce and service delivery in obstetrics and gynaecology. December 2000.
3. Cartwright A. *The Dignity of Labour*. London: Tavistock; 1979.
4. Robinson J. Elective induction of labour. *Lancet* 1975;i:1242.
5. Tennen H, Affleck G. Blaming others for threatening events. *Psychol Bull* 1990;108:209–32.
6. Hall S, Bobrow M, Marteau TM. Psychological consequences for parents of false positive results on prenatal screening for Down's syndrome: retrospective interview study. *BMJ* 2000;320:407–12.
7. MacDonald G. Social work: beyond control? In: Maynard A, Chalmers I, editors. *Non-Random Reflections on Health Services Research*. London: BMJ Publishing Group; 1977. p. 122–46.
8. Davidoff F. Shame: the elephant in the room. *BMJ* 2002;324:623–4.
9. Summerfield, D. Bosnia and Herzegovina and Croatia: the medicalization of the experience of war. *Lancet* 1999;359:771–80.
10. Hodnett E. Attaining and maintaining best practices in the use of caesarean section. Toronto: Ontario Women's Health Council; 2001 [http://www.womenshealthcouncil.on.ca].

SECTION 8

THE ROLE OF MULTI-PROFESSIONAL WORKING

Chapter 31

Midwifery

Christine A Carson

Introduction

Midwives have a unique role to play in maternity care, especially in relation to multiprofessional working. In the UK, midwives provide the majority of care for women during pregnancy, delivery and the postnatal period. Currently midwives are the lead professional for 68.8% of births,[1] while they are also involved in the majority of the remaining 31.2%, which are generally higher-risk pregnancies. In the current climate of radical National Health Service (NHS) reform, midwifery-led care is likely to increase. Obstetric care has a well-established history of progress and innovation. As new technologies continue to develop in fetal and maternal medicine, an opportunity presents itself for midwives to become an important resource in facilitating this progress. Traditionally, the midwife is the provider of individualised care to the mother throughout pregnancy and the puerperium. The most recent triennial report of the Confidential Enquiries into Maternal Deaths (CEMD)[2] highlights a number of key ways in which the midwife can contribute to safer and more holistic maternity care, often acting as an important link between professionals from different disciplines, as well as bridging the primary–secondary care interface. Indeed, of the 378 deaths reported to or identified by the enquiry, 357 of the women had had contact with the midwifery services. The 21 women who had not had contact with a midwife died either before booking or following a miscarriage, ruptured ectopic pregnancy or termination of pregnancy. The relative safety of midwifery-led care is demonstrated by the fact that only eight of the reported deaths were in this category of care.

It is worth noting that the majority of pregnancies can be considered to be a state of normal health for the mother. Even when a mother presents with recognised risk factors, the professionals rarely consider the likelihood of a fatal outcome.[3] From the 1997/99 CEMD report, it is clear that the severity of the mother's condition was underestimated in many cases by the team of professionals involved. Recent research in this area supports this view.[3] This suggests that there is a need to raise awareness regarding this potential outcome. In an attempt to address this, for the first time a copy of the midwifery section including all the recommendations from each chapter of the 1997–99 CEMD report was sent to all registered midwives in the UK.

In recent years, an increasingly significant role has also developed for the midwife, in terms of addressing broad public health issues. This chapter focuses on a number of generic issues in relation to the midwife and multiprofessional working. The areas to be covered are derived directly from the recommendations of the midwifery section of the CEMD report for 1997–99 listed at the end of this chapter.

Individualised care

Current health reforms are driving all disciplines towards the establishment of 'patient pathways' and protocols of service provision. At the time of writing, the English Department of Health (DoH) is developing a maternity module of the Children's National Service Framework. Such long-term strategies now form a statutory part of service provision for any hospital trust, and delivery against milestones is monitored by the Commission for Health Improvement. Such compartmentalisation may appear to detract from individualised care, with the administrative focus being on compliance with pathways and structures. However, the role and importance of an individualised approach to maternity service provision is highlighted by the findings of the 1997–99 CEMD report.[2] The challenge for the future, therefore, must be to match provision of a clearly identified standard of care for all with a flexible plan of appropriate, high-quality care for each individual woman. Compliance with pathways and structures is often monitored through the use of process indicators. All staff involved in the delivery of maternity services must ensure that they are not distracted from the assessment of each mother, at each contact, by the administrative need to collect data. It is well recognised that many clinical situations that use guidelines and standardised instruments for data collection result in boxes being filled in, often without the significance of the data itself being considered. This will be particularly important for midwives, because of their role as the main providers of maternity care.

With regard to a new pregnancy, the usual pathway is likely to involve a mother presenting, via her general practitioner (GP), for booking. An assessment is made of risk factors. This initial assessment is clearly influenced by the quality of information in the referral letter from the GP, as well as any previous obstetric records. A decision on the pattern of care is likely to be made at this point, during which time the midwife will see the mother to take the booking history. This is an opportunity to identify not just physical, medical or other obstetric issues relevant to the current pregnancy but also different social or emotional needs that the mother may have. The pregnancy cannot be viewed in isolation from other important factors that may influence her health or that of her baby. Any new risk factors identified in the booking history need be taken into account in the form of a reappraisal of the pattern of care. Each woman should have a flexible, individual antenatal care plan that reflects her own circumstances and needs. In the majority of cases, the midwife will continue to be the provider of the majority of antenatal care. In so doing, the midwife is well placed to address factors such as health inequalities and health promotion issues. 'Making a difference' suggests that midwives should specifically target vulnerable groups who would not traditionally use the health promotion services.[4]

Risk assessment

The importance of a formal risk assessment at each contact with the mother cannot be overstated. This is of particular relevance to midwives as the main providers of care during pregnancy and the puerperium. It was clear from the 1997–99 CEMD report that risks in relation to specific areas, such as psychiatric illness and thromboembolism, were underestimated. A risk assessment is dependent upon the availability of information. Missing information must be actively sought. Thus, the absence of a urine specimen should trigger a request for the mother to produce one before leaving the clinic. Furthermore, the practice of retaining the hand-held records following transfer home after delivery may result in crucial information about risk factors being unavailable to midwives during the postnatal period. In particular, the absence of information in relation to psychiatric morbidity or the use of the term 'postnatal depression' (or PND) may cause serious underestimation of the severity of a mother's mental state. This can lead to care being delivered reactively rather than proactively, with professionals involved in the care of these women being taken by surprise at the rapid escalation of symptoms.

Further support for stressing the importance of risk assessment is provided by the 1997–99 CEMD finding that clear risk factors were present in 25 of the 31 women who died from venous thromboembolism. In general, once a risk has been identified, appropriate action should be taken. All professionals involved in the care of mothers should be prepared to accept direct referrals from any other professional and should be seen to respond appropriately to the reason for the referral.

Targeting of care and social exclusion

One of the key findings of the 1997–99 CEMD report was that women from the most disadvantaged groups of society are about 20 times more likely to die than women in the highest two social classes. The midwife has a central role to play in appropriate targeting of care. As the main provider of care, the midwife is in a unique position to take an overview of all aspects of the care of the mother, be they physical, psychological or social. The 1997–99 CEMD report has recommended that midwives work proactively with professionals and other agencies to ensure that a flexible approach to care is given at every level of the service, throughout the pregnancy and beyond. While the service has become increasingly responsive to consumer demand of consumers, there is a clear need to ensure that mothers who do not make demands on the service do not miss out on appropriate care. There is a tendency for systems to be inflexible and unresponsive to the needs of those most at risk. For example, mothers who are addicted to Class A drugs may be poor attenders at the antenatal clinic, whereas their compliance with attendance at the community drugs team is likely to be more predictable. This scenario presents an opportunity, perhaps, for the midwife to liaise with the community drugs team in order to provide antenatal care to the mother at the time of her attendance at their clinic.

Twenty percent of the total number of maternal deaths considered by the 1997–99 CEMD involved mothers who either booked after twenty weeks of pregnancy or missed five or more antenatal visits. While it is not possible to follow up women who are unknown to the service, in many instances non-attendance by a woman who has booked generates a routine appointment by post. This could be a purely administrative response or a professional could be involved. Targeting care is about developing services that are effective for all women but particularly for those who would not normally actively seek help and advice. As part of the changes in the delivery of midwifery care, it is crucial that new patterns of antenatal care are developed, particularly for those women who are at the greatest risk. In some instances, this may require individual antenatal care at home. As a minimum, maternity services should provide guidelines for follow-up procedures for women who regularly fail to attend for antenatal care.

When considering all cases from the 1997–99 CEMD report, it was found that nearly half of all mothers who booked after 20 weeks of pregnancy or who were poor attenders at antenatal clinics came from ethnic minority groups. Half of these women did not speak English. In some cases, midwives did go into the community to follow these women up but in others either no active follow-up was undertaken or letters were sent in English, advising the woman to attend her next appointment. It is vital that all midwives should have access to and use culturally sensitive and appropriate services. This should include adequate interpreting services.

Domestic violence is now recognised as being an increasingly important issue. Twelve percent of the maternal deaths reported to the 1997–99 CEMD were associated with recognised domestic violence before the fatal outcome, this subject now meriting a chapter in its own right. The midwife's role in identifying mothers who are subject to domestic violence is key. All mothers should have the opportunity to see a midwife without their partner present at some stage in the pregnancy. All professionals should have a 24-hour help-line number that can be given to women who they have identified as at risk of domestic violence.[5,6] Once this is identified, it behoves the midwife to liaise closely with appropriate local services.

Communication and collaborative working

The importance of communication between midwives and other professionals was highlighted as a recurring theme in the 1997–99 CEMD report. Poor interprofessional communication was a contributory factor in many cases and, in some, communication with the mother was also poor. There were also examples of excellent communication and multidisciplinary working, especially in relation to the care of mothers with cancer.

The midwife is the professional most likely to identify factors that will require medical intervention. Midwives working in primary care appear to have good communication networks with the obstetric services in hospital. However, referrals to professionals working in primary care are infrequent and are generally conducted via the mother. Midwives should feel able to contact a GP directly if this is considered necessary. Moreover, midwives do appear reluctant to refer across specialty boundaries to allied professionals, such as community psychiatric nurses, even when there is a serious risk of mental illness. The midwife should also have the facility to refer women they are concerned about to hospital services directly.

There is a need to work in close partnership with other professionals, even where the midwife is the accountable lead professional, reflecting their membership of a team. The midwife should feel able to approach senior staff directly, even if this involves bypassing a less experienced doctor.

Professional responsibility and accountability

Midwifery care has undergone many changes in the pattern of service delivery over the last decade and these changes are set to continue in the UK in line with developments in government policy and national strategies such as the NHS Plan.[7] Further changes are set to continue with the new Nurses and Midwives Council taking over from the United Kingdom Central Council and the four National Boards from April 2002. Midwives need to reflect on their own practice and develop it, playing an active role in challenging the organisational structure and culture in which they work in order to agree policies that reflect the recommendations in the 1997–99 CEMD report.

The introduction of the consultant midwife in many trusts in the UK will serve to enhance the midwife's professional development. Allied to this is the midwife's role as an advocate, crossing health and social-care boundaries. The midwife should act as an advocate for women, providing a high standard of care in accordance with midwives' rules and code of practice and guidelines for professional practice.[8,9]

Public health role of the midwife

Midwives have had an increasing public health role as part of their practice. Given the current major reorganisation of the NHS, with the development of primary care trusts, midwives are well placed to contribute to the health improvement plans of primary care trusts and trusts providing maternity services. The unique perspective of the midwife, bridging primary and secondary care, will prove invaluable in setting a cohesive strategic direction for these organisations. The main thrust of these strategies must be to ensure that mothers who are well remain so, while also addressing key areas such as breastfeeding policies and support for smoking cessation. Cross-boundary communication must also be addressed in these strategies and the midwife will make an important contribution to referral pathways to health and social care partners. There is a pressing need to work with women and their families to develop maternity services that are flexible and responsive to the needs of each individual.[10] There may be important lessons to learn from colleagues in specific project areas, such as *Sure Start*, so that innovation can be based on clear working examples of best practice.

Conclusion

The goal of minimising maternal mortality will be achieved only by all professionals and agencies involved in the provision of care during pregnancy, delivery and the postnatal period working together rather than perpetuating old rivalries. As clinical governance and reflective, blame-free practice becomes more established, teamwork should be allowed to flourish. The midwife has a key role to play, both as the lead care-provider in the majority of cases and as a provider of pivotal care, addressing not just medical but also psychological and social needs in most other pregnancies. As the health service continues to metamorphose, the public health role of the midwife in contributing to the strategic planning of services to local communities, crossing the primary–secondary care divide, as well as that of health and social care, will be a key development in improving maternal morbidity and mortality.

There needs to be a commitment to providing a modern, flexible framework within the midwifery profession to enable the care to be given to those mothers and their infants who are at greatest risk, those who are least likely to access care.

Recommendations from the midwifery section of the 1997–99 CEMD[2]

Antenatal care

Midwives should be at the forefront of helping to plan new models of service provision. The planning and delivery of maternity services should focus on regarding each woman as an individual person with different social, physical and emotional needs, as well on any specific clinical factors that may affect her pregnancy. Her pregnancy should not be viewed in isolation from other important factors that may influence her health or that of her developing baby.

Each woman should have a flexible, individualised antenatal care plan drawn up at booking that reflects her own circumstances and needs. This should be reviewed regularly throughout her pregnancy.

There may be many reasons why women fail to attend clinic appointments. These women are at higher risk of maternal and fetal complications and death, and the midwife should actively follow up regular non-attendance. If the reasons why she was unable to seek care are ascertained through sympathetic questioning, alternative arrangements should be made that suit the particular circumstances of the woman.

Targeting care is about developing services that are effective for all women but particularly for those women who would not normally actively seek help and advice. As part of the changes in the delivery of midwifery care, it is crucial that new patterns of antenatal care are developed, particularly for those women at the greatest risk. In some instances, this may require individual antenatal care at home.

Interpreters should be provided for women who do not speak English. The use of family members, including the use of children as interpreters, should be avoided if at all possible.

Booking

At booking, a needs and risk assessment should take place to ensure that every woman has a flexible individual plan for her antenatal care, to be reviewed at each visit, that reflects her own particular requirements.

With the growing importance of midwifery-led care, it is vital that midwives undertake a full needs assessment at the booking visit in order to identify women whose medical history or situation may make them unsuitable for this type of care and so that these women can be referred for more appropriate care. Conversely, midwives should be prepared to decline to take responsibility for high-risk cases from an obstetrician, where the involvement of a consultant obstetrician is essential and the reasons for this should be explained to the woman and to the obstetrician.

The GP booking letter is a referral mechanism and should not be relied upon to provide all the information necessary for planning antenatal care.

All mothers should have their body mass index calculated at booking as part of the full risk assessment. Further, they should be offered advice about sensible weight reduction, including diet and exercise, and referred to a dietitian where appropriate. An individual or family history of thromboembolism should be sought and, if present, specialist advice should be obtained.

Midwives are uniquely placed to provide advice and support on healthy lifestyles including:

- diet and exercise
- smoking, alcohol and substance misuse
- safety in the home and workplace
- basic first-aid measures, especially for women with conditions such as epilepsy
- the correct use of car seat belts
- guidance about the warning signs of obstetric complications, such as pre-eclampsia.

All pregnant women should be given advice about the correct use of seat belts as soon as their pregnancy is confirmed. 'Above and below the bump, not over it'.

Three-point seat belts should be worn throughout pregnancy with the lap-strap placed as low as possible beneath the 'bump', lying across the thighs, with the diagonal shoulder-strap above the bump lying between the breasts. The seat belt should be adjusted to fit as tightly as is comfortably possible and, if necessary, the seat should be adjusted to enable the seat belt to be worn properly.

Enquiries about psychiatric history and its severity, the care received and clinical presentation should be made routinely in a systematic and sensitive way at the antenatal booking clinic. Women who have a history of serious psychiatric disorder, postpartum or non-postpartum, should be referred to a psychiatrist and a management plan should be formulated in light of the high risk of recurrence.

The term 'postnatal depression' or 'PND' should be used only to describe a non-psychotic depressive illness of mild to moderate severity with its onset following delivery. It should not be used as a generic term to describe other mental illnesses. The term 'postnatal depression' in the maternity records diminishes the severity of previous illness and the high risk of recurrence and it should not be used unless the illness was minor in nature. Precise details of any previous illness should be sought and recorded in line with the recommendation above.

All pregnant women should be routinely asked about domestic violence as part of their social history and should have the opportunity to discuss their pregnancy with a midwife, in privacy, without their partner present, at least once during the antenatal period.

Continuing care

All providers of maternity services should ensure that there are clear protocols and routes of referral to primary or secondary care when rapid assessment, investigation and treatment are required. This will involve close collaboration with other professionals in both primary and secondary care. When referring a woman to GPs in primary care, midwives should make direct contact with the GP and not ask the woman or her family to do so on her behalf. Midwives should have the facility to refer women about whom they are directly concerned to hospital services. In order to increase the detection of pre-eclampsia, all mothers should have their urine tested at each antenatal contact after 20 weeks of pregnancy.

Individual practice

Midwives must reflect and develop their practice and play an active role in challenging the organisational structure and culture in which they work, to agree policies that reflect the recommendations in this report.

Midwives and other health professionals who work with disadvantaged clients need to be able to understand a woman's social and cultural background, act as an advocate for women with medical staff and colleagues, overcome their own personal and social prejudices and practise in a reflective manner.[11]

Midwives should be prepared to decline to take responsibility for high-risk cases from an obstetrician where the involvement of a consultant obstetrician is essential and the reasons for this should be explained to the woman and to the obstetrician.

Midwives need to make full use of existing systems of statutory supervision to ensure continuing professional development and actively demonstrate evidence-based care.

Continuing professional development should be accepted as the responsibility of the individual practitioner as well as the employer, and knowledge and skills should be regularly updated using current research evidence.

References

1. English National Board for Nursing, Midwifery and Health Visiting. *Report of the Board's Midwifery Practice Audit 1999/2000*. London: ENB; 2001.
2. Lewis G, Drife J, editors. *Why Mothers Die 1997–1999. The Confidential Enquiries into Maternal Deaths in the United Kingdom*. London: RCOG Press; 2001.
3. Mander R. Death of a mother: taboo and the midwife. *Practising Midwife* 2001;4:23–5.
4. Department of Health. *Making a Difference: Strengthening the Nursing, Midwifery and Health Visiting Contribution to Health and Healthcare*. London: DoH; 1999.
5. Department of Health. *Domestic Violence: A Resource Manual for Health Care Professionals*. London: DoH; 2000.
6. Royal College of Midwives. *Domestic Abuse in Pregnancy*. Position paper No 19a. London: RCM; 1999.
7. Department of Health. *The NHS Plan. A Plan for Investment, A Plan for Reform*. London: DoH; 2000.
8. United Kingdom Central Council for Nursing, Midwifery and Health Visiting. *Midwives' Rules and Code of Practice*. London: UKCC; 1988.
9. United Kingdom Central Council for Nursing Midwifery and Health Visiting. *Guidelines for Professional Practice*. London: UKCC; 1996.
10. Kaufmann T. Midwifery and public health. *MIDIRS Midwifery Digest* 2002;12 Suppl 1: S23–S26.
11. Hart A, Lockey R, Henwood F, Pankhurst F, Hall V, Sommerville F. *Researching Professional Education. Addressing Inequalities in Health: New Directions in Midwifery Education and Practice*. London: ENB; 2001.

Chapter 32

Anaesthesia

Griselda M Cooper and Anthony D Wilkey

A historical perspective

The history of deaths resulting from anaesthesia can be traced through the successive reports of the Confidential Enquiry into Maternal Deaths (CEMD) that were initiated in 1952. The preface of this first report[1] in the seminal series drew attention to the major features of anaesthesia as a primary or associated factor of death. Forty-nine deaths were ascribed to anaesthesia, but at least 20 more were identified in which anaesthesia was contributory.

The anaesthetic deaths in each triennium are enumerated in Table 32.1.[1–16] From this table, it is evident that there has been a dramatic reduction in the numbers of deaths from anaesthesia. Until 1981, there were between 30 and 50 deaths in each triennium ascribed directly to anaesthesia. In the 1982–84 triennium, this figure was 19 deaths and the same total number of deaths due to anaesthesia were reported in the years 1985 to 1996, spanning four triennia or twelve years. Indeed, in recent years death from anaesthesia has been a rare occurrence.

However, these raw numbers do not fully illustrate the scale of the improvement. The numbers of maternities have varied over the years (Table 32.2), with a post-war bulge extending into the 1950s and 1960s, but fewer than two million maternities in the triennia spanning 1973 to 1984. Thereafter, the increased maternities are accounted for by the larger population base of the UK, rather than solely England and Wales. Until 1984, the overall maternal death rate had been decreasing by approximately 50% every ten years.[11] This trend is reviewed in the latest CEMD report.[16]

A greater change than in the numbers of maternities is the number of anaesthetics given to pregnant women both in obstetrics and gynaecology. The most common reasons for anaesthesia are caesarean section, retained placenta, vaginal delivery, removing retained products of conception and to treat ectopic pregnancy. In addition, a small proportion of anaesthetics will be given for incidental surgery during pregnancy or for complications around the time of delivery, such as draining wound haematomas or repairing perineal tears. A further aspect is the provision of epidural analgesia for pain relief in labour. Unfortunately there have not been, nor are there now, national (or even comprehensive local) statistics for the numbers of anaesthetics

Table 32.1. The numbers of maternal deaths due to anaesthesia in each triennia; data taken from successive reports of Confidential Enquiries into Maternal Deaths[1–16]; Crown copyright material reproduced with permission of the Controller of HMSO and the Queen's Printer for Scotland

Triennium[a]	Deaths due to anaesthesia (n)
1952–54	49
1955–57	31
1958–60	30
1961–63	28
1964–66	50
1967–69	50
1970–72	37
1973–75	37
1976–78	40
1979–81	29
1982–84	19
1985–87	6 (+2 late)
1988–90	4 (+1 late)
1991–93	8
1994–96	1
1997–99	3

[a] the data from these enquiries relate only to England and Wales until 1985, whereas from the 1985–88 triennium onwards they include the whole of the UK

given for maternity services. The Department of Health does, however, have records of the caesarean rate for most years since 1955. Given knowledge of the numbers of maternities, it has been possible to calculate the numbers of caesarean sections performed. The increasing numbers of anaesthetics given for caesarean section by contrast with the reductions in maternal death from anaesthesia are illustrated in Figure 32.1. Furthermore, from most of the triennial reports it has also been possible to extract the numbers of anaesthetic deaths where anaesthesia was being administered for caesarean section (Table 32.2).

It is noteworthy that although the reports from 1955 until 1963[2–4] did not specify the numbers of anaesthetics given for caesarean sections, a large number of general anaesthetics were given for delivery by forceps. The difficulties presented for anaesthesia would include all those presented by the pregnancy itself, compounded by the positioning of the woman in lithotomy.

The caesarean section data are summarised in Table 32.2. It is possible to calculate a mortality rate for anaesthesia for caesarean section, and this is also displayed in Table 32.2 and Figure 32.2 as a relative risk compared with the mortality rate for anaesthesia in the 1994–96 triennium. This shows that anaesthesia for caesarean section is in the region of 100 times safer now than it was in the 1960s. The three deaths from anaesthesia in the 1997–99 triennium do not necessarily indicate a worsening of the safety of anaesthesia for caesarean section. One of the three deaths clearly happened at the time of caesarean section. The other two women had relatively uneventful anaesthesia for caesarean section but became ill enough to require intensive care because of severe haemorrhage. They subsequently required anaesthesia (one for tracheostomy tube change and the other for removal of abdominal packs) that precipitated their deaths. Accepting this argument brings the relative mortality rate for anaesthesia from caesarean section for the 1997–99 triennium from 2.5 to 0.8. It remains a challenge for the specialty of anaesthesia to maintain this high degree of safety.

Table 32.2. The caesarean section (CS) rate expressed as a percentage of maternities, the calculated numbers of caesarean sections performed, the numbers of anaesthetic maternal deaths where anaesthesia was given for caesarean sections, and the relative risk compared with that occurring in 1994–96

Triennium	Maternities (*n*)	CS[a] (%)	CS (*n*)	Deaths due to anaesthesia (*n*)	Anaesthetic deaths for CS (*n*)	Deaths per CS	Relative risk
1952–54	2 052953	2.2[b]	45165	49	13	1 in 3474	95
1955–57	2 113471	2.2	46496	31	Not given		
1958–60	2 294414	2.6	59655	30	Not given		
1961–63	2 520420	3.0	75613	28	Not given		
1964–66	2 600367	3.4	88412	50	32	1 in 2763	120
1967–69	2 457444	4.0	98298	50	36	1 in 2731	121
1970–72	2 298198	4.6	105717	37	19	1 in 5564	60
1973–75	1 921569	5.4	103765	37	18	1 in 5765	57
1976–78	1 748849	6.9	120671	40	21	1 in 5746	58
1979–81	1 748851	8.8	153899	29	20	1 in 7695	43
1982–84	1 883753	10.1	190259	19	11	1 in 17296	19
1985–87	2 268766	10.9[b]	247295	8	5	1 in 49459	6.7
1988–90	2 360309	11.7	276156	5	4	1 in 69039	4.8
1991–93	2 315204	13.9	321813	8	6	1 in 53635	6.2
1994–96	2 046200	16.2	331484	1	1	1 in 331484	1
1997–99	2 123600	19.0	403484	3	3	1 in 134495	2.5

[a] figures obtained from Department of Health; [b] estimated figure because not available

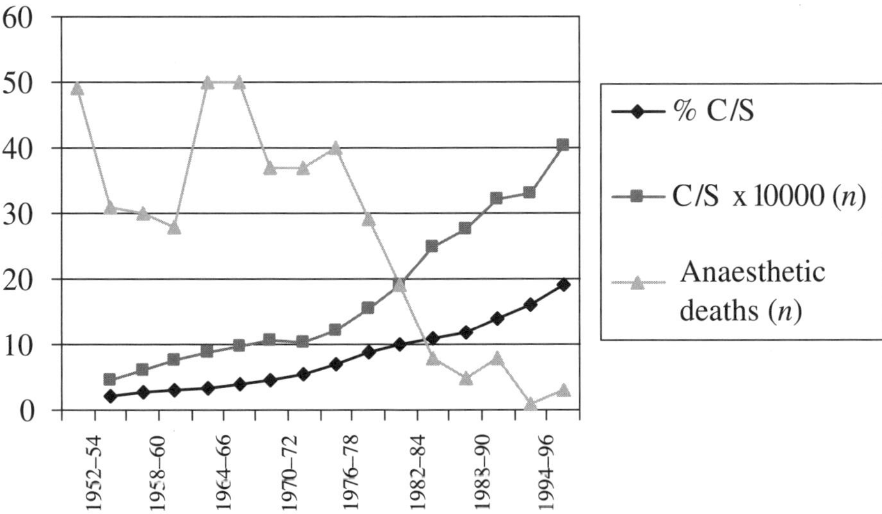

Figure 32.1. The proportion of deliveries by caesarean section, the calculated numbers of caesarean sections (*c/s*) performed and the numbers of maternal deaths from anaesthesia in each triennium; Crown copyright material reproduced with permission of the Controller of HMSO and the Queen's Printer for Scotland

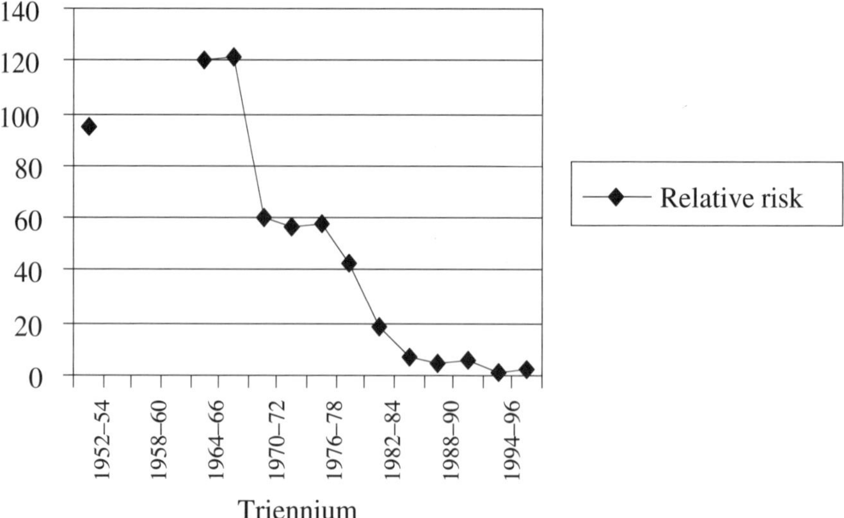

Figure 32.2. The relative risk of dying from anaesthesia for caesarean section, assuming that the risk in 1994–96 is 1

Reasons for improvement in anaesthetic mortality

Why have these improvements occurred? The most common causes of anaesthetic death used to be related to airway management, either through failure to oxygenate the mother while trying to achieve endotracheal intubation or because of aspiration of gastric contents resulting in either immediate asphyxiation or later respiratory failure from acute respiratory distress syndrome. It was a matter of great concern in the reports until the 1980s that there should be so many apparently preventable deaths. It is obvious from reading the older reports that practice was very different from now. Examples that illustrate this include:

'In 5 and possibly 6 cases the anaesthetic was administered by the single-handed obstetrician',[2]

'Anaesthesia (spinal anaesthesia for caesarean section) initially appeared satisfactory but respiratory difficulties occurred before the operation was completed. By this time the anaesthetist was busy elsewhere and not immediately available'.[4]

and: 'One patient during criminal abortion died under chloroform anaesthesia administered by a man with no medical qualification'.[5]

These illustrations speak for themselves, although it is worth noting that abolishing operator-anaesthetists in dentistry did not occur until 1983, enforced by the General Dental Council. Nowadays, it would be unthinkable that the anaesthetist would not be present until the woman was satisfactorily recovering.

One of the key ways of avoiding airway management problems has been the increased use of regional rather general anaesthesia. By 1990, 51% of anaesthetics given for caesarean section were regional anaesthetics[17] and this figure had increased to 76.5% by 1997–1998.[18] The most recent figures for the year 2000 are 91% of elective and 77% of emergency caesarean sections conducted under regional block.[19] Although the increased use of regional block has undoubtedly contributed to the safety of anaesthesia for caesarean section, there are real concerns that this is resulting in anaesthetists being unskilled, inexperienced and frightened of general anaesthesia for obstetrics.[18,20] It is salutary to learn of at least three occasions on which failure of endotracheal intubation by trainee anaesthetists has resulted in maternal death since 1999, particularly as this was absent from the last two triennial reports.[15,16]

The problem of acid aspiration leading to Mendelson's syndrome has been tackled by a series of changes.

The rapid sequence induction involving pre-oxygenation, cricoid pressure, use of suxamethonium and avoidance of mask ventilation before endotracheal intubation was developed in a rather piecemeal fashion, as documented in the first five reports. However, in its complete version, rapid sequence induction provides a vital role of preventing aspiration at induction.

The widespread adoption of the policy of allowing only small amounts of water by mouth during labour has ensured that relatively few women are anaesthetised with a genuinely full stomach. The rarity of aspiration problems has led some midwives to call for an end to such policies and to allow mothers to eat and drink freely during labour. There is some evidence that isotonic drinks may be of benefit without increasing risks but pressure for more liberalisation should be viewed with extreme caution in view of the potential for catastrophic results.[21]

Perhaps the most effective measure has been the widespread administration of drugs to prevent acid secretion from the stomach to women anticipated to need anaesthesia. In the UK, this is achieved in 98% of cases with H_2 blockers such as ranitidine and in the remaining 2% with a proton pump inhibitor (omeprazole), coupled with a drug such as sodium citrate to neutralise any gastric acid already present.[19] As yet not satisfactorily resolved is the prediction of those who will require anaesthesia and hence the need to treat many women who will not require acid prophylaxis.

The requirement for endotracheal intubation for caesarean section in order to reduce aspiration risk had become accepted by the 1960s. This unfortunately led to a marked increase in deaths from failed intubation and oxygenation and other airway problems. Sixteen deaths from these causes were recorded in the 1976–78 report, eight in 1979–81 and ten in 1982–84. This has become unusual in recent reports as a result of better training and assistance, use of failed intubation drills and the use of monitoring by capnography and oximetry throughout induction, maintenance and recovery from anaesthesia. As noted above, a possible increase in deaths from this cause requires all these aspects of care to be rigorously continued. Another criticism of the successive reports has been the lack of consultant involvement. At a time when the specialist input was sparse, the recommendation from the 1964–66 report recognised that 'patients with obstetric emergencies are gravely at risk and require knowledge and skill of an experienced anaesthetist who must be readily available'.[5] The lack of consultant involvement has been less of a feature in later years (although by no means absent) and there have been concerted efforts to improve consultant anaesthetist staffing of obstetric services. It is expected that this in turn has improved the training of anaesthetists new to the discipline of obstetric anaesthesia.

The modern role of anaesthetists in maternal safety

The importance of good teamwork between specialists was not properly recognised until 1979–81, when multidisciplinary working was recommended because of the deaths of three women with severe kyphoscoliosis.[10] The varied skills that anaesthetists have are gained through their training and their work in areas outside obstetric anaesthesia. This is recognised in their key role in the care of many sick mothers, but especially so in the management of women with massive haemorrhage. The use of direct arterial monitoring of blood pressure, central venous and, in some cases, pulmonary artery pressures improves the accuracy of blood and fluid management. These techniques are now being used much more frequently than they were. The 1985–87 report[12] was the first to recommend that expert teams, which included anaesthetists, be established for the management of severe pre-eclampsia.

Maternal morbidity from anaesthesia

The problem for anaesthesia is that it is not an end in itself in the way that delivery of the baby is for the obstetrician. Anaesthesia is an enabling process. This is also balanced against the prevailing view that pregnancy and delivery is a physiological process, although there is a recognition that, if this physiological process is left to its own devices, there is unacceptable morbidity and mortality. However, any adverse effects of anaesthesia are seen as even less acceptable. What therefore is the price to pay for increased safety of anaesthesia?

Near-misses from general anaesthesia

As discussed earlier, the majority of deaths from anaesthesia have been attributable to general anaesthesia. If the mother survives the potentially fatal insult, serious long-term morbidity may result. Pulmonary aspiration of gastric contents has been reported to occur in one in 900 caesarean sections[22] compared with lower figures in general surgery.[23] Short-term morbidity due to pulmonary injury may necessitate intensive care admission, short-term ventilation and prolonged hospitalisation but long-term morbidity is unusual. Avoiding oral intake during labour and antacid prophylaxis have probably helped to maintain a low morbidity.

Any airway crisis, for example failed intubation of the trachea (which occurs in one in 250–300 general anaesthetics),[24,25] airway obstruction or disconnection may result in profound cerebral hypoxia and failure to regain consciousness.[23]

Minor sequelae of general anaesthesia

There are several minor sequelae of general anaesthesia, including nausea and vomiting and sore throat, that are short-lived and self-limiting. Awareness during general anaesthesia, although historically a relatively frequent occurrence has, with modern techniques and monitoring, become unusual but may be associated with psychological consequences if not managed appropriately.

Morbidity from regional anaesthesia

The increase in use of regional anaesthesia has contributed significantly to lower anaesthetic mortality rates but does carry with it a small risk of morbidity including, most seriously, neurological damage.

The most common potentially serious complication is hypotension during the time the block is working. This may occur in any regional anaesthetic, including up to 83% of caesarean sections performed under spinal anaesthetic.[26] Untreated, this may lead to cerebral ischaemia or cardiac arrest in the mother and serious or fatal fetal sequelae. The likelihood of serious hypotension is increased if there is haemorrhage. Meticulous care to avoid aortocaval compression, adequate crystalloid or colloid preload and use of vasopressor drugs will minimise the risk.

Neurological complications after regional block

Overall, severe neurological complications after regional blockade are rare. These were the subject of a detailed review by Loo *et al.*[27] The aetiology of these complications may be difficult to ascertain because labour and delivery may lead to maternal obstetric palsies. Spontaneous complications such as epidural haematoma and abscesses can also occur. The reported incidence of complications in obstetric epidural analgesia in recent reports has been from 0.8–3.5/10 000 blocks[28–30] and 5.4/10 000 for spinal anaesthesia.[31] The majority of these sequelae are not permanent and resolve in a variable period of time.

There is a range of aetiologies to account for these complications. Epidural abscesses occur after 0.2–3.7/10 000 obstetric epidurals.[31,32] The source of infection may be direct contamination or from haematogenous spread from a coexisting infection. Prolonged epidural catheterisation for postoperative pain control may increase the risk but use of a bacterial filter, which is now routine, has been shown to be effective in reducing infection of the catheter tip.[33] Early surgical intervention to treat the epidural abscess has led to good outcomes in most reported cases.

The rare reports of bacterial meningitis are associated with deliberate or inadvertent dural puncture. Isolation of the infective organism suggests that direct contamination is usually the cause and therefore strict aseptic techniques and single-use sterile equipment is vital to minimise the risk. Recovery is the norm in reported cases.

Arachnoiditis is an extremely rare progressive inflammatory disorder that usually leads to permanent disability. Nine cases have been reported after obstetric epidural blocks. The aetiology is unknown but preservatives in the local anaesthetic solutions used may have been responsible in some of the cases.

Spinal haematoma may complicate epidural block in 0.2–3.7/100 000 cases[31,32] but has not been reported after obstetric spinal block. This may be associated with coagulation abnormality and therefore careful history taking, appropriate laboratory investigations and sensible timing of insertion in patients on thromboprophylaxis with a low molecular weight heparin will help to prevent this problem. Prompt surgical intervention has usually been associated with a good outcome, although some residual neurological dysfunction is not uncommon.

Cauda equina syndrome resulting from damage to the nerve roots L2 to S5 has been reported. The association of this syndrome with high concentrations of lignocaine in conjunction with microcatheters has led to the withdrawal of the latter in the USA. There have been no confirmed obstetric cases and the use of the less neurotoxic bupivacaine and more dilute lignocaine solutions ensure that this complication remains extremely unusual.

Neurological sequelae may result from direct trauma from the needle, catheter or injection into a nerve root or spinal cord. This will usually produce pain or paraesthesia during insertion or injection and the subsequent deficit will involve the same distribution. Scott and Tunstall[28] reported 46 cases of single nerve root neuropathy (5.4/10 000 obstetric spinal blocks, 3.5/10 000 obstetric epidural blocks). None of these was permanent and obstetric causes were considered likely in a proportion of cases. Reynolds[34] has recently reported six cases of obstetric patients with spinal cord damage apparently due to direct needle trauma following spinal or combined spinal and epidural anaesthesia. She emphasises the importance of selecting the correct interspace for injection to remain safely below the termination of the spinal cord.

Dural puncture sequelae

Inadvertent dural puncture occurs in approximately 1% of parturients receiving epidural analgesia and is associated with a high incidence of headache (approximately 70%). Deliberate spinal anaesthesia with a small-gauge, atraumatic needle is associated with headache rates of 0.4–5.45%, depending in part on the definition of severity.[35,36] The headache can be severe and debilitating, especially since it occurs at a time when the mother wishes to care for her baby. Fortunately, this normally lasts only a few days and can usually be effectively treated conservatively or with an epidural blood patch. There are, however, reports of longer-term effects, including headache, neckache and backache.[35]

Rarely, more serious neurological problems may result from dural puncture, including cranial subdural haematoma or cranial nerve palsies particularly involving the abducens nerve, which may become stretched as a result of low cerebrospinal fluid pressure.[27]

Summary

The risk of permanent neurological damage after regional block is low. However, screening of patients for sepsis and coagulopathy, meticulous technique and close follow-up are vital to maintain and improve this safety record. The challenge to maintain a high safety record for anaesthesia remains.

References

1. Ministry of Health. *Report on Confidential Enquiries into Maternal Deaths in England and Wales 1952–1954. Reports on Public Health and Medical Subjects No. 97*. London: HMSO; 1957.
2. Ministry of Health. *Report on Confidential Enquiries into Maternal Deaths in England and Wales 1955–1957. Reports on Public Health and Medical Subjects No. 103*. London: HMSO; 1960.
3. Ministry of Health. *Report on Confidential Enquiries into Maternal Deaths in England and Wales 1958–1960. Reports on Public Health and Medical Subjects No. 108*. London: HMSO; 1963.
4. Ministry of Health. *Report on Confidential Enquiries into Maternal Deaths in England and Wales 1961–1963. Reports on Public Health and Medical Subjects No. 115*. London: HMSO; 1966.
5. Ministry of Health. *Report on Confidential Enquiries into Maternal Deaths in England and Wales 1964–1966. Reports on Public Health and Medical Subjects No. 119*. London: HMSO; 1969.
6. Department of Health and Social Security. *Report on Confidential Enquiries into Maternal Deaths in England and Wales 1967–1969. Reports on Health and Social Subjects. No. 1*. London: HMSO; 1972.
7. Department of Health and Social Security. R*eport on Confidential Enquiries into Maternal Deaths in England and Wales 1970–1972. Reports on Health and Social Subjects. No. 11*. London: HMSO; 1975.
8. Department of Health and Social Security. *Report on Confidential Enquiries into Maternal Deaths in England and Wales 1973–1975. Reports on Health and Social Subjects. No. 14*. London: HMSO; 1979.
9. Department of Health and Social Security. *Report on Confidential Enquiries into Maternal Deaths in England and Wales 1976–1978. Reports on Health and Social Subjects. No. 26*. London: HMSO; 1982.
10. Department of Health and Social Security. *Report on Confidential Enquiries into Maternal Deaths in England and Wales 1979–1981. Reports on Health and Social Subjects. No. 29*. London: HMSO; 1986.
11. Department of Health. *Report on Confidential Enquiries into Maternal Deaths in England and Wales 1982–1984. Report on Health and Social Subjects. No. 34*. London: HMSO; 1989.
12. Department of Health, Welsh Office, Scottish Home and Health Department, Department of Health and Social Services, Northern Ireland. *Report on Confidential Enquiries into Maternal Deaths in the United Kingdom 1985–1987*. London: HMSO; 1991.
13. Department of Health, Welsh Office, Scottish Home and Health Department, Department of Health and Social Services, Northern Ireland. *Report on Confidential Enquiries into Maternal Deaths in the United Kingdom 1988–1990*. London: HMSO; 1994.
14. Department of Health, Welsh Office, Scottish Home and Health Department, Department of Health and Social Services, Northern Ireland. *Report on Confidential Enquiries into Maternal Deaths in the United Kingdom 1991–1993*. London: HMSO; 1996.
15. Department of Health, Welsh Office, Scottish Home and Health Department, Department of Health and Social Services, Northern Ireland. *Why Mothers Die. Report on Confidential Enquiries into Maternal Deaths in the United Kingdom 1994–1996*. London: The Stationery Office; 1998.
16. Drife J, Lewis G, editors. *Why Mothers Die 1997–1999. The Confidential Enquiries into Maternal Deaths in the United Kingdom*. London: RCOG Press; 2001.
17. Morgan M. Obstetrical anaesthesia. In: Chamberlain G, Wraight A, Steer P, editors. *Pain and its Relief in Childbirth: The Results of a National Survey Conducted by the National Birthday Trust*. New York: Churchill Livingstone; 1993.
18. Khor LJH, Jeskins G, Cooper GM, Paterson-Brown S. National obstetric anaesthetic practice in the UK 1997/1998. *Anaesthesia* 2000;55:1168–72.
19. J Thomas, S Paranjothy. Clinical Effectiveness Support Unit. *The National Sentinel Caesarean Section Audit Report*. London: RCOG Press; 2001.
20. Tsen LC, Pitner R, Camaan WR. General anesthesia for cesarean section at a tertiary care hospital 1990–1995: indications and implications. *Int J Obstet Anesth* 1998;7:147–52.
21. O'Sullivan G, Shennan A. Labour – a gastronomic experience! *Int J Obstet Anesth* 2002;11:1–3.
22. Soreide E, Bjornestad E, Steen PA. An audit of perioperative aspiration pneumonitis in gynaecological and obstetric patients. *Acta Anaesthesiol Scand* 1996,40:14–19.
23. Warner MA, Warner ME, Weber JG. Clinical significance of pulmonary aspiration during the perioperative period. *Anesthesiology* 1993;78:56–62.
24. Harmer M. Difficult and failed intubation in obstetrics. *Int J Obstet Anesth* 1997;6:25–31.
25. Hawthorne L, Wilson R, Lyons G, Dresner M. Failed intubation revisited: 17-yr experience in a teaching maternity unit. *Br J Anaesth* 1996;76:680–4.
26. Rocke DA, Rout CC. Volume preloading, spinal hypotension and caesarean section. *Br J Anaesth*

1995;75:257–9.
27. Loo CC, Dahlgren G, Irestedt L. Neurological complications in obstetric regional anaesthesia. *Int J Obstet Anesth* 2000;9:99–124.
28. Scott DB, Tunstall ME. Serious complications associated with epidural/ spinal blockade in obstetrics: a two-year prospective study. *Int J Obstet Anesth* 1995;4:133–9.
29. Holdcroft A, Gibberd FB, Hardgrove RL, Hawkins DF, Dellaportas CI. Neurological complications associated with pregnancy. *Br J Anaesth* 1995;75:522–6.
30. Paech MJ, Godkin R, Webster S. Complications of obstetric epidural analgesia and anaesthesia: a prospective analysis of 10 995 cases. *Int J Obstet Anesth* 1998;7:5–11.
31. Crawford JS. Some maternal complications of epidural analgesia for labour. *Anaesthesia* 1985;40:1219–25.
32. Scott DB, Hibbard BM. Serious non-fatal complications associated with extradural block in obstetric practice. *Br J Anaesth* 1990;64:537–41.
33. James FM, George RH, Naiem H, White GH. Bacteriologic aspects of epidural analgesia. *Anesth Analg* 1976;55:187–90.
34. Reynolds F. Damage to conus medullaris following spinal anaesthesia. *Anaesthesia* 2001;56:238–47.
35. Jeskins GD, Moore PAS, Cooper GM, Lewis M. Long-term morbidity following dural puncture in an obstetric population. *Int J Obstet Anesth* 2001;10:17–24.
36. Hopkinson JM, Samaan AK, Russell IF, Birks RJ, Patrick MR. A comparative multicentre trial of spinal needles for caesarean section. *Anaesthesia* 1997;52:1005–11.

Chapter 33

Intensive care

Steve M Yentis

Introduction

Intensive or high-dependency care may be required for the pregnant woman who becomes sick or for the sick woman who becomes pregnant. However, there is also a large population of 'normal' women who require care at a higher level than standard ward care, albeit briefly, after general or regional anaesthesia for procedures such as caesarean section. Routine recovery care merges into high-dependency care, since the absence of the former may well lead to a requirement for the latter.

Discussion of intensive or high-dependency care in obstetrics is hampered by two main interrelated difficulties: first, in collecting and analysing information on the type and severity of disease that leads a pregnant woman to require such care and, second, in determining, encouraging and achieving best clinical practice.

History

Intensive and high-dependency care as a subspecialty is relatively new, and this is reflected in its fairly recent appearance in discussions of maternal morbidity and mortality. The reports on Confidential Enquiries into Maternal Deaths (CEMD) represent a series of chronological snapshots of maternity care, albeit from the extreme aspect of mortality, for over 50 years. For much of this period, mention of critical care in the CEMD reports was only in the context of describing the clinical course of specific cases. It was not until the 1988–90 report that the authors included a chapter on acute respiratory distress syndrome (ARDS) and highlighted deficiencies in monitoring and treatment of severely ill mothers, especially those with complications affecting fluid and electrolyte balance. The authors of the report called for 'a properly equipped, staffed and supervised high-dependency care area in every consultant obstetric unit' and went on to suggest that a consultant anaesthetist should have responsibility for such an area.[1]

The report for 1991–93 includes a chapter devoted to intensive care, in which it is stated that 40% of all direct and indirect maternal deaths involved intensive care treatment at some stage, although there was poor recording on the CEMD forms of the monitoring used and the interventions done.[2] Most deaths were ultimately of multiple organ failure. Again, a lack of appropriate facilities was mentioned. Subsequent reports have continued with a chapter on intensive care: the 1994–96 report states that in 35% of direct and indirect deaths there was a recorded need for intensive care,[3] while in the 1997–99 report 53% of direct and 35% of indirect deaths followed intensive care.[4] The importance of early transfer and treatment is highlighted and the 1997–99 report goes on to identify as major deficiencies the lack of on-site intensive care unit (ICU) facilities, protocols for transfer of critically ill obstetric patients and proper mechanisms for identifying pregnant or recently delivered women on ICUs. The latter report also suggests the morbidity–mortality ratio as a useful outcome measure, given that maternal mortality in developed countries is now generally low.[4]

Interest in obstetric intensive and high-dependency care was also growing from other directions. First, development of obstetric anaesthesia as a separate subspecialty in the latter half of the last century led to increasing numbers of dedicated obstetric anaesthetists with fixed sessions in maternity units, resulting in quicker access to senior anaesthetic cover with expertise in routine and high-dependency acute care. Second, there has been considerable development of intensive care and high-dependency facilities generally over the same period. Since most ICUs were (and still are) run by anaesthetists, cross-fertilisation between the two subspecialties was inevitable. This growing interest is reflected in the increasing number of published reports of obstetric admissions to ICU over the last decade[5–19] and, more recently, obstetric admissions to high-dependency units (HDUs),[20] although extrapolation from most of these studies to the situation in the UK is difficult because of wide variations in resources and in definitions and admission criteria used across the world. Finally, as a result of lower levels of maternal mortality in the UK, there have been calls for a greater focus on morbidity – much of which may involve intensive or high-dependency care – as a better indicator of quality of care and as a means of identifying areas for improvement.[17,21–23]

What is intensive or high-dependency care?

The Department of Health document *Guidelines on Admission to and Discharge from Intensive Care and High Dependency Units*[24] defines different types of high-level care as follows:

- Intensive care: a service for patients with potentially recoverable conditions who can benefit from more detailed observation and invasive treatment than can safely be provided in general wards or high-dependency areas. A minimal nurse–patient ratio of one to one is specified, together with 24-hour dedicated cover by resident trainee medical staff.
- High-dependency care: a level of care intermediate between that on a general ward and that on an ICU. Such care involves the monitoring and support of patients with (or likely to develop) acute or acute-on-chronic single organ failure and ‘step-up’ or ‘step-down’ support between levels of care, although not those requiring multiple organ support or mechanical ventilation. Postoperative care exceeding a

few hours is highlighted as an appropriate indication for (or definition of) high-dependency care. An average nurse–patient ratio of one to two is specified, together with 'continuous availability' of trainee medical staff.

Both types of care require involvement of appropriate senior medical and nursing staff (and in the case of obstetric units, midwifery staff – although obstetric critical care is not considered in the document) and other administrative and educational support. The document stresses that these definitions refer to categories of care, not to geographical areas within which such care is provided; thus, for example, high-dependency care is not restricted to care provided in an HDU.

This document is important because it sets out the levels of support that such units require, although it acknowledges that specialised areas such as renal, coronary care and paediatric units are outside its scope. Interestingly, obstetric critical care is not even mentioned as an area that was excluded from consideration.

In practical terms, the distinction between obstetric intensive and high-dependency care has become blurred because many units are providing high- or intermediate-level care within the maternity suite, often without strictly defined staff–patient ratios. However, progress is slow; for example, a national survey conducted in 1994 found that only 41% of maternity units had designated obstetric HDU beds and 19% did not have an ICU on site.[25] The National Obstetric Anaesthetic Database (NOAD), a multidisciplinary initiative set up in 1998 involving the Obstetric Anaesthetists' Association, the Royal College of Anaesthetists, the Royal College of Obstetricians and Gynaecologists, the Royal College of Midwives and representation from patients' groups and the Department of Health, conducted a national survey of high-dependency care in obstetrics in 2000. The results are still being analysed but they indicate that a majority of maternity units who responded still do not have dedicated obstetric HDU beds. Furthermore, many patients requiring routine postoperative care after caesarean section do not have simple monitoring such as pulse oximetry.

The impact that obstetric HDUs have had on reducing admissions to ICU is difficult to ascertain, since there have been many other changes over this period, most of them (one would hope) improving the overall quality of care. Data from Dublin suggest a sizeable but non-significant reduction of 50% in obstetric admissions to ICU following the setting-up of an obstetric HDU,[20] and this is mirrored by experiences at the Chelsea and Westminster Hospital (24% reduction), the lack of statistical significance representing the small proportion of women requiring intensive care to start with (<1% to 2–3%) and the relatively small sample sizes (123 and 1000 patients respectively). A recent survey of 14 ICUs in the south of England found that a significant proportion of obstetric admissions (35.7%) required minimal care only and, in these cases, admission to HDU would have been more appropriate.[19] Clearly there are factors other than clinical need in admission to ICU.

Who needs obstetric intensive/high-dependency care?

First, there are the women who undergo operative procedures within the maternity unit who may not be overtly ill, although all these patients require careful monitoring and observation for at least a few hours postoperatively in order to detect complications and institute early treatment. In the latest CEMD report, there were three deaths in which substandard postoperative care was highlighted.[4]

Regarding critical care of the sick obstetric patient, there are two main sources of

Table 33.1. Causes of maternal death listed in the Confidential Enquiries into Maternal Deaths for 1991–99 in order of frequency[2–4]

Direct causes	Indirect causes
Thromboembolism	Cardiac
Hypertensive disorders	Neurological
Early pregnancy	Infective
Amniotic fluid embolism	Psychiatric
Haemorrhage	Respiratory
Sepsis	Endocrine, metabolic and immunological
Miscellaneous	Circulatory
Genital tract trauma	Haematological

information on the spectrum of disease that results in the requirement for intensive/high-dependency care: mortality studies and morbidity studies. Each of these is discussed in more detail elsewhere, but the distinction between them is relevant to ICU/HDU admission and outcomes.

Mortality studies

These may be national or local. In the UK, the main national reporting system is the CEMD, now into its fifth triennium of covering the whole of the UK. The implications and contents of these reports are discussed in several chapters but the spectrum of diseases that the CEMD suggests as the main causes of death over the last decade is interesting (Table 33.1), with most resulting from thromboembolism and cardiac disease. As mentioned above, about one-third to one-half of the direct and indirect causes of death have resulted in women requiring intensive care, at least briefly. However, a population study in the US state of Maryland identified 135 deaths out of 822 591 hospital admissions for delivery, of which only 34 died in ICUs (25% of deaths).[26] When considering the main conditions that may result in the requirement for intensive/high-dependency care, it is important not to focus only on the direct causes of death, as has traditionally been the case, but also to look at indirect causes. This has been highlighted in the most recent CEMD, in which indirect causes outnumbered direct causes for the first time.[4]

Morbidity studies

Morbidity studies are more disparate than successive CEMD reports, since the former include series from obstetric units, ICUs, HDUs and specialist units, based in hospitals and countries with widely differing resources, administrations and treatments. This disparity is reflected in the range of admission and mortality rates from such series (Table 33.2). However, different ICUs within the UK are more likely to be similar than those in other countries, as is reflected in a narrower range of mortality rates, and pooling of UK data allows a list of the most common reasons for admission to be drawn up (Table 33.3). The most common causes of obstetric admission to ICU are

Table 33.2. Intensive care unit (ICU) admission and mortality rates for obstetric patients over the last decade

	Reference	Admission rate per 1000 deliveries	Mortality rate per 100 admissions
UK ICU series	Umo-Etuk J *et al.* 1996[11]	0.2–7.6	2.1–4.4
	Wheatley E *et al.* 1996[12]		
	Margarson M *et al.* 1998[16]		
	Hazelgrove JF *et al.* 2001[19]		
Other ICU series	Kilpatrick SJ, Matthay MA 1992[5]	0.1–9.0	0.0–20.0
	Ng TI *et al.* 1992[6]		
	Monaco TJ Jr *et al.* 1993[7]		
	Collop NA, Sahn SA 1993[8]		
	Lewinsohn G *et al.* 1994[9]		
	Lapinsky S *et al.* 1995[10]		
	Bouvier-Colle MH *et al.* 1996[13]		
	el-Solh AA, Grant BJ 1996[14]		
	Lapinsky SE *et al.* 1997[15]		
	Margarson M *et al.* 1998[16]		
	Baskett TF, Sternadel J *et al.* 1998[17]		
	Panchal S *et al.* 2000[18]		

hypertensive disorders and haemorrhage. These conditions are also highlighted in the Intensive Care National Audit and Research Centre (ICNARC) case-mix programme, in which a database of over 46 000 admissions to 91 ICUs in the UK was interrogated in order to identify obstetric admissions in 1995–99. Some of the 393 cases identified may also be included in the series referred to in Tables 33.2 and 33.3; however, the ICNARC team also found that haemorrhage, hypertensive disorders and sepsis accounted for over 60% of admissions and that the ICU mortality rate was 3%.

Taken together, mortality and morbidity studies suggest that the conditions that result in maternal death are not the same as those that cause admission to ICU. The reasons are unclear but this may be because:

- fatal disorders such as pulmonary embolism often take effect rapidly, i.e. before ICU admission
- common conditions such as pre-eclampsia are rarely fatal, although they often result in ICU admission

Table 33.3. Causes of obstetric admissions to ICU in published UK series[11,12,16,19] over the last decade, in order of frequency; direct and indirect causes of death as defined in the Confidential Enquiries into Maternal Deaths[4]

'Direct' causes	'Indirect' causes
Hypertensive disorders	Endocrine, metabolic and immunological
Haemorrhage	Haematological
Miscellaneous	Cardiac
Early pregnancy	Psychiatric
Sepsis	Respiratory
Genital tract trauma	Neurological
Amniotic fluid embolism	Other
Thromboembolism	

- 'medical' disorders are treated on medical wards and do not come to the attention of intensivists, although there is an increasing trend for ICU staff to review seriously ill patients on the wards ('outreach')
- specific disorders, e.g. cardiac or neurological disease, are treated in specialist units
- late deaths are not included in ICU series; for example, a patient with severe ARDS may eventually die in the ICU but only after several months, by which time the fact that she was pregnant within 42 days of admission may have been forgotten.

The morbidity studies may have small numbers, be non-representative series or have poor standardisation; for example, the units may serve different populations or use different admission criteria or standards of care and different disease classifications or definitions. One factor hindering accurate description of case-mix and thus comparison of series is the lack of an 'obstetric severity of illness' score; thus, the scoring systems that have become widespread in the adult ICU population do not perform as well when applied to obstetric patients.[14,19]

Improving the reporting and analysis of mothers requiring intensive/high-dependency care

There is an increasing awareness that more information is needed about what care is being offered to pregnant or recently pregnant women, and where and how it is being provided. The efforts of bodies such as ICNARC and NOAD, supported by the Royal Colleges and the Obstetric Anaesthetists Association, will take time to come to fruition but there has already been some progress. Ultimately, inclusion of pregnancy-related fields in the standard ICU admission database will result in more accurate prospective collection of data rather than the retrospective analyses that are more usual. Regular reporting of standardised data within the UK, akin to the CEMD, would allow trends to be more apparent and provide a useful tool for educating staff. Finally, agreement on strict definitions of conditions and complications (and of admission/mortality rates – e.g. per 100 or 1000 deliveries or maternities) will help to standardise morbidity studies generally, as well as allow comparisons between individual units. However, there is a danger that concentrating on ICU admissions will result in an incomplete picture, so these definitions must also apply to mothers receiving high-dependency care, wherever such care is provided.

Best practice in obstetric intensive/high-dependency care

There are three main difficulties in promoting and achieving best practice. First, there is often poor understanding of the physiological changes of pregnancy, in particular the cardiovascular, respiratory and renal systems. Thus, for example, the crucial importance of avoiding aortocaval compression may not be appreciated by nursing or medical staff in the ICU or HDU that is not situated within the maternity suite (it is hard enough to stress its importance to staff within the labour ward, let alone to intensivists and nurses who only care for the occasional obstetric patient). The fact that the maternal cardiac output and blood volume is greatly increased is also often unappreciated, as is the risk of pulmonary oedema in these patients. Unfamiliarity with maternal respiratory and renal physiology means that ICU staff may underestimate the importance of a laboratory test result that in their usual population would be considered normal or near-normal, e.g. an arterial PO_2 of 5–6 kPa or an increase in plasma urea concentration from 4 mmol/l to 8 mmol/l.

Second, related to this unfamiliarity, is lack of awareness of the needs of the fetus and the physiological changes that occur during and after childbirth. Thus staff may not appreciate the effects of drugs (especially cardiovascular) on the uteroplacental circulation or the significance of postpartum haemorrhage (and the potentially deleterious cardiovascular effects of some of its treatments).[4]

The third major difficulty in obstetric critical care is the relative lack of a sound evidence base for many interventions and treatments. This is also a problem in intensive care generally, although it is one that is increasingly recognised and addressed; thus, there have been many important randomised controlled trials (RCTs) in intensive care but few areas of obstetric critical care have been subjected to this level of investigation. Many RCTs that do exist often rely on surrogate outcomes, for example looking at urine output following dopamine infusion instead of longer-term renal impairment or survival.[27]

Actual practice in obstetric intensive/high-dependency care

It is difficult to be confident of what represents current practice because identification of obstetric patients is so variable, as discussed above. The NOAD project already referred to should provide a glimpse into current practice but this will only be for a minority of cases and may not be representative. Preliminary results from NOAD suggest that duration of high-dependency care varies hugely across all categories; these were widened from the Department of Health's ICU/HDU definitions into: single organ failure; more intensive observation than possible on general wards; step up or down to/from ICU; routine postoperative recovery; prolonged postoperative recovery. Use of invasive monitoring appears to be generally low, perhaps reflecting either a lack of appropriate facilities and/or nursing/midwife expertise or, possibly, a concern about the risks of invasive monitoring in the obstetric population set against its benefits being less certain than in non-pregnant cases.[28–30]

Conclusions and future directions

Assuming that maternal mortality in the UK remains relatively low and even falls further, increasing attention must be paid to morbidity as a representation of underlying trends or (when appropriate) as an indicator of substandard practice or areas for improvement. Many parturients who suffer morbidity will require intensive or high-dependency care – perhaps an increasing number as 'salvage' of severely affected women improves. We can only hope that facilities for providing such high-level care increase correspondingly, but there is little evidence for such a trend currently and existing efforts are hampered by a lack of demographic and clinical information. In conclusion, there are several areas in which we need to act if we are to improve the quality of care offered to the sickest of our pregnant and recently pregnant women:

- to reach agreement on clinical definitions of pregnancy-related conditions requiring intensive or high-dependency care
- to establish systems for routine recording of pregnancy-related morbidity, to include monitoring of admission criteria, treatments and outcomes of women requiring intensive/high-dependency care
- to encourage the setting up and maintaining of HDUs within maternity units as called for by CEMD,[1–4] and the educational/financial support that such units require; this should include provision for women requiring 'routine' postoperative care, either within the same geographical areas or separate recovery areas
- to consider the most pressing research questions regarding obstetric critical care and encourage multicentre studies in these areas, in order to provide the necessary evidence base.

References

1. Department of Health, Welsh Office, Scottish Home and Health Department, Department of Health and Social Services, Northern Ireland. *Report on Confidential Enquiries into Maternal Death in the United Kingdom, 1988–90.* London: HMSO; 1994.
2. Department of Health, Welsh Office, Scottish Home and Health Department, Department of Health and Social Services, Northern Ireland. *Report on Confidential Enquiries into Maternal Death in the United Kingdom, 1991–93.* London: HMSO; 1996.
3. Department of Health, Welsh Office, Scottish Home and Health Department, Department of Health and Social Services, Northern Ireland. *Why Mothers Die. The Confidential Enquiries into Maternal Deaths in the United Kingdom 1994–96.* London: The Stationery Office; 1998.
4. Drife J, Lewis G, editors. *Why Mothers Die 1997–1999. The Confidential Enquiries into Maternal Deaths in the United Kingdom.* London: RCOG Press; 2001.
5. Kilpatrick SJ, Matthay MA. Obstetric patients requiring critical care. A five-year review. *Chest* 1992;101:1407–12.
6. Ng TI, Lim E, Tweed WA, Arulkumaran S. Obstetric admissions to the intensive care unit – a retrospective review. *Ann Acad Med Singapore* 1992;21:804–6.
7. Monaco TJ Jr, Spielman FJ, Katz VL. Pregnant patients in the intensive care unit: a descriptive analysis. *South Med J* 1993;86:414–7.
8. Collop NA, Sahn SA. Critical illness in pregnancy. An analysis of 20 patients admitted to a medical intensive care unit. *Chest* 1993;103:1548–52.
9. Lewinsohn G, Herman A, Leonov Y, Klinowski E. Critically ill obstetrical patients: outcome and predictability. *Crit Care Med* 1994;22:1412–4.
10. Lapinsky S, Kruczynski K, Slutsky AS. Critical care in the pregnant patient. *Am J Respir Crit Care Med* 1995;152:427–55.
11. Umo-Etuk J, Lumley J, Holdcroft A. Critically ill parturient women and admission to intensive care: a 5-year review. *Int J Obstet Anesth* 1996;5:79–84.
12. Wheatley E, Farkas A, Watson D. Obstetric admissions to an intensive therapy unit. *Int J Obstet Anesth* 1996;5:221–4.
13. Bouvier-Colle MH, Salanave B, Ancel PY, Varnoux N, Fernandez H, Papiernik E, *et al.* Obstetric patients treated in intensive care units and maternal mortality. Regional Teams for the Survey. *Eur J Obstet Gynecol Reprod Biol* 1996;65:121–5.
14. el-Solh AA, Grant BJ. A comparison of severity of illness scoring systems for critically ill obstetric patients. *Chest* 1996;110:1299–304.
15. Lapinsky SE, Kruczynski K, Seaward GR, Farine D, Grossman RF. Critical care management of the obstetric patient. *Can J Anaesth* 1997;44:325–9.

16. Margarson M, Dob D, Yentis SM. A retrospective survey of obsetric admissions to the Intensive Care Unit. *Int J Obstet Anesth* 1998;7:205–6.
17. Baskett TF, Sternadel J. Maternal intensive care and near-miss mortality in obstetrics. *Br J Obstet Gynaecol* 1998;105:981–4.
18. Panchal S, Arria A, Harris A. Intensive care utilization during hospital admission for delivery: prevalence, risk factors, and outcomes in a statewide population. *Anesthesiology* 2000;92:1537–44.
19. Hazelgrove JF, Price C, Pappachan VJ, Smith GB. Multicenter study of obstetric admissions to 14 intensive care units in southern England. *Crit Care Med* 2001;29:770–5.
20. Ryan M, Hamilton V, Bowen M, McKenna P. The role of a high-dependency unit in a regional obstetric hospital. *Anaesthesia* 2000;55:1155–8.
21. Harmer M. Maternal mortality – is it still relevant? *Anaesthesia* 1997;52:99–100.
22. Mantel GD, Buchmann E, Rees H, Pattinson RC. Severe acute maternal morbidity: a pilot study of a definition for a near-miss. *Br J Obstet Gynaecol* 1998;105:985–90.
23. Waterstone M, Bewley S, Wolfe C. Incidence and predictors of severe obstetric morbidity: case-control study. *BMJ* 2001;322:1089–94.
24. Department of Health/NHS Executive. *Guidelines on Admission to and Discharge from Intensive Care and High Dependency Units*. London: DoH; 1996.
25. Cordingley JJ, Rubin AP. A survey of facilities for high risk women in consultant obstetric units. *Int J Obstet Anesth* 1997;6:156–60.
26. Panchal S, Arria A, Labhsetwar SA. Maternal mortality during hospital admission for delivery: a retrospective analysis using a state-maintained database. *Anesth Analg* 2001;93:134–41.
27. Mantel GD, Makin JD. Low dose dopamine in postpartum pre-eclamptic women with oliguria: a double-blind, placebo controlled, randomised trial. *Br J Obstet Gynaecol* 1997;104:1180–3.
28. Lo WK, Chong JL. Neck haematoma and airway obstruction in a pre-eclamptic patient: a complication of internal jugular vein cannulation. *Anaesth Intensive Care* 1997;25:423–5.
29. Rodriguez C, Yentis SM. Carotid artery puncture, airway obstruction and the laryngeal mask airway in a pre-eclamptic patient. *Int J Obstet Anesth* 1996;5:194–7.
30. Nolan TE, Wakefield ML, Devoe LD. Invasive hemodynamic monitoring in obstetrics. A critical review of its indications, benefits, complications and alternatives. *Chest* 1992;101:1429–33.

Chapter 34

Pathology

Harry Millward-Sadler

During a period in which considerable media attention – much of it critical – has been paid to the autopsy, it is appropriate to examine the role of the autopsy in maternal deaths. A recent study[1] found significant clinical discrepancies in approximately 15% of all autopsies despite improvements in diagnostic imaging and other techniques, suggesting that autopsy is still important for reviewing and confirming clinical diagnoses. It is my belief that the value of the autopsy in maternal deaths has also been repeatedly demonstrated. By definition, this group of deaths is occurring in a young population and is frequently unexpected. Each has a considerable impact on the family and any autopsy in this situation should command a thorough and detailed investigation with careful clinicopathological correlation. A good autopsy should include a review of the circumstances before death, establish the cause of death and exclude other causes, as well as confirm ancillary diagnoses and identify unexpected pathology. It is not appropriate to cover the entire spectrum of diseases that contribute to maternal death in this review, but selected clinical examples are given to illustrate these various points.

Review of circumstances

The pathologist is one of the few professional staff dealing with the death who has not been directly involved in the clinical care. It is therefore important that an objective review of the case notes is provided with the report. The recently described association between antipsychotic drug therapy and idiopathic venous thromboembolism serves to emphasise the critical importance of a review of the clinical history. This confirmed that the mother had also died from primary pulmonary hypertension. Tissues from the maternal death were then referred to a specialist centre, where the genetic mutation for familial primary pulmonary hypertension was confirmed. The recently described association between antipsychotic drug therapy and idiopathic venous thromboembolism serves to emphasise the critical importance of a review of the clinical history even in deaths from pulmonary embolus.[2]

While appropriate in hospital deaths, a history is of even greater significance in deaths occurring in the community. The most recent Confidential Enquiries into Maternal Deaths (CEMD) report[3] has identified a distressing number of suicides within the first year of childbirth. Probably many similar deaths have previously been unreported and it is likely that the current systems do not comprehensively identify all such deaths. It is important therefore for the pathologist to take an active role in identifying any maternal death to the Confidential Enquiry and provide, with the coroner's or the procurator fiscal's consent, such clinical details as are available.

Standards:

- review clinical history
- use clinical history to direct further investigation
- proactively identify maternal deaths.

Pulmonary thromboembolism

Death from pulmonary thromboembolism remains one of the most common causes of direct maternal death in the UK. This is not usually a difficult diagnosis to establish at autopsy and it often excludes other causes of sudden unexpected death. However, the history frequently includes episodes of chest pain and/or breathlessness that had been attributed clinically to a variety of diagnoses, including anxiety states and chest infections in the weeks before death. As non-fatal pulmonary emboli become progressively more adherent to the arterial wall and are then organised, it becomes possible to identify such prior episodes and distinguish them from the terminal event. It is rare for the autopsy report to investigate these previous clinical episodes and identify their cause. It is even less common for the nature of the embolus to be confirmed. The 1991–93 CEMD report[4] included a death from pulmonary embolism where the embolus was choriocarcinoma. This is esoteric but not unique. A young woman in Southampton underwent a right lower lobe lobectomy for a pulmonary abscess (Figure 34.1). Histology demonstrated that the abscess formed within areas of infarction caused by tumour emboli from a choriocarcinoma (Figure 34.2). On subsequent investigation, the patient had high β human chorionic gonadotrophin (βhCG) blood levels (6000 iu). The only clinical history was of a missed menstrual period approximately three months earlier.

Standards:

- identify ages of emboli
- establish nature and source of emboli.

Pre-eclampsia

Pre-eclampsia is still one of the most common causes of direct maternal death. In the last report, 15 deaths were directly attributed to pre-eclampsia. Cerebral haemorrhage was the cause of death in six of the ten cases that came to autopsy. Despite the clear clinical features and in many instances the obvious cause of death in such patients, careful autopsy is still of value. It is probable that some cases of fulminating

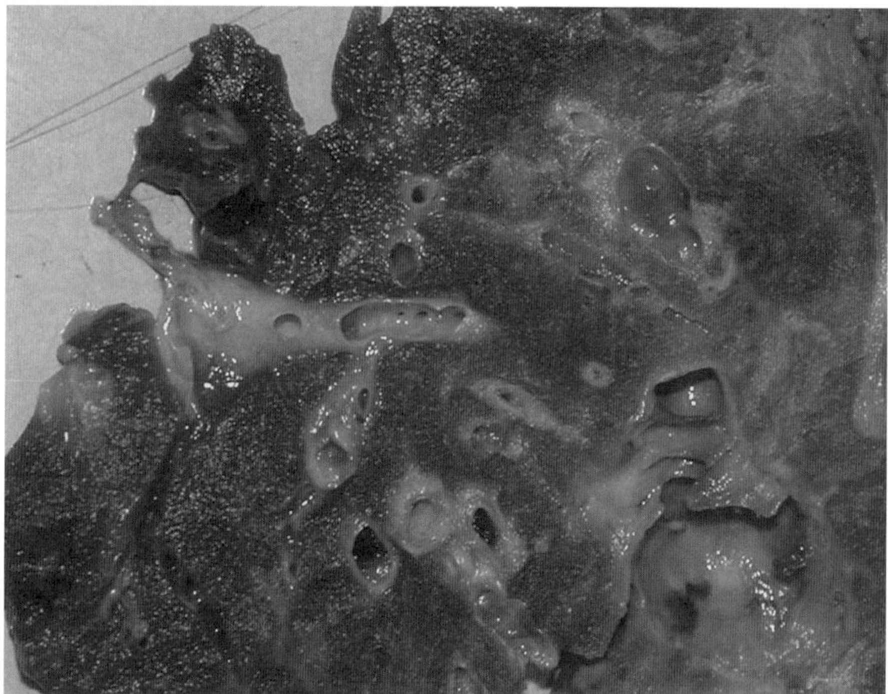

Figure 34.1. Right lower lobe of lung contains a cavitating abscess with areas of surrounding consolidation; macroscopically many pulmonary arteries are patent but some small arteries do contain a granular brown thrombus (courtesy of Professor W R Roche)

pre-eclampsia can present and cause death in the interval between antenatal clinical visits and without a preceding clinical detection. In the latest CEMD report,[3] a young primiparous woman had slight puffiness of the hands at 33 weeks of gestation but there were no other features of pre-eclampsia. Two weeks later, she had a fit at home and was dead on arrival at the hospital. It was thought that death might have been caused by an eclamptic fit, but the autopsy had been delayed for six days, was performed in a public mortuary distant from the hospital and no histology was taken, so the putative diagnosis could not be confirmed. With an autopsy of such poor quality, it is difficult to be confident that alternative causes of death have been satisfactorily excluded. Conversely, an extremely good autopsy can exclude some conditions and suggest alternative diagnoses. One such autopsy suggested to the central assessors that sleep apnoea was a possible cause of death. The patient was an obese grande multiparous woman with diabetes and chronic hypertension. She had developed mild pre-eclampsia and had been admitted to hospital for observation and treatment but was found dead in bed one morning. In the days prior to death, she had had mild dyspnoea attributed to asthma and her obesity. Histology confirmed the presence of pre-eclampsia in the kidneys and excluded malignant hypertension: there was no significant pathology in the heart, brain or liver. However, there was evidence of a bronchiolitis from a viral pneumonia in the lungs. Although this did not appear to be severe enough to have caused death in itself, it is conceivable that it could do so in conjunction with sleep apnoea.

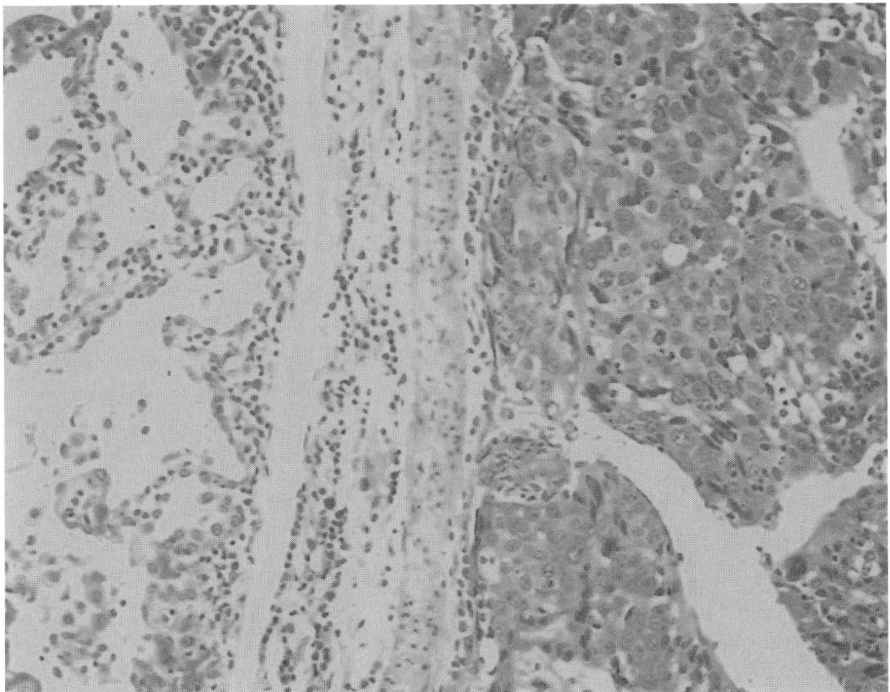

Figure 34.2. A tumour composed of large pleomorphic cells fills pulmonary artery lumen on the right. The majority of the cells are cytotrophoblast but the more hyperchromatic syncytial trophoblast can also be identified. Unremarkable lung parenchyma is present on the left (H and E x 25)

It is also possible that deaths from pre-eclampsia are being underestimated. Several deaths from cerebral haemorrhage in pregnancy occurred in neurosurgical units. Because of the clear demonstration of the cerebral haemorrhage by imaging techniques, autopsy had not been performed and therefore the underlying cause of the haemorrhage had not been ascertained.

Standards:

- fluid balance review
- exclude other causes of hypertension
- confirm pre-eclampsia histologically.

Amniotic fluid embolism

Classically amniotic fluid embolism (AFE) is diagnosed by the finding of fetal squames in the lungs at autopsy. More recently, however, the definition has been extended to include deaths with a clinical diagnosis of AFE that is not necessarily confirmed by autopsy. The reasons are multifactorial but poor autopsy technique and difficulty in identifying squames should no longer be justified reasons. The previous

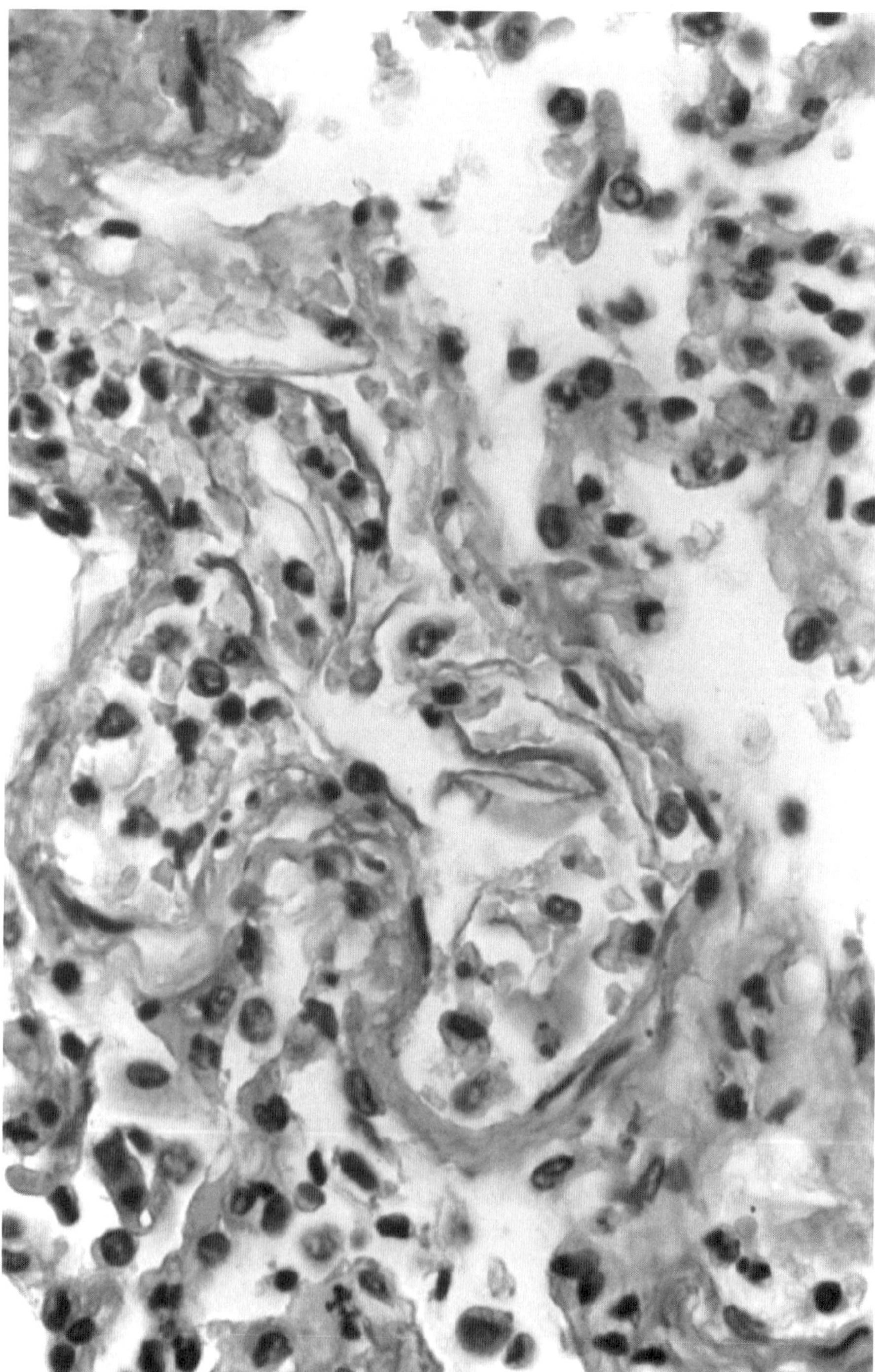

Figure 34.3. Amniotic fluid embolism; it is difficult to identify the fetal squames and differentiate them from fibrin even using special histochemical techniques (MSB x 40)

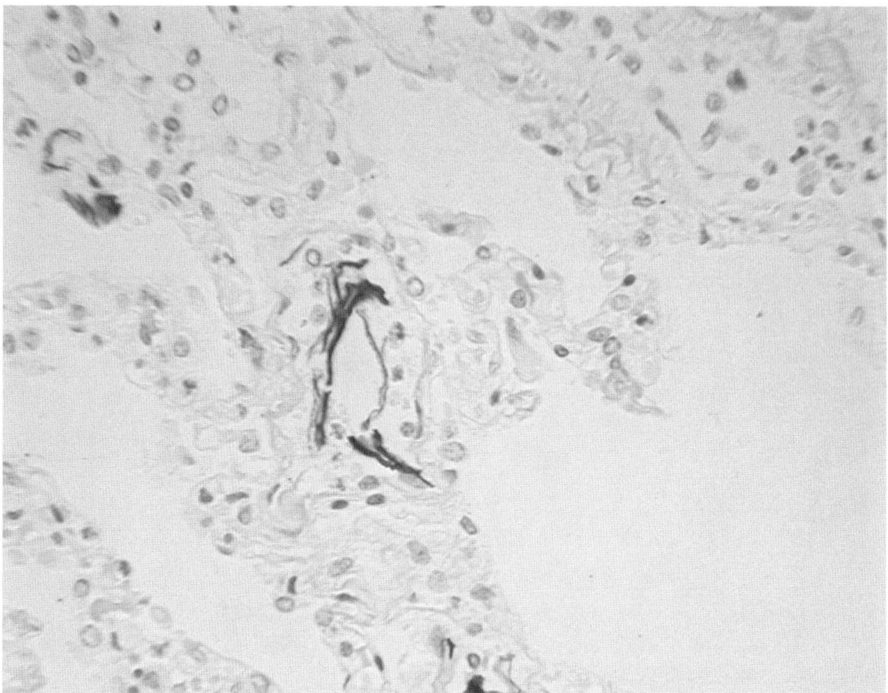

Figure 34.4. Immunocytochemical staining with LP34 clearly demonstrates the brown stained fetal squames within the pulmonary capillaries; note the lack of background staining of alveolar pneumocytes; immunocytochemistry x 40

histochemical methods for detecting fetal squames lacked both specificity and sensitivity but immunocytochemistry antibodies such as LP34 can highlight fetal squames with a minimum of background staining of other tissue components (Figures 34.3 and 34.4). However, these new techniques do raise different questions. With survival now being prolonged in intensive care units, it is not known how long fetal squames persist in the maternal pulmonary circulation. Also, given that fetal red cells routinely escape into the maternal circulation during parturition, it is conceivable that fetal squames could do likewise. These may be insufficient in number to precipitate overt clinical problems but could in theory be detectable using these modern immunocytochemical methods.

Standard:

- search for AFE using immunocytochemical methods.

Genital tract sepsis

Classic cases of group A beta haemolytic streptococcal infection in the genital tract causing death still occur but fortunately these are rare. There were five cases of streptococcal septicaemia in the latest CEMD report[3] but not all of these originated as

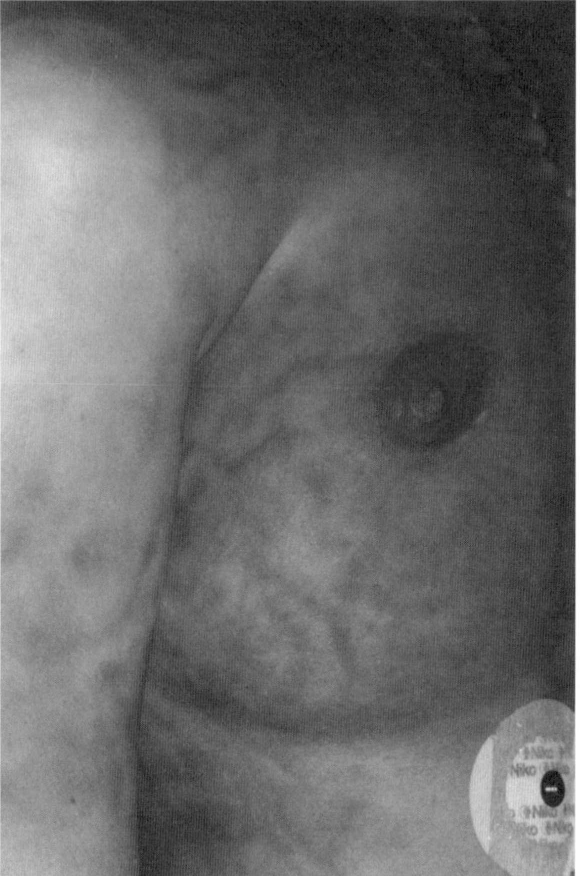

Figure 34.5. Streptococcal septicaemia: the blotchy erythroderma and the early marbling of the skin from haemolytic staining of the skin veins is evident

genital tract infections. More recently, one woman who died had been admitted in the early evening with a history of sore throat, diarrhoea and vomiting since mid-morning. Although on admission she was conscious and coherent, within two hours she had collapsed and died. Cardiac resuscitation was ineffective. At the autopsy performed the next day, there was a dramatic blotchy purple erythroderma over the whole body, with marked haemolytic staining of the small venules in the skin that produced a marbling effect (Figure 34.5). Cultures confirmed a pure growth of beta haemolytic streptococci from all organs sampled. There had been no history of genital tract intervention and there was no clinical suspicion of the diagnosis until immediately before death. Such cases emphasise the need for high index of clinical suspicion and the need for rapid coordinated investigation and treatment.

Standard:

- microbiological culture of several organs and genital tract.

Cardiac deaths

A full spectrum of cardiac pathology is seen in the maternal deaths that have been reported to the Confidential Enquiry but it is in the cardiomyopathies that there is the greatest need for accurate and detailed autopsy studies. The differentiation of the puerperal cardiomyopathy from hypertrophic and congestive cardiomyopathies is difficult and often impossible. A young multiparous woman suddenly collapsed a few days after a normal full-term vaginal delivery. She survived for four days in intensive care, during which time an echocardiogram demonstrated an enlarged heart consistent with hypertrophic cardiomyopathy. The cardiomegaly was confirmed at autopsy but the characteristic myocardial fibre disarray of hypertrophic cardiomyopathy was not present on histology. Expert cardiac pathological opinion was sought and it was confirmed that the findings were atypical and could not be characterised as puerperal, dilated or hypertrophic cardiomyopathy. A category of pseudohypertrophic cardiomyopathy was suggested that did not have the same familial implications as hypertrophic cardiomyopathy.

The familial and genetic basis for hypertrophic cardiomyopathies is now well-established and, in the past ten years, genetic abnormalities in some of the dilated cardiomyopathies have also been identified.[5] Accurate diagnosis obviously has implications for counselling of the family. Also, the worse prognosis of a peripartum cardiomyopathy compared with a dilated cardiomyopathy suggests that more work separating and defining these conditions is required.[6] Unfortunately, the problems now experienced with organ retention indicate that in many cases there will be great difficulty in obtaining the necessary expert cardiac opinion.

Standards:

- careful examination with histology
- expert cardiac pathology opinion for cardiomyopathies.

Epilepsy

The overall effect of pregnancy on epilepsy is unknown. In some instances epilepsy improves during pregnancy, whereas in others there is increased risk of fitting. A variety of reasons has been proposed for the latter, including a haemodilution that occurs particularly in the last trimester, failure to adjust drug levels and even non-compliance with drug therapy because of its potential teratogenic effects. Unexpected deaths that are attributed to epileptiform seizures have also been recorded in pregnant women with no history of fits for over two years and occasionally with no history of fits at all. Such diagnoses obviously require a careful and detailed autopsy to exclude other causes of fits such as eclampsia. While in known epilepsy the problem is controlled by the clinical response to the drug therapy, it is also valuable at autopsy to have drug levels estimated. In such circumstances, non-compliance with therapy or a rapid change in drug levels can be documented and the appropriate analysis of the death can be achieved.

In many instances in these reports, death from epilepsy has been associated with drowning in the bath. Therefore, although the risks are low the recommendations made

Table 34.1 Grading of autopsy reports in the latest triennial report

Area	Excellent	Good	Adequate	Deficient	Appalling
London	0	4	7	2	6
Other UK	13	25	14	9	1

in the report are that the woman should only bathe in shallow water or take a shower. This should be undertaken preferably when another adult is in the house.

Standards:

- careful exclusion of other causes, e.g. pre-eclampsia by histology
- postmortem drug levels of anticonvulsants.

Quality of the autopsy

Many of the points made emphasise the need for a high-quality autopsy service but review of the autopsies shows that this standard, while achieved in many instances and improving, is patchy. Particularly notable in this regard is the poor quality of the autopsy report performed for medico-legal purposes in many of the London and Home County areas. An analysis of direct maternal deaths for the latest CEMD report[3] graded the autopsy reports into five categories of excellent, good, adequate, deficient and appalling (Table 34.1). From the London and Home Counties area, eight out of the 19 direct deaths were considered to be appalling reports or thought to have significant deficiencies. This compared with ten of 62 direct maternal deaths in the remainder of the UK.

There are multifactorial reasons for this difference. However, in the London area, even for hospital deaths bodies are transferred to a distant public mortuary so that liaison between clinical staff and the pathologist is minimal, and the pathologist conducting the autopsy is not necessarily local to the area or from a nearby hospital. Public mortuaries are not linked to any laboratory service and consequently histology of tissues, bacteriological cultures and drug assays are rarely undertaken for non-forensic causes. There have been instances where the autopsy has been delayed for up to six days while awaiting the visiting pathologist.

Further factors that adversely affect the quality of the autopsy include the apparent reluctance of many coroners to pay for histopathological investigations necessary to investigate clinical problems but not related to the immediate cause of death. The retention of tissues and organs creates problems of which the most obvious examples are in the appropriate investigation of cardiac and brain diseases. All these issues are then further compounded by the current profound shortage of histopathologists throughout the UK.

Future actions

It is perhaps stating the obvious but most pathologists will provide a more detailed and thorough autopsy if there is known to be some clinical interest and this is best achieved if obstetricians and/or anaesthetists can attend the autopsy in person. Medical records do not always identify or give appropriate emphasis to the clinical problems and much added value can be gained from direct clinicopathological communication – a point that has been made in many of the previous CEMD reports.

Many of the issues relating to the quality of the autopsy must be addressed by a programme of education and information. This is partly achieved through the publication of the CEMD report but it must be supplemented by presentations at meetings such as this and also in fora of more immediate relevance to hospital pathologists. There has been no significant review of maternal death pathology for over 20 years.[7] Updated information through the auspices of the Royal College of Pathologists Bulletin and updates in the pathology annuals would therefore be both appropriate and timely.

The majority of the maternal death autopsies are conducted under the auspices of Her Majesty's Coroner and there is a similar need to keep them informed about the importance of the autopsy to the CEMD. Also, any actions requested of them must have the support of the medical profession, have clarity and focus and be appropriate to their functions.

Currently, most maternal death autopsies are randomly distributed between practising pathologists, without reference to their skills, interests or experience in this field. It would be helpful to have a dedicated group of pathologists to examine all maternal deaths who would be prepared to seek the relevant further expert opinion as appropriate. The potential sources for such a cadre of pathologists are the paediatric pathologists, the forensic pathologists and pathologists nominated by regional pathology assessors. These groups may not be mutually exclusive and there are advantages and disadvantages associated with each group.

The number of paediatric pathologists is diminishing not increasing. Historically, there has been difficulty recruiting to this specialty. Within the current environment, recruitment is even more difficult and several established consultants have taken early retirement or obtained alternative employment.

In forensic pathology, the numbers are small. They operate an active on-call rota that is rarely better than one in two, they rarely practice hospital pathology and a significant number are independent of the universities and the NHS. Nonetheless, they investigate a small but not insignificant proportion of maternal deaths and they would be acceptable to HM Coroners.

A small group of selected pathologists identified through regional pathology assessors for the Confidential Enquiry is attractive but requires organisation, commitment, training and renewal. It would be on a volunteer basis and therefore might not have an even geographical spread; such pathologists would need acceptance by the local coroners.

Proposals:

- educational programme for clinicians, pathologists and coroners
- develop 'key pathologists' theme.

References

1. Sonderegger-Iseli K, Burger S, Muntwyler J, Salomon F. Diagnostic errors in three medical eras: a necropsy study. *Lancet* 2000;355:2027–31.
2. Zornberg GL, Jick H. Antipsychotic drug use and risk of first-time idiopathic venous

thromboembolism: a case-control study. *Lancet* 2000;356:1219–23.

3. Drife J, Lewis G, editors. *Why Mothers Die 1997–1999. The Confidential Enquiries into Maternal Deaths in the United Kingdom*. London: RCOG Press; 2001.
4. Department of Health, Welsh Office, Scottish Home and Health Department, Department of Health and Social Services, Northern Ireland. *Report on Confidential Enquiries into Maternal Death in the United Kingdom, 1991–93*. London: HMSO; 1996.
5. Suomalainen A, Paetau A, Leinonen H, Majander A, Peltonen L, Somer H. Inherited idiopathic dilated cardiomyopathy with multiple deletions of mitochondrial DNA. *Lancet* 1992;340:1319–20.
6. Bernstein PS, Magriples U. Cardiomyopathy in pregnancy: a retrospective study. *Am J Perinatol* 2001;18:163–8.
7. Rushton DI, Dawson INP. The maternal autopsy. *J Clin Pathol* 1982;35:909–21.

Chapter 35

The role of multi-professional working

Discussion

Discussion following Mrs Carson's submitted paper (chaired by Professor MacLean)

MacLean: Does anyone wish to make any comments about the submission on midwifery care?

Robson: It would be a shame if the midwifery group as a whole were not given the opportunity of making slightly more focused recommendations about one or two areas of practice that clearly might impact upon maternal mortality. There are issues such as the awareness of the risks of thromboembolism and postnatal depression.

Robinson: There is one section that we have already contacted the Department of Health about, to which both we and the National Childbirth Trust (NCT) take the strongest possible exception and we think it increases risk. That is the recommendation on page 370 (Chapter 31) that: 'midwives should be prepared to decline to take responsibility for high-risk cases from an obstetrician where the involvement of a consultant obstetrician is essential and the reasons for this should be explained to the woman and to the obstetrician.'

Women for whom obstetric care or hospital care is unacceptable, for any reason, will then be giving birth at home, alone and unattended. We are seeing an increase in those cases in high-risk women. Trusts will see this as an excuse to justify their refusal to supply a domiciliary midwife, which they are already doing. We see this as increasing the risk of maternal death. We and the NCT object to this most strongly.

Having talked to the Department and to the person who drafted this, we understand how it happened, in that sometimes the obstetrician had wrongly referred the person back for community care. However, this will be read by trusts and midwifery managers as giving them the complete right to refuse a midwife's care because the midwife can decline responsibility. That means that the woman receives no maternity care in labour at all, and we will not accept that. We will criticise it strongly and publicly if it is included.

MacLean: There is a statutory obligation that midwives must provide care. There is no obligation that obstetricians should, but there is a statute.

Robinson: There is no legal obligation to provide care in the home, but there is an obligation for the trust to provide maternity care. Now everybody has taken legal advice on this, and they have to provide maternity care but they do not legally have to provide it in the home. This is the growing dilemma that we are seeing in case after case. We – total amateurs with no qualifications – are the only people supporting very high-risk women giving birth alone at home, and it is terrifying.

MacLean: This is not related specifically to the home. It may, for instance, be applicable to people who choose to deliver in a birthing centre, where the selection of patients is thought by the midwife to be inappropriate.

Cooper: It related to high-risk cases where the obstetrician had referred them back to the midwife but the midwife did not feel able to say to the obstetrician, 'Look, chaps, this is a case that you should be looking after.'

Robinson: But this is not how it comes across, and it is not how it is being interpreted.

Cooper: But the sentiment has to prevail.

Robinson: The other point is that, in terms of helping the very high-risk women who are late bookers and reducing psychiatric morbidity, we feel that caseload midwifery, where the midwife has her own caseload and the woman has continuity of care, is the best possible way to provide the service. With the so-called 'team midwifery', there are eight midwives and you never see the same one twice, which is no improvement on whatever there was before and is sometimes worse.

Marteau: I would endorse Dr Robson's comment that midwifery should make specific recommendations. I would like to touch on two points from the chapter. One of the recommendations is about the use of interpreters and, from the evidence we have heard, should be strengthened. It says that the use of children as interpreters 'should be avoided if at all possible', but I think we should say that this is not acceptable.

The other point relates to smoking. We have heard that smoking is a possible co-factor, but nonetheless is quite important. This recommendation is rather vague – it just says that midwives are uniquely placed to provide advice, and indeed they are, but the trial evidence is that it is not effective advice. We therefore need to do something about smoking, and we should do more than just say that midwives could do it. We need to talk about effective smoking cessation services.

Cooper: The other point about interpreters is that they should be available around the clock. When the acute problems occur, that is when you cannot get hold of an interpreter.

Marteau: Absolutely, but we should say that family members are not acceptable as interpreters.

MacLean: Except that, when there is no one else available, then clearly they should be able to use those people who are there. I agree that it is not optimal, but to say that it will never be acceptable excludes that as a means of being able to communicate with a patient.

Marteau: Given the evidence we have heard about the high rates of maternal mortality and morbidity in families where appropriate interpreters are not provided, it is rather like saying that if you do not have a clean knife to do the operation, then you should use a dirty one. There are certain standards that we apply in specific circumstances and if we leave a loophole, saying 'where possible', we will not achieve those standards. Perhaps this will be a matter for debate later on.

Bewley: I would support Professor Marteau on that point. If you do not understand that something is unacceptable, then you do not do anything about it. If you say that it is unacceptable – of course we would use a child at three o'clock in the morning if there were no one else, but we fill in a risk management form and we report it. In my hospital, we are currently reporting all incidences of unavailability of interpreters, because otherwise we cannot argue with the trust that there is a real, serious problem locally because they have cut the services.

As a study group we can say that we have a standard that is slightly different from that expressed in one of the chapters of the book. I would support Ms Robinson on some of the comments that she has been making about the misunderstanding. I have listened to the discussions in the maternity care working party about midwives' legal obligations. People are under pressure, these are very stressful situations and, like you, I thought that there was a legal obligation to attend. It is a central part of midwives' core beliefs and it is being eroded because it turns out that it might not be so. As a study group, we should support the right of all women in labour to a skilled attendant, which is a global right that women should have. This means that, if a woman is at home despite being high-risk, and the midwife has told her this and declined to treat her, all women in labour nevertheless have the right to a skilled attendant.

Discussion following the papers by Dr Cooper, Dr Yentis and Professor Millward-Sadler (chaired by Dr Lewis)

Bewley: I wanted to ask why anaesthetists are apparently not concerned about the rise in the caesarean section rate. I am slightly concerned that the National Sentinel Audit did not report that four percent of babies in this country are stillborn under general anaesthetic, which is a morbidity for the mother and baby themselves. Clearly, whatever your complication rates of general and epidural anaesthesia – which are decreasing substantially – the fact that the caesarean section rate is going up must be of concern because of the complications. Nobody would have an epidural or a general anaesthetic without a reason, because of the complications – particularly in pregnancy. Your comment that women want elective caesarean sections because the safety of anaesthesia is unjustified – nobody would want that. It is not the safety issues that are making them want it.

Cooper: I obviously worded that badly. What I mean is that, if it were not so safe, they certainly would not be requesting it.

Robinson: I cannot let go this question of eating during labour because it is a very hot consumer issue. We desperately need more research on this because there are indications, from such research as exists, that not being allowed to eat during labour may affect its progress and thereby increase the chance of a caesarean section being necessary. You are not supposed to eat in case you need a caesarean section, but not eating probably increases your risk of needing one. We need more research on this: women are calling for it. I have never yet met a woman who wanted curry and chips in labour.

When women labour at home, they are free to eat what they want when they want.

In the general chat, I always ask them whether, when and what they chose to eat. They all choose to eat and, in the early stages of labour, they find it particularly helpful if they have the presentation, or size of baby or whatever, that will lead to a long and exhausting labour. They are able to compare this with outcomes of earlier labours in hospital, when they were not allowed to eat. This is one of the factors in choosing home births. They choose to eat things such as yoghurt, soup, sometimes sandwiches, but certainly never curry and chips.

We understand why you are saying this. We are extremely grateful for what the anaesthetists have done with regard to the safety record. This is an area that we have to watch. We can understand why you are saying it and we respect your concerns, but there are also concerns in the other direction. We just do not have adequate research yet on eating in labour, and this is a great gap.

Lewis: I would just like to say that curry and chips was the standard food at University College Hospital, London, when I did obstetrics!

Cooper: It is clear that anaesthetists rarely have to anaesthetise women with a full stomach at present. Our backs are against the wall: we do not want to delay because the woman has a full stomach and put the baby at risk. However, we have to deal with this and what we do not want is more maternal deaths. I agree with you that we need some further research, but not against solid food that blocks the trachea. That is pertinent to whether you use regional or general anaesthesia. There is a perception among midwives that, because a woman is having regional anaesthesia, this is not a problem and the woman may have a full stomach.

Nelson-Piercy: I would like to reassure Ms Robinson and remind Dr Cooper that there is currently a randomised controlled trial going on at Guy's and St Thomas's Hospital Trust, London, for eating in labour. This randomises primiparous women to eating and not eating. Your questions and your concerns will be answered.

Cooper: We may well be joining that trial. Geraldine O'Sullivan, Consultant Obstetric Anaesthetist from St Thomas's Hospital, has asked if we would, because of the slow recruitment.

Nelson-Piercy: This question is not on intensive care, and it is really to Dr Yentis and Dr Cooper together as I wanted to give them both the opportunity to comment on this. Dr Yentis did not mention the increased role of anaesthetists in assessing women before delivery who have the potential for complications with regional or general anaesthesia. Could I prompt you to add to, or modify, one of your two recommendations to state that this should be included – if, indeed, you believe that would be useful and worthwhile.

Cooper: That is actually one of the recommendations that will be coming out.

Nelson-Piercy: I do not remember an assessment before labour being mentioned.

Yentis: Are we talking about antepartum or antenatal clinics, or the labour ward?

Nelson-Piercy: No, I do not mean on the labour ward. I mean when the woman is 30 weeks pregnant and has had a previous tracheal stenosis.

Cooper: That is included in our recommendations.

Yentis: Could I just add to that – in fact, it is not in the sheet we have been given but the National Institute for Clinical Excellence is looking at antenatal care. The Obstetric

Anaesthetists Association (OAA) is now one of the stakeholders and it has already stated that this should take place. I think the OAA was rather stung by being left out of the guidelines on intrapartum monitoring, which gave completely the wrong message about epidurals, so we were particularly keen to become involved for this one.

Cooper: It is in Chapter 36, under 'Health policy and education', number 29. Is that what you mean? 'With regard to anaesthesia, the lessons of history should not be forgotten. These include the need to train anaesthetists in obstetric anaesthesia, adequate staffing and equipping and early consultation in high-risk cases'.

Pattinson: On the question of anaesthetics, a large number of women who die have had an anaesthetic at some point, although it might not have been related. Do you assess those anaesthetics in any way?

Cooper: We have a low number of deaths that we decide are to be ascribed to anaesthesia. However, for all the women who had any form of anaesthetic involvement – which might just have been resuscitation in the Accident and Emergency department – the notes go to the anaesthetic assessor. Several recommendations in the chapter concern aspects of care that might have been better or anaesthetic involvement that was necessary but did not occur. This encompasses quite a large number of cases – about 150 of the 398 or so.

Lewis: Is there anything on pathology?

Bewley: Did I understand correctly that you were thinking of regional assessors for maternal deaths, to whom the coroner would then refer the deaths, before liaising as appropriate with the forensic people?

Millward-Sadler: Basically, this is just an embryonic idea of mine that has not been discussed with the coroners. We have regional pathology assessors and they are in the best position to know which pathologist in their area would take an interest and be available to perform an autopsy. Then, having got that, I think it would be my job – I hope with the help of Professor Drife and Dr Lewis – to beard the lions in their den at the Coroners' Society and try to persuade them of the value of this.

Bewley: Hearing it again at the end, about people burning the midnight oil for nothing, I just wonder whether you should not undertake an assessment of the actual costs of the Confidential Enquiry in terms of time that is being volunteered. These are opportunity costs to the NHS. If someone is at a committee meeting rather than their clinic, and if they are working at midnight on goodwill, that will not last in the 21st century. We ought to put real costings on the present system.

Lewis: I will reply to that shortly.

Nelson-Piercy: I have an anecdote for Professor Millward-Sadler. We had a maternal death in which the views of both the pathologist and the clinicians caring for the woman changed quite radically when they all met for a case discussion. This is really a plea for a recommendation that the clinicians caring for the women should ideally attend postmortems and, at the very least, speak to the pathologist before, during or after the postmortem. In that problem, the fault lies with the clinicians as much as with the pathologists, I suspect. If the pathologist is in a remote area, then it is very difficult.

This recent case taught us so much about what pathologists can learn from clinicians and vice versa. It is particularly pertinent when a woman dies in an intensive therapy unit (ITU). The intensivist may go to the autopsy, but the account of the events leading up to ITU admission is not given to the pathologist; how is he or she supposed to reach a conclusion without the information, which is often not in the notes?

Millward-Sadler: I could not agree with you more. When I do an autopsy, I always make sure that local obstetricians know what time I am proposing to come and do it. If it is in Portsmouth, however, I am not usually there until seven o'clock in the evening.

Lewis: If there are no further questions for Professor Millward-Sadler, let me come back to Dr Bewley on the real costs of running this Enquiry. We have to demonstrate to its new masters exactly how many hours we all put in. Everyone knows that I work far too hard, as do Professor Millward-Sadler and everyone else. Perhaps it behoves us to try to cost out how many real hours of work we do because this Enquiry has run for too long on the goodwill of health professionals who have wanted, from their own hearts, to improve care for pregnant women. It is all too easy for us just to keep going because we are being told to do so, without actually sitting back and looking at it. You are right: as part of our recommendations, we need to say that we should put a true cost on what it is currently costing us, and also indicate what improvements we would like to make.

On a personal note, there is something else that I had not thought about until you mentioned the word 'costs'. There are other costs. I am a hard-bitten old civil servant and doctor of many years. I read these reports, and I have to put them all on the database. I can get through five or ten quite easily, for a week, and then one hits me, and another one hits me and I cry – usually at three o'clock in the morning, all alone at home. We underestimate the effect that running an Enquiry can have – particularly one with so much detail. The suicide note made me cry, Dr Oates. We ought to be realistic about the cost to ourselves, but it shows at the end of the day that it is real women we are trying to help.

SECTION 9

RECOMMENDATIONS

Chapter 36

Recommendations arising from the 43rd Study Group: Maternal Morbidity and Mortality

Recommendations fall into three categories:

1. Recommendations for **clinical practice** (principally aimed at Fellows and Members of the Royal College of Obstetricians and Gynaecologists) based upon research evidence (where available) and the consensus view of the Group. The clinical practice recommendations have been graded from 'A' to 'C' according to the strength of evidence on which each is based (Table 36.1). The scheme for the grading of recommendations is based on the system adopted by both the NHS Executive and the Scottish Intercollegiate Guidelines Network.
2. Recommendations for **future research** in those clinical areas where the Group identified a need for further evidence on which to base practice.
3. Recommendations relating to **health education** and **health policy**.

Recommendations for clinical practice

1. Active management of the third stage of labour reduces blood loss. (Grade A)
2. The uterotonic for active management involves trade-offs between oxytocin and Syntometrine® (Alliance Pharmaceuticals). (Grade A)

Table 36.1. Grading of recommendations

Grade	Recommendation
A	Requires at least one randomised controlled trial as part of the body of literature of overall good quality and consistency addressing the specific recommendation.
B	Requires availability of well-conducted clinical studies but no randomised clinical trials on the topic of recommendation.
C	Requires evidence from expert committee reports or opinions and/or clinical experience of respected authorities. Indicates absence of directly applicable studies of good quality.

3. Routine episiotomy should be abandoned. (Grade A)
4. Saline plus oxytocin infusion into the cord vessels reduces the need for manual removal of placenta. (Grade A)
5. Patients with cardiac disease must be assessed at primary and secondary levels. Those with high risk (any of the risk factors of the Toronto study (Chapter 22[40]) plus disease-specific risks must be managed in a tertiary centre. (Grade B)
6. Women who have had cancer treated recently may wish to become pregnant. Discussion between oncologist and obstetrician is better before conception. In some cancers, such as breast and melanoma, pregnancy should be deferred for two to three years after treatment. (Grade B)
7. Good-quality information about the health of mother and fetus should be provided using multiple media, accessible to all users of a service, at all stages of pregnancy. (Grade C)
8. All women should be offered screening for anaemia on at least one occasion during pregnancy. (Grade C)
9. Repeat screening for anaemia early in the third trimester is recommended to assess the effect of supplementation and/or treatment of underlying disease. (Grade C)
10. Iron supplements (together with folic acid) should be offered to all pregnant women with anaemia. In areas with high prevalence of malaria, prophylaxis or presumptive treatment for malaria should be provided in addition to these supplements. (Grade C)
11. All women should be screened for hypertension and proteinuria at each antenatal clinic visit – those at highest risk require more frequent screening (especially between 24–32 weeks). (Grade C)
12. Tertiary centres managing pregnant cardiac patients should have a multidisciplinary team that includes at least a specialist obstetrician, a cardiac physician with knowledge of obstetrics, an anaesthetist, a haematologist and a high-risk midwife. (Grade C)
13. Patients with epilepsy should be offered timely and appropriate counselling concerning teratogenic risks of anti-epilepsy drugs, strategies to minimise risk, importance of antenatal care and contraception issues. (Grade C)
14. General practitioners, neurologists, general physicians, obstetricians and midwives should be encouraged to volunteer such advice at any appropriate opportunity to any women with epilepsy within or approaching childbearing years. (Grade C)
15. Women with major convulsive seizures should deliver in hospital. (Grade C)
16. It is unnecessary to screen all pregnant patients for thrombophilias but patients with a significant personal or family history should be assessed. (Grade C)
17. If low molecular weight heparin is to be given to women with thrombophilia or those with a history of idiopathic venous thromboembolism, it should be started early in pregnancy. (Grade C)

18. Clinical consultation with the obstetric anaesthetist during antenatal assessment of patients with co-existing medical conditions can anticipate problems and reduce morbidity. (Grade C)
19. Management protocols for women with a past history of serious mental illness should be in place, including identification of local psychiatrist/team with special interest. (Grade C)
20. If patients are seen during pregnancy with unusual or common but persistent symptoms, the possibility of cancer must be considered and appropriate examination, imaging and biopsy should be performed. (Grade C)
21. Clinicians and medical students must be made more aware of atypical clinical presentations of ectopic pregnancy and the option of beta human chorionic gonadotrophin testing in women with unexplained abdominal pain of recent onset. (Grade C)
22. Laparoscopic surgery for ectopic pregnancies should only be undertaken by appropriately trained surgeons; laparoscopic surgery may be inappropriate in haemodynamically unstable women. (Grade C)
23. Septic miscarriage should be recognised as a potentially serious complication requiring experienced obstetric input; surgical evacuation of the uterus may be best performed around one hour after intravenous antibiotic treatment. (Grade C)

Research

1. Concerted efforts are needed to improve routine data sources and enquiry methods on a global scale for determining inequalities and inequities in maternal health.
2. The global persistence of significant levels of substandard care as avoidable factors in maternal mortality requires fresh perspectives.
3. Greater attention should be paid to the indirect causes of maternal mortality, which may reflect different socio-economic inequalities from those linked with direct causes.
4. The use of haemoglobin as a ‘marker of morbidity’ should be evaluated.
5. There is a need for improved knowledge of factors contributing to anaemia in different regions of the world. This knowledge should form the basis for regional guidelines for the prevention and treatment of anaemia.
6. Trials are needed to evaluate whether iron should be given in combination with other micronutrients, for example as a multivitamin preparation.
7. There is a need to examine more carefully the interaction between micronutrient deficiency and infection in pregnancy.
8. The estimated contribution of malaria to maternal morbidity in developing countries is considerable. These estimates should be studied in relation to malaria prevalence, which is available for many developing countries.

9. Evidence is required from intervention studies, using appropriate health packages, to determine their effectiveness in reducing malaria-related outcomes. This is especially relevant in high-risk groups such as adolescents.
10. Research is required to elucidate whether malaria contributes to the pathogenesis of pre-eclampsia.
11. In order to improve mortality ascertainment, improved monitoring and evaluation is required through sentinel sites. This is also necessary to determine the contribution of HIV infection and drug-resistant malaria to malaria-related mortality.
12. It is necessary to address and focus on those areas and interventions in which funding, time and human resources should be invested to ensure sustainable and long-term impact against HIV infection.
13. There is a significant link between maternal mortality and a history of psychiatric illness and domestic violence. Research is necessary on how to elicit the key elements of such history without compromising the relationship between patient and caregiver.
14. Future research should focus on whether 'aggressive' anti-hypertensive therapy reduces the risks of maternal mortality and serious morbidity.
15. A carefully designed randomised controlled trial (RCT) is necessary to determine the safety of allowing patients home after an admission with an antepartum haemorrhage and a diagnosis of placenta praevia.
16. For the treatment of postpartum haemorrhage, high-dose (800–1200 μg) misoprostol should be evaluated in appropriately designed RCTs.
17. There should be further funding to allow the development and implementation of a national maternity minimum data set.
18. Further pilot studies are needed to define useful and applicable definitions of maternal morbidity.
19. The RCOG should be working, in collaboration with the Royal College of Midwives, Obstetric Anaesthetists Association and possibly others, on a few representative performance measures that could be used nationally and reflect overall services and individual clinician performance.
20. Systems should be established for recording pregnancy-related morbidity requiring intensive/high-dependency care, to include monitoring of admission criteria, treatments and outcomes.
21. Further information is needed on how uncertainty about the wellbeing of the fetus, the pregnancy and the birth can most effectively be provided to all women to minimise anxiety and give reassurance, while facilitating informed choices.
22. If the term 'debriefing' is to be used in maternity services, a consensus needs to be reached on its definition.
23. Qualitative research is needed to explore frequency, timing, setting and content of debriefing and who is the appropriate person to conduct that session.
24. Postmortem studies should be undertaken to determine how frequently fetal material is found in the maternal lungs.

25. When cancer occurs during or soon after pregnancy, appropriate tissue samples should be banked to allow research and understanding in the future.

Health policy and education

1. This Study Group endorses the Recommendations contained within the latest Confidential Enquiry into Maternal Deaths.
2. The value of the Confidential Enquiry into Maternal Death cannot be underestimated or presumed. Adequate funding and professionally led expertise must be ensured to allow further investigation into the areas of highest mortality.
3. Estimating the maternal mortality ratio is an essential component of health care for women.
4. The avoidability of the majority of maternal deaths in all countries should be acknowledged as a human rights issue.
5. In judging the success of intervention strategies in reducing maternal mortality, it is crucial that not only clinical effectiveness and cost-effectiveness are considered, but also the implications for equity goals.
6. There is a need to increase political awareness, financial investment and commitment to maternal health and safe motherhood.
7. There should be promotion, dissemination and implementation of key interventions that are known to be evidence-based and cost-effective to reduce maternal and newborn morbidity and mortality.
8. There should be increased collaboration with the WHO Making Pregnancy Safe Initiative and other institutions to improve professionals' role in supporting maternal and newborn health programmes.
9. Where human or financial resources are limited, detailed analysis of maternal mortality should be focused on major remediable problems.
10. In countries with high HIV/AIDS rates, we must encourage availability of funding to test pregnant women for HIV, provide anti-retroviral drugs and offer hope to HIV-positive mothers.
11. Continuity of carer leads to better labour outcome and lower intervention rates. Therefore, there must be more investment in maternity services, especially in the recruitment, retention and continuing development of midwives.
12. The RCOG should address the exploitation of healthcare workers immigrating to the United Kingdom from developing countries and explore the role of developed countries in reversing this trend.
13. Reductions in maternal mortality in the UK can be achieved by improving access to care. This includes making services more acceptable, tailored to each woman, stressing the importance of early booking, providing suitable translation services, overcoming dismissive staff attitudes and engaging representatives of vulnerable groups in the planning of services.

14. If possible, partners, friends, family members and children should not be used to interpret for women unable to speak English. An interpreter should be provided.
15. Antenatal services should be flexible enough to meet the needs of all women, bearing in mind that the needs of those from the most disadvantaged, vulnerable and less articulate groups in society are of equal if not greater importance. Many women who died found it difficult to establish or maintain access with the services, and follow-up mechanisms for those who failed to attend were poor. Women who regularly fail to attend clinics should be actively followed up.
16. We must enhance the status of listening to all women and explore ways to provide all women with the opportunity to discuss their experience (e.g. link workers, appropriate interpreters, special needs practitioners).
17. There should be local training programmes for midwives and obstetricians in 'listening skills'.
18. Sufficient time must be costed for providing to patients the information generated as part of antenatal care.
19. There is evidence that, where women can choose, it is medically better to have children between the ages of 20–35 years. All healthcare professionals should give consistent medical advice that pregnancy is more adverse at the extremes of reproductive life.
20. It is recognised that unplanned pregnancy and the deferral of childbearing are culturally determined. Older childbearing may be related to financial security. The RCOG and Department of Health should advise government how social policy impacts negatively or positively on women's health and wellbeing.
21. Primary care nurse, midwifery or general practice preconceptional services should be developed, with secondary support from genetics, obstetrics, mental health and medical services.
22. Commissioners should ensure that all women have access to a local mental health team with a special interest in perinatal psychiatric disorders.
23. Women requiring psychiatric admission following delivery should be admitted to a specialist mother and baby unit.
24. An effective anti-hypertensive agent and magnesium sulphate should be available to all women when appropriate.
25. All regions should have guidelines for the management of women with pre-eclampsia and stipulate indications for referral to tertiary centres.
26. As women with epilepsy may sometimes be from socially deprived populations, every effort should be made to ensure that they receive and understand the need for regular multidisciplinary antenatal care.
27. Cases of amniotic fluid embolism (AFE) should be reported to a national register.
28. There are still uncertainties about the behaviour of cervical and breast cancer during pregnancy. Collection of data by establishing a register in the UK would appear desirable.
29. With regard to anaesthesia, the lessons of history should not be forgotten. These

include the need to train anaesthetists in obstetric anaesthesia, adequate staffing and equipping of maternity units and early consultation of high-risk cases.

30. Obstetric anaesthetists should be involved in the policy making of individual maternity units.

31. Women having caesarean section require the same standard of postoperative care as those undergoing non-obstetric surgery.

32. Multidisciplinary agreement on clinical definitions of pregnancy-related conditions requiring intensive or high-dependency care is urgently required.

33. High-dependency units must be set up and maintained within maternity units, as called for by the Confidential Enquiry into Maternal Deaths, including the educational and financial support that such units require.

34. The contribution of the autopsy findings to understanding maternal death is dependent on the quality of the autopsy examination: this should be achieved by identifying small teams of pathologists for each region.

35. It is important that autopsy examinations in cases of maternal death are conducted in a time and a place such that the clinicians involved can attend.

36. The experience, past and present, of assessing maternal mortality in developed countries may be helpful to developing countries.

37. Recommendations for improvements in maternal health care may be based on observational studies and informed professional opinion, where RCT data are not available.

38. Maternal deaths have an over-representation of certain ethnic groups, women who did not speak English or who were illiterate.

39. Overall, 30% of women who died from direct or indirect causes were poor attenders. Late bookers tend to be poor subsequent attenders.

40. There is a need to agree on definitions of a direct and indirect malaria death in pregnancy.

41. Patients with cardiac disease and their general practitioners and obstetricians should be made aware of the risks of pregnancy.

42. Antepartum haemorrhage remains an important contributor to maternal mortality and morbidity.

43. Clinicians should be aware of the presentations of AFE and the importance of early multidisciplinary care.

44. Obstetricians and midwives need training in how to ask patients in a systematic fashion, at booking, about a history of psychiatric disorder.

45. Specific written and verbal advice should be offered to mothers with epilepsy concerning practical measures to minimise the risk of harm to the baby.

46. There is a need for evidence-based training in effective and sensitive communication of risk and other information during pregnancy.

Index